THE TEACHING CASES FROM ANNALS OF ONCOLOGY

THE TEACHING CASES FROM ANNALS OF ONCOLOGY

The clinical cases collected in the present book have all been previously published in the 'Clinical case' series in the journal *Annals of Oncology*, from April 1993 to April 1996. *Annals of Oncology* is devoted to the rapid circulation of scientific communications concerning oncology, particularly medical oncology. Its character, however, is multidisciplinary, in reflection of the proliferation of activities and interests in Europe, and contributions on clinically oriented laboratory research, surgery and radiotherapy are assured by the presence of representatives of these disciplines on the Editorial Committee and Board.

The Teaching Cases from Annals of Oncology

Edited by

R. L. SOUHAMI

Department of Oncology, University College London Medical School,
The Middlesex Hospital, London, UK

KLUWER ACADEMIC PUBLISHERS
DORDRECHT / BOSTON / LONDON

Library of Congress Cataloging-in-Publication Data

A C.I.P. Catalogue record for this book is available from the Library of Congress.

ISBN 0-7923-4373-5 (HB)
ISBN 0-7923-4117-1 (PB)

Published by Kluwer Academic Publishers,
P.O. Box 17, 3300 AA Dordrecht, The Netherlands.

Kluwer Academic Publishers incorporates
the publishing programmes of
D. Reidel, Martinus Nijhoff, Dr W. Junk and MTP Press.

Sold and distributed in the U.S.A. and Canada
by Kluwer Academic Publishers,
101 Philip Drive, Norwell, MA 02061, U.S.A.

In all other countries, sold and distributed
by Kluwer Academic Publishers Group,
P.O. Box 322, 3300 AH Dordrecht, The Netherlands.

Printed on acid-free paper

Table of contents

Preface

The Teaching Cases Series of *Annals of Oncology* was started in April 1993. The aim was to use clinical cases as a means of teaching the principles of diagnosis and management of cancer. We kept in mind the educational needs of doctors in training, and of other health care professionals. We planned that the cases would cover a wide range of clinical diagnosis and diagnostic problems and treatment decisions.

In choosing the authors I have emphasized expertise and enthusiasm. I attempted to invite cases from as wide a range of contributors as possible to reflect different opinions in the European countries. The contributors have responded magnificently to my requests for changes, my constant reminders, and my adaptation of their prose.

The interest in the cases and the enthusiastic response of readers of *Annals of Oncology* led me to suggest to the editor and publisher of *Annals* that the first series of cases should be published in book form.

Looking back over the first three years of cases, it is clear that a wide range of cancer medicine has been covered to a very high standard. Taken together, the cases are a valuable and a convenient source of information. For this book the text and references have been updated where necessary.

I hope that readers of *Annals of Oncology* and others will find it a useful addition to their libraries. I am grateful to Franco Cavalli for having invited me to be the first editor of this series which I am sure will continue to flourish.

R. L. Souhami

R. L. Souhami (ed.) The Teaching Cases from Annals of Oncology, 1–4, 1997.
© 1997 *Kluwer Academic Publishers. Printed in the Netherlands.*

Fever and neutropenia during intensive chemotherapy

J. Klastersky

Service de Médecine Interne et Laboratoire d'Investigation Clinique H. J. Tagnon, Institut Jules Bordet, Centre des Tumeurs de L'Université Libre de Bruxelles, Bruxelles, Belgium

Key words: guidelines for febrile episodes, neutropenia, acute leukemia, abdominal symptoms

A 52-year-old man was admitted to the Institut Jules Bordet for consolidation therapy of acute leukemia. He was a high school teacher; he did not smoke, did not drink alcohol in excess or use narcotic drugs. His past medical history was unremarkable except for painful haemorrhoids to which he applied a topical preparation.

Three months prior to his admission he developed repeated episodes of upper respiratory tract infection. At that time, blood tests demonstrated an acute non-lymphoblastic leukemia, which was subsequently classified as M4, following the FAB classification. At the time of the diagnosis, his white blood cell count was 37,900 with 22% blasts. Induction therapy was started with cytosine arabinoside and daunomycin and a complete remission was obtained. During the period of aplasia which followed that treatment, he had fever with no clinical signs of infection. A blood culture was positive for *Staphylococcus epidermidis* and the patient received piperacillin, amikacin and vancomycin for 15 days. At the end of induction treatment, he developed erythema nodosum for which local corticosteroids were prescribed.

One month later, he was readmitted for consolidation therapy with high-dose cytosine arabinoside and amsacrine. From day 7 to day 22 after chemotherapy, he developed severe mucositis which markedly limited his food intake. He also had persistent diarrhea. Cultures of the stools were negative for the usual pathogens and for *Clostridium difficile*. Investigation for *Clostridium difficile* toxin was negative.

On day 30, the patient suddenly became tachypneic and his temperature rose to 40 °C. Within less than 2 hours, he became obtunded, agitated and his systolic blood pressure dropped to 60 mmHg. He was transferred to the medical intensive care unit. On admission to the unit, he was found weak but responsive. His blood pressure was 80/50 mmHg while receiving fluids and dopamine and his heart rate was 120/minute but regular. His temperature was 38.7 °C and he had constant chills. The physical examination revealed nothing remarkable except for a very swollen and exquisitely painful haemorrhoid. Rectal examination was very painful. The stools were negative for occult blood.

Dopamine was continued and the blood pressure stabilized at 100/60 and the urinary output was 30 ml/hour. At that time hemoglobin was 7 g/dl, the white cell count was 200/ml without neutrophils and the platelets were 26,000. Serum creatinine was 2 mg/dl, serum urea was 36 mg/dl; serum sodium, chloride and bicarbonate were within the normal limits; the serum potassium was 2,3 mEq/l; the liver function test results were normal; the prothrombin time was 64%, fibrinogen was 694 mg/dl and the search for fibrin split products was negative. The patient received 3 units of packed red blood cells and 5 mg morphine subcutaneously every 6 hours. Ticarcillin (4 × 5 g/24 hours) and amikacin (2 × 500 mg/24 hours) were administered with supplements of KCl (40 mEq/24 hours).

During the next few hours, the patient complained of severe pain located in the left inguinal and scrotal area which was increasing from hour to hour. It was present at rest but was greatly increased when the area was touched. The dose of morphine was increased. After 3 hours, the left inguinal area became red, hot and swollen and an important painful swelling was observed all over the scrotum (Fig. 1). Over the succeding hours, foci of necrosis appeared over this whole area and the skin began to ulcerate. No crepitation was noted. Otherwise, the physical examination was nor-

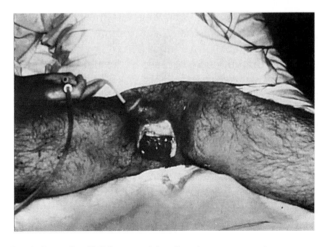

Fig. 1. Scrotal cellulitis caused by *Pseudomonas aeruginosa*: note the swelling, the erythema and the necrotic patches.

mal. A chest x-ray was unremarkable and an electrocardiogram showed ST segment depression, suggestive of myocardial ischemia, in V4, V5 and V6.

The following day the blood cultures, which had been obtained prior to the administration of empiric antibiotic therapy, were reported positive for *Pseudomonas aeruginosa*. The same antimicrobial therapy was continued. Clinically, the patient was stable with a blood pressure at 110/60 mmHg and a heart rate at 80/minute; his temperature was 38.2 °C and the physical examination was unremarkable except for the extensive inguinal and scrotal lesions which now were progressing to the anterior abdominal wall and to the rest of the perineum. Several necrotic areas were noted over the scrotum, which was dramatically swollen and tender. Culture of biopsy and swab of necrotic areas yielded *P. aeruginosa*. An ultrasound examination of the scrotum showed an extensive cellulitis involving all the structures around the testicles which, themselves, appeared normal. A granulocyte transfusion (1×10^{10} cells) was administered.

During that day, the patient started to complain of abdominal pain, which was diffuse but moderate. The abdomen was distended and tympanic; no ascitic fluid was demonstrable. A plain film of the abdomen, showed a major dilatation of the entire colon and a few dilated loops of the small bowel with air-fluid levels. No bowel sounds were heard and the rectal examination was normal. A sigmoidoscopy to 30 centimeters showed no stenosis. The mucosa was very congested but no specific lesions were seen.

At that time, the hemoglobin level was 9.7 g%/dl, the white blood cell count was 300 without neutrophils and the platelet count 55,000. Serum creatinine was 2.7 mg/dl, sodium was 136 mEq/l, potassium 1.9 mEq/l, bicarbonate 20 mEq/l; the other biochemical parameters were normal. By the end of that day, the sensitivity of the *Pseudomonas aeruginosa* was reported: the MIC for ticarcillin was 64 microgm/ml and the MIC for amikacin was 4 microgm/ml. The bactericidal titer in the serum, obtained just prior to the administration of ticarcillin plus amikacin, was 1/2.

On this basis, the following modifications of the therapy were made: firstly, ceftazidime was administered at the dose of 4 g 3 times per 24 hours, and ticarcillin was discontinued, because of the resistance of the *Pseudomonas aeruginosa*. This was associated with a considerable increase in the serum bactericidal titer; the trough level was 1:32. Supplements of potassium were given with serial controls of the serum level and cardiac monitoring. The administration of morphine was discontinued. Within the next 24 hours, the patient became afebrile, and the skin lesions (ecthyma gangrenosum) ceased progressing. At the same time that the potassium level normalized in the serum, the pseudo-obstruction of the colon resolved with no other therapeutic measures.

The patient remained severely neutropenic for six additional days but afebrile. Antimicrobial therapy was continued for a total of 16 days, until healing of the skin lesions was well under way. A complete remission was achieved which lasted for 18 months.

Comments

Therapy of acute leukemia and other neoplastic diseases often involves a transient period of severe medullary aplasia which may persist for several days. The consequences of neutropenia and thrombocytopenia are, respectively, infection and hemorrhage. To some extent, platelet transfusion can control bleeding unless the patient is alloimmunized, but infection remains a considerable problem and a major cause of mortality.

Granulocyte colony-stimulating factor (G-CSF) and granulocyte-macrophage colony-stimulating factor (GM-CSF) are hemopoietic growth factors, now commercially available for use in patients, which might change our concepts and attitudes about the management of febrile neutropenia. The predominant effects of G-CSF are to stimulate the survival, proliferation, differentiation and function of neutrophil granulocyte precursors and mature cells. GM-CSF acts not only on cells of the neutrophil lineage, but also on cells of the eosinophil and monocyte/macrophage lineages. The properties of the respective agents have been recently reviewed [1].

Neutropenia predisposes to severe and rapidly progressing infection by bacterial and fungal pathogens; it also interferes with the usual clinical manifestations of sepsis. Therefore, empirical antibiotic therapy has become an accepted practice and has been designed to cover the most likely pathogens, namely, Gram-negative rods and especially *P. aeruginosa* [2]. Of course, besides 'microbiologically defined infections', in some patients no microbiological nor clinical cause for the infection will be found ('unexplained fever'); in others, only clinical clues will lead to a presumptive diagnosis of infection ('clinically defined infection'). The criteria for these categories have been established and are widely accepted [3].

During the two past decades, we have witnessed, in granulocytopenic patients, a progressive reduction of Gram-negative infections and a gradual rise of those due to Gram-positive organisms, especially those caused by *Staph. epidermidis* and the streptococci.

Although Gram-negative infections represent only 30% of the pathogens currently responsible for sepsis in granulocytopenic patients, these infections can be fulminant, especially if *P. aeruginosa* is involved. This is well illustrated in the case reported here which emphasizes a characteristic skin lesion, named ecthyma gangrenosum, pathognomonic of *P. aeruginosa* infection, in the perineum [4].

Empiric therapy of febrile neutropenia therefore includes broad spectrum antibiotic coverage against Gram-negatives. If neutropenia is severe and expected to be prolonged, a combination of a cephalosporin with an aminoglycoside is superior to single-drug therapy [5]. The EORTC group has recently reported the successful use of ceftazidime or ceftriaxone with amikacin. Because the aminoglycoside carries a risk of oto- and nephrotoxicity, especially when other toxic agents are used, it should not be continued beyond a few days unless microbiological investigations strongly support its use.

The question of whether Gram-positive organisms should be covered from the start is as yet unsettled. Most studies used vancomycin or teicoplanin. Some authors claim that infections caused by *Staph. epidermidis* are quite indolent and carry a very low mortality rate, and thus, do not require empiric therapy prior to their micriobiological documentation. Others have stressed the high morbidity and serious mortality (± 15%) of streptococcal infections [6], and recommended either prophylaxis or empirical therapy under circumstances where streptococcal infection is likely.

Failure to respond to empirical therapy occurs in about 30% of cases. As in our patients, this may be associated with a clearly progressing infection and/or persisting bacteremia. Under these circumstances, it is essential to monitor the serum bactericidal titer, since it has been found that a trough titer of 1/8 is required, in neutropenic patients, to predict safely a favorable outcome [7]. Here, the titer was obviously inadequate, owing to the intrinsic resistance of the *Pseudomonas aeruginosa* to both drugs that had been prescribed empirically, and required a change in therapy, whose effectiveness was subsequently demonstrated by the rise of the serum bactericidal titer and control of the infection. A microbiologically documented failure would also be a good indication for therapeutic administration of CSFs. A granulocyte transfusion was administered to our patient, but at the same time other significant modifications to his treatment were made. This makes it difficult to interpret its role in the overall outcome.

Fungal infection can be documented in 5% of the patients as the cause of the initial febrile neutropenia. This figure has not changed much for years. Bacterial and fungal sepsis may coexist and under these circumstances bacteremia might overshadow the more difficult-to-document fungal infection. The latter may then manifest itself as a persisting or recurring fever after the eradication of bacteremia by empirically prescribed antibiotics. This explains why it has become accepted to administer amphotericin B empirically to those granulocytopenic patients who remain febrile after a few (4–7) days of broad-spectrum antimicrobial therapy and in whom no bacteria can be documented [8].

The other interesting feature of our patient is his abdominal symptoms and signs. He had a major distention of the colon and radiological signs of obstruction at the small bowel level. Since no mechanical obstruction could be documented at the lower level and because the entire colon was distended, it is a case of intestinal 'pseudo-obstruction' or paralytic ileus.

Among the many possible causes the following are likely in this patient: an acute autonomic neuropathy related to the chemotherpy which he received, hypokalemia, and the administration of morphine. The therapy which was administered here is not known to be neurotoxic and the time between the administration of chemotherapy and the appearance of the neuropathy was long. On the other hand, hypokalemia and the administration of morphine might have played a synergistic role in the development of this intestinal pseudo-obstruction. The role of hypokalemia is probable. It can be caused by a loss of potassium within the intestinal tract, as a result of the mucositis related to chemotherapy. In our patient, a chronic diarrhea had been documented and his food intake had been poor, leading to potassium deficiency, inadequately compensated for, since the level of serum potassium was 2.3 mEq/l at the time of the appearance of the vasomotor collapse. Supplementation with potassium was made difficult because of the renal function impairment and the vasomotor instability. Later, the level of potassium decreased further and additional urinary loss as a result of the administration of ticarcillin was suspected. It is well-known that penicillins, when administered in high doses, can play the role of non-resorbable anion in the kidney and are excreted with potassium which is exchanged with sodium [9].

Another possible cause of the abdominal symptoms is necrotizing colitis, which occasionally complicates aggressive chemotherapy, especially in acute leukemia. The pathogenesis of this intestinal lesion, which is primarily localized in the colon, is not well understood. It may be the result of cytotoxic chemotherapy and in particular, cytosine arabinoside. The role of leukopenia, which is almost always present, is not clear. It is possible that multiple factors play a role in its development. It is also well known that necrotizing colitis predisposes to bacterial sepsis of intestinal origin, and many patients die in vasomotor collapse due to polymicrobial bacteremia. This was not the case with our patient, however, since the usual presentation of the latter condition consists of abdominal pain, bloody diarrhea, extensive mucosal edema and damage, which result in a characteristic swelling of the colonic wall on x-rays. The mucosa was nearly normal in our patient.

The management of fever in granulocytopenic patients requires a high level of expertise and close collaboration between clinician and microbiologist. Guidelines for its management are shown in Fig. 2, but it must be underscored that constant re-evaluation of clinical progress and treatment is essential.

Acknowledgment

Drs M. Aoun, D. Bron and J. P. Sculier were kind enough to help with the preparation of this manuscript.

4

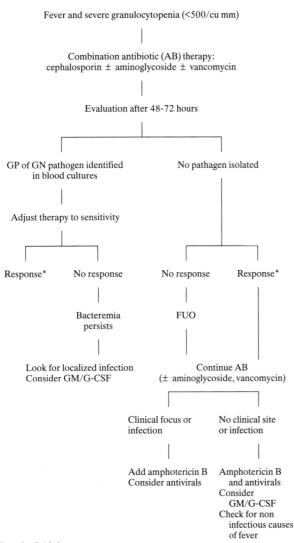

Fever and severe granulocytopenia (<500/cu mm)

Combination antibiotic (AB) therapy:
cephalosporin ± aminoglycoside ± vancomycin

Evaluation after 48-72 hours

GP of GN pathogen identified
in blood cultures

No pathagen isolated

Adjust therapy to sensitivity

Response*   No response   No response   Response*

Bacteremia
persists

FUO

Look for localized infection
Consider GM/G-CSF

Continue AB
(± aminoglycoside, vancomycin)

Clinical focus or
infection

No clinical site
or infection

Add amphotericin B
Consider antivirals

Amphotericin B
and antivirals
Consider
GM/G-CSF
Check for non
infectious causes
of fever

* Treat for 7-10 days

Fig. 2. Guidelines for the diagnostic and therapeutic approach of febrile episodes in granulocytopenic patients.

References

1. Lieschke GJ, Burgess JD. Granulocyte colony stimulating factor and granulocyte-macrophage stimulating factor. N Engl J Med 1992; 327: 28–55 and 99–106.
2. Klastersky J. Empiric antimicrobial therapy for febrile granu-locytepenic cancer patients: lessons from four EORTC trials. Eur J Cancer Clin Oncol 1988; 24 (Suppl 1): S35–S45.
3. Pizzo PA, Armstrong D, Bodey G et al. The design, analysis, and reporting of clinical trials on the empirical antibiotic manage-ment of the neutropenic patient. Report of a consensus panel. J Inf Dis 1990; 161: 397–401.
4. Greene SL, Su WPD, Muller SA. *Ecthyma gangrenosum*: report of clinical histopathologic, and bacteriologic aspects of eight cases. J Am Acad Dermatol 1984; 11: 781–7.
5. EORTC International Antimicrobial Therapy Cooperative Group. Ceftazidime combined with a short or long course of amikacin for empirical therapy of gram negative bacteremia in cancer patients with granulocytopenia. N Engl J Med 1987; 317: 1692–8.
6. Awada A, Van der Auwera P, Meunier F et al. Streptococcal and enterococcal bacteremia in patients with cancer. Clin Infect Dis 1992; 15: 33–48.
7. Sculier JP, Klastersky J. Significance of serum bactericidal activ-ity in Gram negative bacillary bacteremia in patients with and without granulocytopenia. Am J Med 1984; 76: 429–35.
8. EORTC International Antimicrobial Therapy Group. Empiric antifungal therapy in febrile granulocytopenic patients. Am J Med 1989; 86: 668–72.
9. Klastersky J, Vanderkelen B, Daneau D et al. Carbenicillin and hypokalemia. Ann Intern Med 1973; 78: 774–5.

R. L. Souhami (ed.) The Teaching Cases from Annals of Oncology, 5–9, 1997.

Tamoxifen and hypercalcaemia

G. Daugaard

Department of Oncology, Rigshospitalet, Copenhagen, Denmark

Key words: tamoxifen, hypercalcaemia, hormone-flare syndrome, polyuria

Case report

A 72-year-old woman with metastatic infiltrating ductal cancer of the breast was admitted for further treatment. She had undergone a right radical mastectomy in January 1989; no tumour was found in sampled lymph nodes. Oestrogen receptor status was unknown. The patient had severe lumbar back pain. Chest x-ray was normal. Plain x-rays and isotope showed evidence of osteolytic metastases involving the skull, the lumbar and thoracic spine, left side of the pelvis, upper part of the left femur, left shoulder and arm and several ribs (Fig. 1 and 2).

The alkaline phosphatase level was 706 U/l (normal 50–275 U/l), the serum ionised calcium level was 1.38 mmol/l. (normal 1.30–1.50 mmol/l) and the serum creatinine 80 μmol/l (normal 40–110 μmol/l). Treatment with tamoxifen 30 mg daily was started followed by radiation therapy from the 12th thoracic to the 1st sacral vertebrae 4 days later. Four days after starting on the tamoxifen the bone pain increased severely and over the following three days the patient became somnolent and poorly orientated. At this time her serum ionised calcium had increased to 2.90 mmol/l (total calcium 5.5 mmol/l) and her serum creatinine was 163 mmol/l. Vigorous hydration with 4L of isotonic saline was started together with clodronate 300 mg i.v. This treatment was repeated over the next 3 days with correction of serum potassium and serum magnesium. Small doses of loop-diuretics (20–40 mg) were administered to prevent congestive heart failure.

The serum calcium level decreased steadily. Despite normalization of the serum calcium level, she remained somnolent until the third hospital day, when she became rousable although confused and combative. A lumbar puncture performed during this time showed no evidence of infection or carcinomatous involvement.

Gradually, her confusion cleared and she became fully oriented. Her serum calcium level continued to decrease and stabilized in the normal range. After one week, treatment with megestrol acetate was instituted without recurrence of hypercalcaemia.

Discussion

The hypothesis that oestrogens play a role in the regulation of growth of mammary cancer is supported by

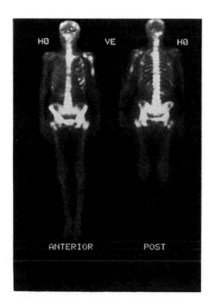

Fig. 1. ⁹⁹Tc bone scan showing numerous areas of increased uptake in the skull vertebrae, ribs and pelvis.

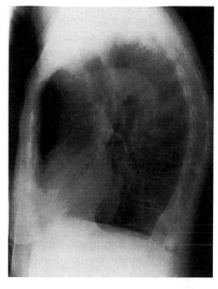

Fig. 2. x-ray of the thoracic spine showing vertebral collapse (arrowed).

the clinical remissions achieved with various ablative procedures (oophorectomy, adrenalectomy, and hypophysectomy) that are presumed to lower tissue oestrogen levels or reduce oestrogen production. Although oestrogen secretion diminishes considerably after any of these procedures, the levels fluctuate, and oestrogen secretion may not stop completely even after hypophysectomy [1–3]. The persistence of oestrogens after oophorectomy is due to conversion of androgens of adrenal origin to estradiol, which can take place in peripheral tissue and even in breast cancer tissue [4].

As a result of the binding of the hormone to the specific receptor the secretion of growth factors exerting autocrine or paracrine control of growth is stimulated. Antioestrogens exert their action through a competitive inhibition of this binding [5]. It has been suggested that the antioestrogen tamoxifen might exert part of its action by decreasing the secretion of transforming growth factor-beta (TGF-B) [6]. The presence of hormone receptors in the tumour tissue predicts the probability of responding to endocrine therapy. Thus, in receptor-positive tumours approximately 50%–60% of the patients with receptor-positive tumours will respond compared to less than 10% of those with receptor-negative tumours [7].

Tamoxifen has played a prominent role in the successful treatment of oestrogen-sensitive breast tumours. One of the major attractions of tamoxifen is its relative lack of toxic effects. The side effects reported most frequently are hot flushes (14%) and nausea (10%), while mild leuko- and thrombo-cytopenia have been observed in 5%–10% of reported cases. Less frequent side effects include vaginal bleeding (5%), erythematous skin rashes, hypercalcaemia and transient increases in tumour pain similar to the 'flare' noted with oestrogens and androgens.

The reported incidence of hypercalcaemia induced by hormone therapy varies between 5% and 10% [8–10]. Since hypercalcaemia occurs spontaneously in 10%–25% of breast cancer patients, particularly when osteolytic bone metastases are present, the distinction between 'spontaneous' hypercalcaemia and hormone-induced hypercalcaemia is sometimes difficult. Hormone-induced hypercalcaemia has a rapid onset characteristically occurring within five to ten days after start of hormonal therapy, and the serum calcium levels return to normal when the offending agent is withdrawn. Spontaneous hypercalcaemia is generally slower in onset and accordingly, the symptoms develop gradually.

Hormone-flare syndrome

The hormone-flare syndrome is characterized by hypercalcaemia, inflammation of skin metastases and increased pain caused by bone metastases during the first two to three weeks of therapy with tamoxifen [11]. The tamoxifen-flare syndrome appears to be due to an initial agonist effect followed by an antagonistic effect.

At low concentrations (10^{-7} to 10^{-9}M) and in the absence of estradiol, tamoxifen stimulates the proliferation of oestrogen receptor-positive cell lines in vitro [12]. This low-dose stimulation may be responsible for the tumor flare phenomenon when tamoxifen serum levels are gradually rising during the first weeks of therapy [13]. The temporal relationship in the present case report of the patient's hypercalcaemia to the initiation of tamoxifen therapy indicates an association of her profound hypercalcaemia with the medication.

In a study by Legha et al. [14] tamoxifen-induced hypercalcaemia was observed in 10 of 470 patients (2.3% of all patients, 4% of those with bone metastases) with metastatic breast cancer. Hypercalcaemia developed after a median period of seven days (range 4–11 days). All patients reported in the literature with tamoxifen-induced hypercalcaemia have had evidence of bone metastases [14–19]; hypercalcaemia has generally developed within the first two weeks after initiation of tamoxifen therapy. Tamoxifen therapy has been continued without interruption in some patients [14, 15], interrupted and reinstituted in some patients [14, 16, 19] and discontinued permanently in some patients [14, 17–19]. The serum calcium level can decrease despite continued tamoxifen treatment. When tamoxifen is reinstituted, recurrence of hypercalcaemia is uncommon. If the hypercalcaemia is mild, tamoxifen therapy can be continued together with appropriate treatment of the hypercalcaemia. If the hypercalcaemia is severe a brief interruption in the tamoxifen treatment is necessary.

Tamoxifen-induced hypercalcaemia occurs in only a small portion of patients with malignant disease and hypercalcaemia. About 10%–20% of all patients suffering from malignancy experience episodes of hypercalcaemia during their disease. The risk of developing hypercalcaemia, however, varies among the different types of malignancy. Among the solid tumours the common lung and breast cancers, squamous cell carcinomas of the head and neck and the rare cholangio-carcinomas are fairly often complicated by hypercalcaemia, while other common tumours such as carcinomas of the colon and the female genital tract are rarely associated with hypercalcaemia. Among the haematologic disorders multiple myelomas and lymphomas are most often associated with hypercalcaemia.

Pathophysiology of hypercalcaemia

The pathophysiology of hypercalcaemia of malignancy is complex. Increased bone reabsorption is involved in most cases, caused either by extensive direct local bone destruction or by humoral factors which may operate at a distance. Tumor extracts from patients with humoral hypercalcaemia of malignancy (HHM) often contain parathyroid hormone (PTH)-like bioactivity. This activity appears to be due to PTH-related peptide (PTH-rP). The N-terminal amino acid sequence of this protein shows considerable homology with human PTH. However, other bone resorbing factors including prostaglandins, transforming growth factors, colony-stimulating factors, leukocyte cytokines and 1,25-di-hydroxyvitamin D may be involved in different types of malignancy.

The effects of synthetic PTH-rP are similar to those of PTH, although differences in potency may exist. The peptide stimulates renal reabsorption of calcium [20] and increases bone reabsorption in vitro and in vivo [20]. Despite the homology with PTH and the binding to PTH receptors in kidney and bone, many aspects of PTH-rP action in these tissues show differences from the action of PTH. In bone a negative balance due to increased bone reabsorption and profound depression of bone formation develops in most cases of HHM [21]. This picture is different from the normal balance between reabsorption and formation observed in most cases of primary hyperparathyroidism [22]. Another difference is the suppression of renal 1-α-hydroxylase by PTH-rP [23]. In primary hyperparathyroidism the production of 1, 25(OH)$_2$D$_3$ is usually increased [24]. Finally, alkalosis is prominent in HHM rather than the slight hyperchloremic acidosis in primary hyperparathyroidism. The mechanisms behind these differences are still obscure, but may involve binding to different domains of the PTH-receptor or modification of PTH-rP action by other factors.

In breast cancer direct bone reabsorption by tumor cells has been demonstrated and constitutes a process that operates independently of osteoclastic bone reabsorption [25] (Table 1). Osteoclast activation by TGF-α, TGF-β, and possibly prostaglandins play a significant role [26]. The role of lymphokines and other locally acting agents remains to be established. Increased renal tubular calcium reabsorption may also contribute to hypercalcaemia in breast cancer patients, although the mechanism responsible is unknown. The majority of breast cancers do not produce PTH-rP, and hypercalcaemia is due to bone metastases. The clinical features of hypercalcaemia related to malignancy are listed in Table 2.

Hypercalcaemia reduces the ability of the kidney to concentrate the urine, probably due to inhibition of the effect of ADH as a direct effect of hypercalcaemia on the distal renal tubule. The resulting polyuria often induces dehydration with reduced extracellular volume (ECV), diminished renal perfusion and glomerular filtration rate (GFR). The reduction in GFR decreases the filtered load of calcium. Moreover, the contracted ECV enhances the proximal tubular reabsorption of sodium and calcium [27]. The resulting increase in

serum calcium will further compromise renal function.

The symptoms are often very troublesome and unpleasant, with persistent nausea and vomiting, confusion and disturbing nightmares. They vary considerably from patient to patient and it is often difficult to differentiate between symptoms caused by advancing malignant disease, cytotoxic drug therapy or radiation therapy and those induced by complicating hypercalcaemia. The neuro-psychiatric symptoms in hypercalcaemia may mimic cerebral metastases. Anorexia and vomiting often complicate chemotherapy or the malignant disease *per se* and bed rest, inactivity, anorexia and dehydration promote constipation. Impaired glomerular function may be explained by causes other than hypercalcaemia such as Bence-Jones nephropathy in myeloma or obstructive uropathy in other tumours.

Management

Because of these pathophysiological mechanisms, rehydration is a major step in the treatment of hypercalcaemia. The best way to restore adequate hydration and increase renal calcium output is to infuse normal saline. The amount depends on the degree of dehydration and the tolerance of the patient's cardiovascular system to extracellular volume replacement. The administration of 3 to 6 liters of saline will often be sufficient to break the previously described vicious cycle of polyuria, vomiting, dehydration, reduced ECV, reduced GFR, decreased urinary output, decreased renal calcium excretion and rising serum calcium. Other electrolyte abnormalities should be corrected as well. Hypokalemic alkalosis is frequently seen in severe hypercalcaemia and the administration of large amounts of saline potentiates renal potassium and magnesium losses.

Loop-diuretics have been shown to induce calciuresis [28], and they might be needed in order to prevent congestive heart failure in elderly patients. Routine use of loop-diuretics may be harmful unless their administration is delayed until volume expansion is achieved. Thiazides decrease renal excretion of calcium and should be avoided in any hypercalcaemic patient.

Table 2. Symptoms and signs of hypercalcaemia of malignancy.

Neurological
depression, irritability, disturbed sleep, lethargy, confusion, stupor, coma, muscle weakness hypotonia, absent deep-tendon reflexes

Cardiovascular
shortening of QT interval, broadening of T-wave, heart block, asystole, ventricular arrytmias, increased sensitivity to digoxin

Gastrointestinal
anorexia, vomiting, gastric atony, constipation, acute pancreatitis

Renal
polyuria, polydipsia, dehydration, impaired glomerular filtration, nephrocalcinosis

Table 1. Pathogenetic mechanisms underlying hypercalcemia in breast cancer.

1. Osteoclast activation
2. Direct reabsorption of bone by tumour cells
3. Increased renal tubular calcium reabsorption

8

The bisphosphonates are analogues of pyrophosphate. They are stable in vivo because no enzyme in the body can hydrolyze these compounds. They have a high affinity for bone, especially hydroxyapatite, in skeletal areas of increased bone turnover, such as those occurring near metastatic bone lesions. The precise effects of bisphosphonates on bone and bone cells are not known in detail. However, they are thought to be taken up by osteoclasts and appear to inhibit the action of these cells.

Each bisphosphonate appears to have its own mechanism of osteoclast inhibition. The absorption of these compounds from the gastrointestinal tract is generally poor, averaging less than 10%, and is particularly poor when they are given with food. The intravenous administration of bisphosphonates has proved to be effective therapy for acute hypercalcaemia.

There are three bisphosphonates available: etidronate, pamidronate and clodronate. In addition to these three compounds, a new generation of bisphophonates is currently under investigation.

Of the three drugs, pamidronate is probably the most potent [29, 30]. A single-dose regimen has been reported to lead to normalization of serum calcium concentration in 70% to 100% of patients [29–30]. The intravenous route is preferred in view of the limited gastrointestinal tolerance of many patients with hypercalcaemia and the gastrointestinal side effects that may be associated with oral administration of the drug. The adverse effects of parenteral pamidronate are limited to a mild, transient increase in temperature (less than 2°C), transient leukopenia, and a small reduction in serum phosphate levels.

Treatment with glucocorticosteroids in patients with hypercalcaemia and solid tumours has generally been disappointing [31]. Nevertheless, a recent randomized study performed in patients with breast cancer showed some beneficial effect of glucocorticoids [32]. The fact that the potential response to glucocorticoid therapy may be delayed up to one week or more makes it imperative that more effective means of lowering serum calcium levels be used in symptomatic patients.

On a theoretical basis, the inhibitory effect of calcitonin on bone reabsorption and blood-bone barrier makes it the ideal agent for treating hypercalcaemia. The recommended dose of calcitonin is 4–100 IU in half a liter of saline infused over 3 to 6 hours. Unfortunately, most patients treated with calcitonin show only a limited and transient effect [33]. Calcitonin can be used in patients with renal and cardiac failure. It is often associated with nausea and vomiting, but otherwise the treatment is safe, with only minimal short-term toxicity.

Mithramycin, an inhibitor of RNA synthesis in osteoclasts, is also an effective treatment for hypercalcaemia. It is given intravenously in a dose of 25 μg per kilogram over a period of four to six hours. The dose can be repeated several times at intervals of 24 to 48 hours. The serum calcium concentration begins to decrease as early as 12 hours after administration of the drug, and the maximal reduction occurs in 48 to 72 hours.

Mithramycin has several side effects. Nausea, irritation and cellulitis with extravasation of the drug, hepatic toxicity, nephrotoxicity and thrombocytopenia can occur. The effectiveness of bisphosphonates means that mithramycin and calcitonin are now seldom necessary.

Summary

The present case demonstrates the importance of close observation, also of serum calcium, when initiating tamoxifen therapy, especially in patients with known osseous metastases. Hypercalcaemia should also be considered as a possible cause of CNS symptoms in patients newly started on endocrine treatment. Hydration with saline is the first step in the management of hypercalcaemia. In patients with a serum calcium level >3.50 mmol/l (serum ionised calcium ≈ 2.00 mmol/l) hydration should be combined with bisphosphonates.

References

1. Dao TL-Y. Estrogen excretion in woman with mammary cancer before and after adrenalectomy. Science 1953; 118: 21–2.
2. Bulbrook RD, Greenwood FC. Persistance of oestrogen excretion after oophorectomy and adrenalectomy. Br Med J 1957; 1: 662–6.
3. Greenwood FC, Bulbrook RD. Effect of hypophysectomy on urinary oestrogen in breast cancer. Br Med J 1957; 1: 666–8.
4. Miller WR, Forrest APM. Oestrodiol synthesis by a human breast carcinoma. Lancet 1974; 2: 866–8.
5. Jordan VC. Biochemical pharmacology of antiestrogen action. Pharmacol Rev 1984; 36: 245–76.
6. Dickson RB, Lippman ME. Growth factors and oncogenes. In Powels TJ, Smith IE (eds): Medical Management of Breast Cancer. Martin Dunitz: London 1991; 5–18.
7. Rose C, Mouridsen HT. Combined cytotoxic and endocrine therapy in breast cancer. In Bresciani F, King RBJ, Lippman ME (eds): Progress in Cancer Research and Treatment. Raven Press: New York 1984; 269–96.
8. Davis HL, Wisely AN, Ramirez G et al. Hypercalcemia complicating breast cancer. Oncology 1973; 28: 126–37.
9. Beckett VL. Hypercalcemia associated with estrogen administration in patients with breast carcinoma. Cancer 1969; 24: 610–6.
10. Kennedy BJ, Tibetts DM, Nathanson IT et al. Hypercalcemia, a complication of hormone therapy of advanced breast cancer. Cancer Res 1953; 13: 445–59.
11. Howell A, Dodwell DJ, Anderson H et al. Response after withdrawal of tamoxifen and progestogens in advanced breast cancer. Ann Oncol 1992; 3: 611–7.
12. Reddel RR, Sutherland RL. Tamoxifen stimulation of human breast cancer cell proliferation in vitro: A possible model for tamoxifen tumour flare. Eur J Cancer Clin Oncol 1984; 11: 1419–24.
13. Clarysse A. Hormone induced tumor flare. Eur J Cancer Clin Oncol 1985; 21: 545–7.
14. Legha SS, Powell K, Buzdar AU et al. Tamoxifen-induced hypercalcemia in breast cancer. Cancer 1981; 47: 2803–6.
15. Pritchard KI, Clark RM, Fine S et al. Tamoxifen and hypercalcemia. Ann Intern Med 1978; 89: 423.

16. Minton MJ, Cantwell BMJ, Knight RK et al. Safety of tamoxifen. Lancet 1978; I: 396–7.

17. Larsen W, Fellowes G, Rickman LS. Life-threatening hypercalcemia and tamoxifen. Am J Med 1990; 88: 440–2.

18. O'Connell TX. Hypercalcaemia induced by tamoxifen. Am J Surg 1981; 141: 277–8.

19. Spooner D, Evans BD. Tamoxifen and life-threatening hypercalcemia. Lancet 1979; II: 413–4.

20. Yates AJP, Gutierrez GE, Smolens P et al. Effects of a synthetic peptide of a parathyroid hormone related peptide on calcium homeostatis, renal tubular calcium reabsorption and bone metabolism. J Clin Invest 1988; 81: 932–8.

21. Insogna KL, Broadus AE. Hypercalcaemia of malignancy. Annu Rev Med 1987; 38: 241–56.

22. Eriksen EF, Mosekilde L, Melsen F. Bone remodeling and balance in primary hyperparathyrcodism. Bone 1986; 7: 213–7.

23. Stewart AF, Mangin M, Wu T et al. Synthetic human parathyroid hormone-like protein stimulates bone reabsorption and causes hypercalcaemia in rats. J Clin Invest 1988; 81: 596–600.

24. Stewart AF, Horst R, Deftos LJ et al. Biochemical evaluation of patients with cancer associated hypercalcaemia: Evidence for humeral and nonhumeral groups. N Engl J Med 1980; 303: 1377–83.

25. Eilon G, Mundy GR. Effects of inhibition of microtubule assembly on bone mineral release and enzyme release by human breast cancer cells. J Clin Invest 1981; 67: 69–76.

26. Salomon DS, Zweibel JA, Bano M et al. Presence of transforming growth factors in human breast cancer cells. Cancer Res 1984; 44: 4069–77.

27. Lins RE. Renal function in hypercalcaemia. Acta Med Scand Supp 1979; 632: 1–12.

28. Suki WN, Yium JJ, Von Minden M et al. Acute treatment of hypercalcaemia with furosemide. N Engl J Med 1970; 283: 836–9.

29. Ralston SH, Gallacher SJ, Patel U et al. Comparison of three intravenous bisphosphonates in cancer-associated hypercalcaemia. Lancet 1989; II: 1180–2.

30. Gucalp R, Ritch P Wiernik PH et al. Comparative study of pamidronate disodium and etidronate disodium in the treatment of cancer-related hypercalcaemia. J Clin Oncol 1992; 10: 134–42.

31. Percival RC, Yates AJP, Gray JES et al. Role of glucocorticoids in management of malignant hypercalcaemia. Br Med J 1984; 289: 7.

32. Kristensen B, Ejlertsen B, Holmegaard SN et al. Prednisolone in the treatment of severe malignant hypercalcaemia in metastatic breast cancer: A randomized study. J Intern Med 1992; 232: 237–45.

33. Bienstock ML, Mundy GR. Effects of calcitonin and glucocorticoids in combination on the hypercalcaemia of malignancy. Ann Intern Med 1980; 93: 269.

R. L. Souhami (ed.) The Teaching Cases from Annals of Oncology, 11–15, 1997.
© *1997 Kluwer Academic Publishers. Printed in the Netherlands.*

Tumour-induced hypoglycaemia: A case report

K. Hoekman,[1] J. van Doorn,[2] T. Gloudemans,[3] O. S. Hoekstra,[4] J. A. Maassen,[5] J. B. Vermorken,[1] J. Wagstaff[1] & H. M. Pinedo[1]

[1]*Department of Oncology, Free University Hospital, Amsterdam;* [2]*Laboratory of Endocrinology, Wilhelmina Children's Hospital, Utrecht;* [3]*Laboratory of Physiological Chemistry, University of Utrecht;* [4]*Department of Nuclear Medicine, Free University Hospital, Amsterdam;* [5]*Sylvius Laboratory, Department of Medical Biochemistry, Leiden, The Netherlands*

Key words: sarcoma, hypoglycaemia, insulin-like growth factors

Case report

A 50-year-old Caucasian man was admitted unconscious to the hospital in the early morning. His medical history began 10 years earlier, when he was treated for an haemangiopericytoma in the cerebellum. The tumour was resected and post-operative radiotherapy (56 Gy) was given. Two years later a thyroid metastasis was treated by a hemi-thyroidectomy followed again by radiotherapy (60 Gy). Eight years later the patient received 5 cycles of doxorubicin 90 mg/m^2 plus granulocyte-macrophage colony-stimulating factor (GM-CSF) because of metastases in both lungs, the left lobe of the liver and in the left adrenal gland. A minor anti-tumour response was observed. Three months after chemotherapy he was admitted to the hospital in coma.

Physical examination showed only an enlarged liver. There were no focal neurological signs. Computerised tomography (CT) of the brain showed only post-operative changes, which could not explain his reduced level of consciousness. His serum glucose level was 1.1 mmol/L and he rapidly regained consciousness after glucose infusion. Glycosylated haemoglobin (HbA$_{1c}$), which is an index for the integral glucose variations in the previous 2 or 3 months, was 1.3% (N: 4.5–6.5%).

His family then mentioned repeated episodes of odd behaviour over the past months, especially early in the morning, which disappeared after food intake. The patient was not taking medication, did not drink alcohol and had previously been in reasonably good physical condition.

During the admission, the hypoglycaemia could easily be re-induced by a few hours of fasting. The very low levels of serum glucose were accompanied by an undetectable serum insulin level and very low levels of c-peptide, the connecting peptide of pro-insulin. These results are pathognomonic of a completely suppressed endogenous insulin production. Following an increase in the glucose levels to normal values, the serum insulin and c-peptide concentrations were appropriate. This result is indicative of an adequate reaction of insulin production to circulatory glucose levels, which excludes an insulinoma.

Evaluation of the tumour status showed a slow progression. The patient was then treated with 2 cycles of ifosfamide 5 g/m^2 with no anti-tumour response.

The hypoglycaemic episodes in this patient were initially controlled by dietary measures. Half a year later, he was readmitted because of intractable hypoglycaemias, which occurred especially in the early morning. Treatment with somatostatin 2 × 150 µg/d s.c. had no effect on insulin-like growth factor (IGF, see below) or glucose concentrations. Dexamethasone 6 mg/day taken orally prevented severe hypoglycaemias for about 3 months. When the episodes of hypoglycaemia again increased in frequency and seriousness the patient was treated with glucagon 6–12 mg/day by continuous infusion via a Port-a-Cath system in combination with dexamethasone 3 mg/day. This resulted in a more or less normal pattern of serum glucose levels throughout the entire day. After 3 months of treatment the severity of the hypoglycaemias increased and a decision was made to reduce the tumour volume by surgery. A resection of the metastasis in the left lobe of the liver and the left adrenal was performed and immediately thereafter serum glucose increased to normal levels. The liver metastasis contained a central area of fluid (Fig. 1), and 50 ml of this fluid was collected for further analysis. One day post-operatively the patient was receiving only intravenous saline solutions and had normal serum glucose concentrations. In the succeeding months only one serious hypoglycaemic episode was documented. Half a year later the patient died of sepsis. Post mortem analysis was not performed.

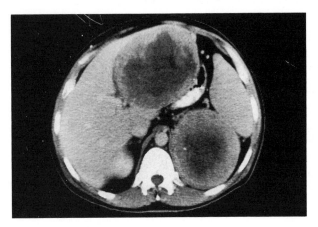

Fig. 1. Metastases from the haemangiopericytoma in the left lobe of the liver and the left adrenal gland.

Additional investigations

Concentrations of insulin-like growth factors (IGF) in blood and tumour fluid

The concentration of plasma IGF-I was very low (14–21 ng/ml) and IGF-II was within the normal range (515–800 ng/ml) in this patient. These values were not significantly different whether the patient was normo- or hypoglycaemic. Sampling of the hepatic, renal and femoral veins did not demonstrate increased IGF-II levels. After surgery, which was an incomplete debulk- ing, the level of IGF-I increased and the level of IGF-II decreased, but only by a small amount. Tumour fluid contained no insulin, a very low level of IGF-I (8 ng/ ml) and a strongly elevated concentration of IGF-II (2200 ng/ml).

Analysis of the IGF-I and IGF-II genes

Genomic DNA and RNA was isolated from frozen tumour tissue for Southern and Northern blot analysis. Southern blot analysis of tumour DNA revealed no amplification or rearrangements in the IGF-II gene. Messenger RNAs for IGF-I were not detected in tumour tissue but the level of expression of the IGF-II gene was about fifty times higher than in normal adult tissue. No aberrant IGF-II gene transcripts were found.

Analysis of IGF protein and interactions with IGF-bind- ing proteins (IGFBP)

Acid gel filtration was used to investigate IGF-II size heterogeneity. In normal human serum, 90% of IGF-II was present in the mature 7.4 kD form. In contrast, preoperative patient serum had most ($\approx 80\%$) of the IGF-II as a broad peak of 10–20 kD ('big' IGF-II), de- creasing to $\approx 50\%$ after surgery. In tumour fluid >90% of IGF-II appeared as big IGF-II.

The different molecular-size classes of endogenous IGFBP-IGF complexes in serum and tumour fluid were resolved by neutral gel filtration. In normal human serum, IGF-I appeared to be exclusively present as a 150 kD complex, which also contained most of the IGF-II ($\geqslant 60\%$). The remaining portion of IGF-II com- plexes eluted slightly later than serum albumin (60 kD). In the patient's serum, the peak of IGF-II corresponded to a molecular weight of about 60 kD with a minimal contribution from the 150 kD complex. In tumour fluid, most of the IGF-II was present as a 60–65 kD complex. The conclusion is, therefore, that IGF-II was present in both the patient's serum and tumour fluid as big IGF-II, associated with a small IGFBP complex.

Counter-regulatory mechanisms

The humoral responses to hypoglycaemia, induced by fasting, were studied in this patient. In normal persons, hypoglycaemia induces a strongly increased production of glucagon, catecholamines, growth hormone (GH) and cortisol, which stimulate endogenous glucose re- lease by the liver and/or inhibit glucose utilisation by insulin-sensitive tissues [8].

Hypoglycaemia in this patient was accompanied by a serum GH concentration which was always below the level of detection. Stimulation with 30 grams of argi- nine did not induce a GH response. Growth hormone- releasing hormone (100 μg i.v.) induced a weak GH response with a maximum value of 4.1 μg/l at 30 mi- nutes (T_{30}), whereas the glucose levels remained be- tween 2.1 and 3.2 mmol/l during the two hours of this observation period.

During hypoglycaemia, serum glucagon increased to slightly (and inappropriately) enhanced levels (104– 249 ng/l), serum cortisol remained normal (400–575 nmol/l), as did serum catecholamines [(nor)-adrenaline <3.5 nmol/L].

Glucagon 1 mg i.v. during a hypoglycaemic episode induced an increase of serum glucose from 1.8 mmol/l to a maximum of 4.0 mmol/l at T_{30}, but the glucose level at T_{90} was once again 1.9 mmol/l. The daily corti- sol concentration curve was low and flat. Stimulation with synthetic ACTH demonstrated a normal cortisol response (maximum 960 nmol/L). These studies sug- gest that the normal counter-regulatory responses to hypoglycaemia, especially the GH response, were sup- pressed.

Metabolic studies

Calculated resting energy expenditure (REE), an index of the basal metabolism, was 2285 kcal/24h, which was 136% of the predicted value for the height and weight of this patient. The respiratory quotient was 0.94, indi- cating a preferential glucose utilisation. Basal glucose oxidation was 8.7 μmol/kg/min. Fasting glycerol con- centrations were between 70–95 μmol/L, free fatty acids (FFA) < 0.10 mmol/L and β-hydroxybutyrate (βOH-B) < 0.01 mmol/L. The latter values are very low and correspond to an inhibited lipolysis. Both the increased glucose turnover and the inhibited lipolysis suggest an enhanced insulin-like activity.

Glucose-scan

18F-fluoro-deoxyglucose (18FDG) scintigraphy was performed with a conventional gamma-camera, equipped with a collimator specially designed for 511 keV photons (Nuclear Fields, Boxmeer, The Netherlands). The 18FDG scan showed a normal 18FDG distribution as well as an abnormal accumulation in the upper abdomen, reflecting the hepatic and adrenal metastases. The 18FDG tumour uptake was, however, less than we commonly observe in other tumours such as lymphomas, which are not associated with hypoglycaemias. This suggested that the hypoglycaemias were not primarily induced by an increased glucose consumption by the tumour.

Stimulation of insulin and IGF-I receptors by serum and tumour fluid

The metabolic effects of IGF-II are mediated through both the insulin and IGF-I receptor [9]. The in vitro ability of serum and tumour fluid to stimulate partially purified insulin and IGF-I receptors was, therefore, examined [10]. Control and patient serum had no effect, but tumour fluid stimulated the insulin receptor as strongly as 75 nM insulin (normal serum values <0.5 nM) whilst the IGF-I receptor was stimulated to the same degree as by 60 nM ($\approx$ 450 ng/ml) free IGF-II. These findings show an enormous insulin-like activity in tumour fluid but not in the patient's serum.

Discussion

Pathophysiology of tumour-induced hypoglycaemia

Hypoglycaemia induced by a tumour-related mechanism is a rare phenomenon [4]. It has been associated with tumours producing insulin (insulinomas), antibodies against insulin or insulin receptors [5, 6] and tumours producing an insulin-like growth factor. These IGFs are small peptides of 70 (IGF-I) and 67 (IGF-II) aminoacids, respectively, with homology to proinsulin. Their properties include both mitogenic and metabolic activity. IGF-I is the mediator of many of the effects of growth hormone whereas IGF-II is involved in embryogenesis but has no well defined function in the adult life. A great variety of tumours have been shown to be able to induce an IGF-mediated hypoglycaemia. Among them are primary liver cell carcinomas (the most frequent reason for tumour-induced hypoglycaemia in the eastern part of the world), adrenal and neuroendocrine tumours, Wilms' tumour and sarcomas. In nearly all cases, the sarcomas which show this syndrome are large and slow-growing, and the hypoglycaemia is a late event in the disease history.

Table 1. The causes of tumour-related hypoglycaemia.

Enhanced transcription of the IGF-II gene in tumour tissue
Secretion of big (immature) IGF-II by the tumour
Suppression of the production of mature IGF-II and GH-IGF-I-IGFBP-3 in normal tissues
Sequestration of big IGF-II in small IGFBP-complexes
Facilitated transcapillary transport resulting in enhanced bioavailability of tumour derived IGF-II

Tumour-induced insulin-like activity
 increased glucose turnover
 instability of glucose balance due to insufficient counter regulation
 inhibited lipolysis

In the group of sarcomas, haemangiopericytomas are frequently associated with hypoglycemias. The causes of tumour-induced hypoglycaemia are shown in Table 1.

Tumour-derived IGF-II is thought to be largely responsible for the hypoglycaemia induced by sarcomas, although increased circulatory concentrations of IGF-II are exceptional in these patients. The evidence for an IGF-II-mediated mechanism is the finding that these sarcomas invariably show an enhanced expression of the IGF-II gene [7]. This results in a tumour product which is present in the circulation as a high-molecular-weight (10–20 kDa) protein ('big' IGF-II) [8]. This protein represents abnormally or incompletely processed IGF-II, resulting in the appearance of a mixture of precursors of IGF-II. The production of mature 7.5 kDa IGF-II by normal tissues is suppressed.

The association of big IGF-II with the IGF-binding proteins (IGFBPs) is abnormal. In normal human serum both IGFs are complexed with IGFBPs which regulate their access to target tissues as well as their clearance rates [9]. Less than 5% of the IGFs appears in the free form. Six IGFBPs have been characterised so far. IGFBP-3 is the most abundant IGFBP, existing in a ternary complex of 150 kDa, which, besides an IGFBP-3 (β-subunit), also contains an acid-labile 85 kDa glycoprotein (α-subunit) and either IGF-I or IGF-II (γ-subunit). Both IGFs are associated with IGFBP-3 in normal adult serum and these 150 kDa IGF-BP complexes are too big to cross the capillary barrier.

In contrast to normal 7.5 kDa IGF-II, tumour-derived big IGF-II circulates in a 60 kDa complex [10]. This is caused by a decreased concentration of circulatory IGFBP-3 and the acid-labile component together with a reduced ability of the α-subunit to combine with the $\beta\gamma$-complex [11]. This impaired formation of normal IGFBP complexes may be indirectly affected by the excess of IGF-II, which inhibits the production of GH, IGF-I and the IGF-I-dependent IGFBP-3 [12] and by an abnormal structural appearance of the $\beta\gamma$-complex when it includes big IGF-II. It has been postulated that these small tumour-derived IGF-II-IGFBP complexes have an easier transcapillary transport and result in an enhanced bioavailability of tumour derived IGF-

14

II. There has as yet, however, been no direct demonstration of the insulin-like activity of a tumour product.

In this patient an enhanced expression of the IGF-II gene in tumour tissue, an increase of IGF-II in tumour fluid, the appearance of big IGF-II in patient serum and tumour fluid and the association of IGF-II with small IGFBP complexes were all observed. In addition, it has been demonstrated for the first time that tumour fluid possessed enormous insulin-like activity in vitro. The finding that tumour fluid, but not patient serum, had this capacity confirms the above hypothesis of increased IGF-II bioavailability. In addition, it was demonstrated that glucose consumption by the tumour itself was not of great importance for the hypoglycaemias in this patient. Finally, the normal counter-regulatory responses against hypoglycaemia, namely, increased glucagon, GH, cortisol and catecholamine levels were shown to be insufficient to prevent hypoglycaemic episodes in this patient. These perturbations in counter-regulatory responses are the consequence of abnormal IGF-II activity on the one hand and the prolonged periods of hypoglycaemia on the other [14]. These facts are important in explaining the pathophysiology of tumour-induced hypoglycaemia [13] and are illustrated by the preferential occurrence of hypoglycaemias in the early morning. The increased insulin-like activity due to an IGF-II excess and the insufficient counter-regulatory responses easily explain the severe hypoglycaemias observed in this patient (see Table 1).

Insulin-like growth factors and sarcomas

The involvement of IGFs in tumour biology has been demonstrated for many tumour types [15–17]. Observations which indicate this include enhanced concentrations of IGFs and IGF receptors in tumours, the effect of IGFs on the proliferation of tumour cells and the anti-proliferative effects of IGF receptor inhibition in vitro. The data do, however, show considerable variability. Recently, IGF-II expression in leiomyosarcoma [18] and rhabdomyosarcoma [19] cells and the stimulatory effect of IGF-I on the growth of sarcoma cells [20] has been reported. The role of IGFBPs in tumour biology has not been investigated thoroughly thus far. This work should be undertaken because of the dominant effect of IGFBPs on the biological activity of IGFs. In addition, it is important to mention that a standard RIA cannot discriminate between normal and tumour-derived IGF-II. Column chromatography can demonstrate the presence of big IGF-II. Recently, a RIA has been developed [21] which detects the E-region of the molecule, this being the carboxy-terminal extension of the IGF-II precursor. This RIA can directly show the presence of tumour-derived IGF-II precursors in biological fluids.

Soft tissue sarcomas are frequently associated with areas of 'necrosis', which can be easily detected by standard radiological techniques. These areas may be of great interest because of the fact that they contain enhanced concentrations of tumour products, as has been demonstrated in the present case. Aspiration of tumour-derived fluid is an easy procedure which may be of great help in the investigation of tumour biology.

Management of tumour induced hypoglycaemia

Any excessive insulin-like activity can be detected by measuring the glucose concentration in a blood sample taken after fasting when hypoglycaemia will be present. In such a situation measurable levels of both insulin and c-peptide are indicative of an insulinoma. Unmeasurable levels of these proteins suggest that other insulin-like mechanisms are operating. This is decisive for the discrimination between insulin and insulin-like mechanisms of tumour-induced hypoglycaemia. A further indication for an IGF-II-induced mechanism is the ratio of IGF-I/IGF-II which is low in these patients [22] due to normal or slightly elevated IGF-II levels and low IGF-I concentrations.

The best therapy for tumour-induced hypoglycaemia is reduction of the tumour load. In the case of bulky mesenchymal tumours a partial removal of tumour may be worthwhile, as demonstrated here. Symptomatic treatment consists of dietary guidelines, including strategies to prevent long periods to fasting and advice for the patient and his family of what to do in case of an imminent hypoglycaemia. In addition, drugs can be used which stimulate endogenous glucose production. These medications include glucagon [23], growth hormone [24] and corticosteroids. Somatostatin was not successful in reducing IGF-II production or the frequency of hypoglycaemic episodes in this patient. Treatment with IGFBP-3 is a theoretical possibility, which has not previously been attempted.

The study of the role of IGFs, their binding proteins and IGF-receptors in the biology of sarcomas may offer a new understanding of and new treatment modalities for this type of tumour.

References

1. Cryer PE. Glucose counter regulation: Prevention and correction of hypoglycaemia in humans. Am J Physiol 1993; 264: E149–55.
2. Sinha MK, Buchanan C, Raineri-Maldonado C et al. IGF-II receptors and IGF-II stimulated glucose transport in human fat cells. Am J Physiol 1990; 258: E534–42.
3. Maassen JA, Klinkhamer MP, Odink MP et al. Improper expression of insulin receptors on fibroblasts from a leprechaun patient. Eur J Biochem 1988; 172: 1321–30.
4. Marks V, Teale JD, Tumours producing hypoglycaemia. Diabetes/Metabolism Rev 1991; 7: 79–91.
5. Redmon B, Pyzdrowski K, Elson MK et al. Brief report: Hypoglycaemia due to a monoclonal insulin-binding antibody in multiple myeloma. New Engl J Med 1992; 326: 994–8.
6. Braund WJ, Naylor BA, Williamson DH et al. Autoimmunity to insulin receptor and hypoglycaemia in a patient with Hodgkin's disease. Lancet 1987; 237–40.
7. Lowe WL, Roberts CT, LeRoith D et al. Insulin-like growth factor-II in nonislet cell tumours associated with hypoglycae-

mia: Increased levels of messenger ribonucleic acid. J Clin Endocrinol Metab 1989; 69: 1153–9.

8. Shapiro ET, Bell GI, Polonsky KS et al. Tumour hypoglycaemia: Relationship to high molecular weight insulin-like growth factor-II. J Clin Invest 1990; 85: 1672–9.

9. Sara VC, Hall K. Insulin-like growth factors and their binding proteins. Physiol Rev 1990; 70: 591–615.

10. Daughaday WH, Kapadia M. Significance of abnormal serum binding of insulin-like growth factor II in the development of hypoglycaemia in patients with non-islet-cell tumours. Proc Natl Acad Sci 1989; 86: 6778–82.

11. Baxter RC, Daughaday. Impaired formation of the ternary insulin-like growth factor-binding protein complex in patients with hypoglycaemia due to nonislet cell tumours. J Clin Endocrinol Metab 1991; 73: 696–702.

12. Ceda GP, Davis RG, Rosenfeld RG et al. The growth hormone (GH)-releasing-hormone (GHRH)-GH-somatomedin axis: Evidence for rapid inhibition of GHRH-elicited GH release by insulin-like growth factors I and II. Endocrinology 1987; 120: 1658–62.

13. Ron D, Powers AC, Pandian MR et al. Increased insulin-like growth factor II production and consequent suppression of growth hormone secretion: A dual mechanism for tumour-induced hypoglycaemia. J Clin Endocrinol Metab 1989; 68: 701–6.

14. Mitrakou A, Fanelli C, Veneman T et al. Reversibility of unawareness of hypoglycemia in patients with insulinomas. J Engl J Med 1993; 329: 834–9.

15. Daughaday WH. The possible autocrine/paracrine and endocrine roles of insulin-like growth factors of human tumours. Endocrinology 1990; 127: 1–3.

16. Chen S, Chou C, Wong F et al. Overexpression of epidermal growth factor and insulin-like growth factor-I receptors and autocrine stimulation in human esophageal carcinoma cells. Cancer Res 1991; 51: 1898–903.

17. Furnaletto RW, Harwell SE, Baggs RB. Effects of insulin-like growth factor receptor inhibition on human melanomas in culture and in athymic mice. Cancer Res 1993; 53: 2522–6.

18. Gloudemans T, Prinsen I, van Unnik JAM et al. Insulin-like growth factor gene expression in human smooth muscle tumours. Cancer Res 1990; 50: 6689–95.

19. Yun K. A new marker for rhabdomyosarcoma: Insulin-like growth factor II. Lab Invest 1992; 67: 653–64.

20. Pollak MN, Polychronakos C, Richard M. Insulin-like growth factor I: A potent mitogen for human osteogenic sarcoma. J Natl Cancer Inst 1990; 82: 301–5.

21. Daughaday WH, Trivedi B. Measurements of derivates of proinsulin-like growth factor-II in serum by a radioimmunoassay directed against the E-domain in normal subjects and patients with nonislet cell tumour hypoglycaemia. J Clin Endocrinol Metab 1992; 75: 110–5.

22. Teale JD, Maks V. Inappropriately elevated plasma insulin-like growth factor II in relation to suppressed insulin-like growth factor I in the diagnosis of non-islet cell tumour hypoglycemia. Clin Endocrinol 1990; 33: 87–98.

23. Samaan NA, Pham FK, Sellin RV et al. Successful treatment of hypoglycaemia using glucagon in a patient with an extrapancreatic tumour. Ann Intern Med 1990; 113: 404–6.

24. Teale JD, Blum WF, Marks V. Alleviation of non-islet cell tumour hypoglycaemia by growth hormone therapy is associated with changes in IGF binding protein-3. Ann Clin Biochem 1992; 29: 314–23.

R. L. Souhami (ed.) The Teaching Cases from Annals of Oncology, 17–21, 1997.
© 1997 Kluwer Academic Publishers. Printed in the Netherlands.

Metastatic tumor of unknown primary site

A. Piga, V. Catalano, N. Cardarelli & R. Cellerino

Medical Oncology and Postgraduate School of Oncology, University of Ancona, Ancona, Italy

Key words: unknown primary tumors, spinal cord compression, management, case report

Case history

A 67-year-old woman presented in April 1992 with a two-month history of paresthesia of her lower limbs with progressive weakness and impairment of ambulation. MRI of the thoracic vertebrae showed extradural neoplastic tissue with compression and lateral dislocation of the spinal cord at T2 (Figs. 1 and 2). A month later a percutaneous fine needle aspiration led to the cytological diagnosis of metastatic carcinoma, with immunocytochemistry positive for cytokeratins. The patient underwent a number of diagnostic procedures including chest X-ray, abdomino-pelvic ultrasonography, bone scintiscan, thorax and abdomen computed tomography (CT), gastrointestinal tract X-ray, barium enema, scintigraphy and ultrasonography of thyroid. The results of all of these procedures were inconclusive, and those of routine blood tests were negative.

In June 1992 the patient was submitted to posterior hemilaminectomy of T2-T3, but it was possible to excise only part of the tumor mass. Histology was of a malignant epithelial tumor with no other morphological specification; immunohistochemistry showed positivity for cytokeratins (AE1–AE3), and neurone-specific enolase (NSE). In August 1992, four months after the initial diagnosis, the patient was first seen in our department. The diagnosis was metastatic carcinoma of unknown primary site (UPT, unknown primary tumor) with neuro-endocrine differentiation, with residual dis-

ease after surgical excision. For this group of UPT it is our policy to begin with chemotherapy. Three courses were given of carboplatin, 400 mg/sqm i.v. day 1, doxorubicin 50 mg/sqm i.v. day 1, etoposide 100 mg/sqm i.v. days 1–3; all drug doses of the first course were

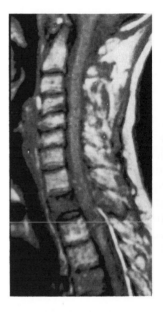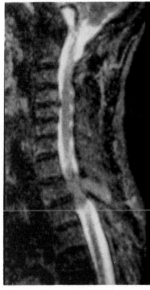

Fig. 1. Sagittal MRI of the column. Left: T1-weighted image showing involvement of T2, which appears darker than the rest of the column. Right: T2-weighted image showing cord displacement around T2.

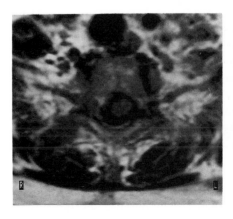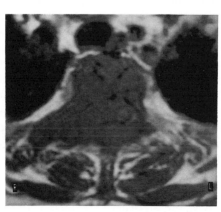

Fig. 2. T1-weighted spinal MRI, cross sections at T1 (left) and T2 (right), the latter showing epidural proliferation of neoplastic tissue originating in the right half of the vertebral body, invading the dural sac, and causing compression and lateralization of the spine.

reduced by 25%. Courses were repeated every 21 days. MRI after three courses, in October 1992, showed at T2 dyshomogeneous tissue possibly of fibrotic nature, with no evidence of neoplasia. Local radiation treatment was given on T1-T4, to a total of 50 Gy, and chemotherapy was restarted aiming at three additional courses; however, after two courses marked myelosuppression (Hb 5.5 g/dl, WBC 500/mm^3, platelets 3000/mm^3) led to hospital admission, supportive treatment and cessation of chemotherapy. Subsequent follow-up has shown neither local relapse nor appearance of the primary tumor; the patient is therefore NED 44 months after diagnosis, and 37 months after completion of treatment.

Discussion points

Tumors of unknown origin

UPT are commonly defined as tumors with histology that is incompatible with the site of biopsy (e.g., adenocarcinoma in a lymph node) and which cannot be definitively diagnosed on the basis of clinical history, physical examination (including gynecological and rectal exploration), chest X-ray, hematochemistry, or blood in urine or stool. Despite extensive diagnostic procedures, a diagnosis of origin in these patients is often not established prior to their deaths. UPT are relevant from an epidemiological point of view, since in various clinical series they represent approximately 5%–10% of all tumors [1–5]. Their incidence may vary widely depending on the definition of UPT and on the type of institution/department where they are observed (e.g., general hospital vs. referral center). In residents of SEER (Surveillance, Epidemiology, and End Results) areas, about 2% of cases observed in the period 1973–1987 were UPT [6], with little variation over time.

UPT usually occur in the elderly, with a peak of incidence around 60 years and a slight preponderance in males [1, 5–9].

The most commonly involved sites are mediastinal and retroperitoneal nodes, lung, and liver. Half of the patients may present with widespread metastatic disease. The histology of the tumor is of major importance for prognosis and possibly for selection of treatment. Well-differentiated adenocarcinoma is the most frequently-occurring histological type, representing approximately two thirds of all cases, with the rest accounted for by poorly-differentiated adenocarcinoma and carcinoma; squamous cell carcinomas and undifferentiated neoplasms represent only a minority of these tumors.

A small proportion of patients with UPT will have a diagnosis of origin established during life. Conversely, in most of the cases in which autopsy is performed the site of origin will be discovered: the majority turn out to be of lung or gastrointestinal origin. However, tumors responsive to chemotherapy (e.g., breast, ovary, prostate carcinoma, small-cell lung cancer), or even curable (e.g., germ cell tumors, Hodgkin's disease and non-Hodgkin's lymphomas) might be discovered in a very small but extremely important proportion of UPT.

Several different categories are now being defined within UPT. From a prognostic point of view the most important distinction concerns isolated lateral cervical lymph node involvement by epidermoid or undifferentiated carcinoma, which should be viewed as regional extension of head and neck tumors. This subgroup of UPT has a prognosis, and calls for diagnostic procedures and treatment distinct from those of other sites or histology [10].

The prognosis of the other groups of UPT is otherwise grave with median survival ranging from 3 to 6 months. Approximately 20%–25% of patients are alive at 1 year and less than 10% at 5 years [1, 3–5, 8, 11, 12].

Diagnostic approach to UPT

Before initiating the diagnostic workup in a patient with UPT it is worthwhile to consider the amount of benefit to be expected from reaching diagnostic conclusions. The possibility of attaining a diagnosis of origin in these patients is poor, usually below 10%, despite the employment of a number of diagnostic procedures. As a rule, the site of origin in these cases is discovered only at necropsy, and even then the origin might not be discovered in as many as 27% [3–5, 13–15]. The traditional approach to UPT has been one of extensive, useless and costly diagnostic procedures aimed at determining the primary site, usually repeated and protracted for a period which may represent a significant proportion of the residual life expectancy of the patient and with the result that the start of treatment is needlessly delayed. A reasonable approach to UPT would be to avoid an excess of diagnostic procedures, without compromising the possibility of finding the primary site, weighing the overall cost of diagnostic procedures with their diagnostic efficacy and clinical (therapeutical) usefulness [16–18].

Hematological and biochemical investigations should include determination of tumor markers, especially those with higher specificity and tests which will have distinct therapeutic consequences (e.g. βHCG, PSA). The routine use of a panel of tumor markers may not offer any diagnostic or prognostic assistance [19]. Urine and stool should be examined for the presence of blood. Chest X-ray will help exclude a lung primary. CT and MRI have not been extensively evaluated, but especially CT should be considered a routine procedure for its ability to search different anatomic sites for the primary tumor, and at the same time gather information on the extent of the disease [20]. Bone scintiscan might also be used to assess the extent of the disease, while other tests should be used only if clinically indicated.

Given the presence within UPT of a proportion of patients with curable or treatable diseases, diagnostic procedures should not be protracted at the expense of prompt institution of treatment. The rapid deterioration of performance status and clinical condition in most of these patients could soon compromise the possibility of even moderately intensive chemotherapy.

On the other hand major efforts should be addressed to histopathology, including repetition of biopsy if necessary and possible. If adequate tissue is available, the pathologist might be able to provide information helpful in treatment planning, such as determination of hormone receptors or special histochemical techniques. The routine use of immunohistochemistry and electron microscopy will often give a better definition of the likely site of origin of the tumor. More recent advances in molecular pathology and genetics may contribute to a more precise diagnosis of these neoplasms in the near future [21]. However, it must be said that when the diagnosis is moderately differentiated adenocarcinoma it is often difficult to determine which of the many primary sites is the most likely one. Histological review using special stains is the most useful single diagnostic procedure.

Prognosis of UPT

Identification of histotype is especially important in UPT, since some tumors might be curable diseases [22–24]. Well-differentiated adenocarcinomas generally have poor prognoses since in most cases this reflects a metastases of gastrointestinal tract origin. Less well differentiated tumors such as undifferentiated neoplasms, poorly-differentiated carcinoma, but also poorly-differentiated adenocarcinoma have somewhat better prognoses and may be responsive to chemotherapy.

In recent years subgroups of patients with a relatively favorable prognosis and responsiveness to treatment have been defined. These are women with peritoneal carcinomatosis, young patients with lymphadenopathies of the midline and tumors with clinical features suggestive of extragonadal germ cell tumors such as midline mediastinal tumors, and tumors with neuroendocrine differentiation.

Extent of the tumor strongly influences prognosis and the possibility of control of UPT. There are at present no specific staging systems for UPT. By using the TNM system, all UPT might be classified as $T_xN_xM_1$, since they present as metastases. The usual way to define extent of the disease is to determine spread in relation to the diaphragm. Patients presenting with the disease confined to one side of the diaphragm have better prognoses than those with dissemination to both sides. The former reflects both lower tumor burden and the possibility of obtaining satisfactory local control of the disease. In all reported series, number of sites is one of the most important prognostic factors; limited involvement and the possibility of local control are associated with better prognosis [1, 4, 5, 9, 25–27]. Previously identified relevant prognostic factors were validated in recently published papers [9, 28], and new prognostic variables proposed; molecular and genetic studies might in the future assist both in prognosis and in prediction of response to treatment [29].

Treatment of UPT

It is of course essential not to overlook the proportion of patients with a curable to treatable tumor. Our present approach is to reduce the diagnostic phase to a minimum, favoring rapid institution of the treatment. With this approach and the use of an intensive regimen of chemotherapy we are now obtaining approximately 40% of responses (complete + partial) and better survival than in historical controls [30].

The presence of a hidden primary site should not preclude attempts to achieve local control at known sites of disease. The natural history of these tumors shows that only rarely does the primary tumor become manifest; patients may die with widespread disease while the primary goes undetected.

In the presence of UPT of limited extent the combination of radiotherapy and chemotherapy may ensure local control and improve survival. Prognosis might be particularly favorable if the involved sites are nodes rather than viscera [5, 9].

Chemotherapy is the treatment of choice for widespread disease. Various subgroups of UPT (e.g., germ cell tumors, lymphomas, SCLC, etc.), which normally belong to poorly-differentiated histotypes, are responsive to chemotherapy. The most effective treatment for these has not been defined but combinations containing platinum and etoposide give satisfactory results; the various series show complete remission in 12%–31% of patients, with some long-lasting remissions [27, 31–34]. Non-responsive tumors (such as ones originating from lung or gastrointestinal tract) are often found among UPT with histology of well-differentiated adenocarcinomas, and their treatment with platinum-based regimens may be less justified. For this category of UPT a possible origin in breast or prostate should be considered, since these tumors exhibit some degree of hormone responsiveness.

Management of cord compression

Cord compression occurs in approximately 5% of patients with neoplasms, and more frequently in those with lung, breast or prostate cancers, unknown primary tumors, lymphomas, myelomas or soft tissue sarcomas [35]. Spinal involvement is usually of extradural origin, developing from bone (vertebral) metastases; it may less often originate from intraspinal extension of perispinal tumors such as lymphomas or neuroblastomas that reach the vertebral canal through intervertebral foramina or by direct metastasis to the spine. Although uncommon, spinal cord compression is an oncologic emergency because of the severity of functional compromise it may cause and because recovery depends strictly on the rapidity with which treatment is initiated [36, 37].

Early signs and symptoms of cord compression include spinal and possibly radicular pain exacerbated by movement, sensory loss, limb weakness, and abnormal tendon reflexes. Symptoms may progress until ataxia, paraplegia, or loss of sphincter control occur. Irreversible loss of neurologic functions is usually caused by delay in institution of treatment.

The onset of paraparesis leaves a maximum of 24 hours within which to start treatment if permanent neurologic damage is to be averted.

Even before a diagnosis has been made, clinical suspicion should indicate immediate treatment with steroids to antagonize the inflammatory component of the compression. MRI will in most instances accurately diagnose a cord compression; the more invasive myelography should be reserved for cases in which MRI does not provide a definite diagnosis.

Surgery consists of laminectomy in instances of posterior compression, and vertebral body resection for anterior compression. Surgery is especially useful when a histological diagnosis is needed when the tumor is expected to be radio-resistant or progresses during radiotherapy, or when the stability of the spinal column is compromised. Since surgery rarely results in eradication of tumor radiation treatment will usually follow. In general radiotherapy alone should be used for radiosensitive neoplasms to preserve the stability of the column. Chemotherapy has only a minor role as primary treatment, except in responsive tumors of childhood or as a palliative measure in instances of relapse after local treatments.

In case of UPT, as described here, surgical decompression is the treatment of choice both to relieve cord compression and to establish the diagnosis. In our case the neuro-endocrine phenotype indicated the need for both chemotherapy and local radiotherapy to minimise the risk of local recurrence.

Conclusion

The patient described here had a tumor with neuro-endocrine differentiation, presenting with spinal involvement as the only site of disease. The primary treatment was surgery which partially eradicated the disease and provided clearer definition of histology. Results of diagnostic procedures, as expected, were inconclusive, as to the site of origin. When the patient first came to our attention a combined chemoradiotherapeutic approach was decided upon based on the expected responsiveness to chemotherapy of this subset of UPT, and on the single site of involvement which suggested the possibility of eradication by the adjunct of local treatment.

The patient is now being followed with 6-monthly clinical and instrumental procedures which include chest X-ray and MRI of spine, and is free of disease 26 months after diagnosis.

References

1. Didolkar MS, Fanous M, Elia EG et al. Metastatic carcinomas from occult primary tumors. A study of 254 patients. Ann Surg 1977; 5: 625–30.
2. Karsell PR, Sheedy PF, O'Connel MJ. Computed tomography in search of cancer of unknown origin. JAMA 1982; 248: 340–3.
3. Hamilton CS, Langlands AO. ACUP (adenocarcinoma of unknown primary site). A clinical and cost benefit analysis. Int J Rad Oncol Biol Phys 1987; 13: 1497–503.
4. Kirsten F, Chi CH, Leary JA et al. Metastatic adeno or undifferentiated carcinoma from unknown primary site. Natural history and guidelines for identification of treatable subsets. Q J Med 1987; 238: 143–51.
5. Piga A, Bascioni R, Vissani L et al. Unknown primary tumors. A clinical retrospective study of 136 patients. J Exp Clin Cancer Res 1992; 11: 63–8.
6. Muir C. Cancer of unknown primary site. Cancer 1995; 75: 353–6.
7. Stewart JF, Tattersall MHN, Woods RL et al. Unknown primary adenocarcinoma: Incidence of over-investigation and natural history. Br Med J 1979; 1: 1530–3.
8. Altman C, Cadman E. An analysis of 1539 patients with cancer of unknown primary site. Cancer 1986; 57: 120–4.
9. Abbruzzese JL, Abbruzzese MC, Hess KR et al. Unknown primary carcinoma: Natural history and prognostic factors in 657 consecutive patients. J Clin Oncol 1994; 12: 1272–80.
10. de Braud F, Al-Sarraf M. Diagnosis and management of squamous cell carcinoma of unknown primary tumor site of the neck. Semin Oncol 1993; 20: 273–8.
11. Markman M. Metastatic adenocarcinoma of unknown primary site: Analysis of 245 patients seen at Johns Hopkins Hospital from 1965 to 1979. Med Pediatr Oncol 1982; 10: 569–74.
12. Le Chevalier T, Cvitkovic E, Chille F et al. Early metastatic cancer of unknown primary origin at presentation. A clinical study of 302 consecutive autopsied patients. Arch Intern Med 1988; 148: 2035–9.
13. Osteen RT, Kopf G, Wilson RE et al. In pursuit of unknown primary. Am J Surg 1978; 135: 494–8.
14. Nystrom JS, Weiner JM, Meshmik Wolf R et al. Identifying the primary site in metastatic cancer of unknown primary origin. Inadequacy of roentgenographic procedures. JAMA 1979; 241: 381–3.
15. Gaber AO, Rice P, Eaton C et al. Metastatic malignant disease of unknown origin. Am J Surg 1983; 145: 493–7.
16. Abbruzzese JL. An effective strategy for the evaluation of unknown primary tumors. Cancer Bull 1989; 41: 157–61.
17. Abbruzzese JL, Abbruzzese MC, Lenzi R et al. Analysis of a diagnostic strategy for patients with suspected tumors of unknown origin. J Clin Oncol 1995; 13: 2094–103.
18. Schapira DV, Jarrett AR. The need to consider survival, outcome, and expense when evaluating and treating patients with unknown primary carcinoma. Arch Intern Med 1995; 155: 2050–4.
19. Pavlidis N, Kalef-Ezra J, Briassoulis E et al. Evaluation of six tumor markers in patients with carcinoma of unknown primary. Med Pediatr Oncol 1994; 22: 162–7.
20. Leonard RJ, Nystrom SJ. Diagnostic evaluation of patients with carcinoma of unknown primary tumor site. Semin Oncol 1993; 20: 244–50.
21. Daugaard G. Unknown primary tumors. Cancer Treat Rev 1994; 20: 119–47.
22. Azar HA, Espinoza CG, Richman AV et al. Undifferentiated large cell malignancies: An ultrastructural and immunocytochemical study. Hum Pathol 1982; 13: 323–33.
23. Gatter KC, Alcock C, Heryet A et al. Clinical importance of analysing malignant tumours of an uncertain origin with immunohistochemical techniques. Lancet 1985; 1: 1302–5.
24. Hales SA, Gatter KC, Heryet A et al. The value of immunocytochemistry in differentiating high-grade lymphoma from

other anaplastic tumours: A study of anaplastic tumours from 1940 to 1960. Leuk Lymph 1989; 1: 59–63.

25. Pasterz R, Savaraj N, Burgess M. Prognostic factors in metastatic carcinoma of unknown primary. J Clin Oncol 1986; 4: 1652–7.

26. Kambhu SA, Kelsen D, Fiore J et al. Metastatic adenocarcinoma of unknown primary site. Am J Clin Oncol 1990; 13: 55–60.

27. Hainsworth JD, Johnson DH, Greco FA. Treatment of poorly differentiated carcinoma and poorly differentiated adenocarcinoma of unknown primary site with cisplatin based chemotherapy: Results of a twelve year experience. J Clin Oncol 1992; 10: 912–22.

28. Van der Gaast A, Verweij J, Planting AS et al. Simple prognostic model to predict survival in patients with undifferentiated carcinoma of unknown primary site. J Clin Oncol 1995; 13: 1720–5.

29. Motzer RJ, Rodriguez E, Reuter VE et al. Molecular and cytogenetic studies in the diagnosis of patients with poorly differentiated carcinomas of unknown primary site. J Clin Oncol 1995; 13: 274–82.

30. Piga A, Cardarelli N, Catalano V et al. Cancer of unknown primary site: A collaborative study on diagnosis and treatment. Proc ASCO 1994; Abs 1380.

31. Van der Gaast A, Verweij J, Henzen-Logmans SC. Carcinoma of unknown primary: Identification of a treatable subset. Ann Oncol 1990; 1: 119–23.

32. Raber MN, Faintuch J, Abbruzzese JL. Continuous infusion of 5-fluorouracil, etoposide and cis-diamminedichloroplatinum in patients with metastatic adenocarcinoma of unknown primary origin. Ann Oncol 1991; 2: 519–20.

33. Greco FA, Johnson DH, Hainsworth JD. Etoposide/cisplatin-based chemotherapy for patients with metastatic poorly differentiated carcinoma of unknown primary site. Semin Oncol 1992; 19: 14–8.

34. Pavlidis N, Kosmidis P, Skarlos D. Subset of tumors responsive to cisplatin or carboplatin combination in patients with carcinoma of unknown primary site. Ann Oncol 1992; 2: 631–4.

35. Bruckman JE, Bloomer WD. Management of spinal cord compression. Semin Oncol 1978; 5: 135.

36. Delaney TF, Oldfield EH. Spinal cord compression. In De Vita VT, Hellman S, Rosenberg SA (eds): Cancer: Principles & Practice of Oncology. Philadelphia: J. B. Lippincott Co., 4th ed. 1993; 2118–27.

37. Souhami R, Tobias J. Cancer and its Management, 2nd ed. Oxford: Blackwell Science Ltd 1995; 154–5.

R. L. Souhami (ed.) The Teaching Cases from Annals of Oncology, 23–28, 1997.

Paraneoplastic neurologic syndromes

J. Bauer,[1] T. Kuntzer[2] & S. Leyvraz[1]

[1]Centre Pluridisciplinaire d'Oncologie; [2]Neurology Department, Centre Hospitalier Universitaire Vaudois, Lausanne, Switzerland

Key words: Lambert-Eaton myasthenic syndrome, paraneoplastic neurologic syndrome

Introduction

Paraneoplastic neurologic syndromes (PNS) are remote, nonmetastatic complications of systemic cancer. Clinically they are characterized by subacute, progressive neurologic deficits that usually result in profound disability and eventually death. PNS may be present as long as 2 to 4 years before diagnosis of the associated tumor, but it can develop after diagnosis or when the cancer is thought to be in remission. Serum and cerebrospinal fluid (CSF) from many patients with PNS contains antineuronal antibodies which recognise antigens within the tumor. This suggests that PNS are autoimmune disorders in which the immune response, elicited by the patient's tumor, cross-reacts with specific neuronal proteins.

The incidence of clinically relevant PNS is low: less than 1%–3% of patients with cancer present with or subsequently develop one of these syndromes.

This review will focus on the major PNS with special emphasis on the most common and best understood, the Lambert-Eaton myasthenic syndrome (LEMS).

Case history

A 68-year-old man, a former smoker with chronic obstructive pulmonary disease, reported with a two-month history of cough, worsening dyspnea and progressive weakness. His main complaints, however, were of neurological origin, namely increasing weakness of the legs and sudden, transient flexion of the left knee, walking strain, difficulty in raising both arms, transitory episodes of ptosis and diplopia, dry mouth and decrease in sweating. Clinical examination revealed moderate muscle wasting with an assymetric proximal tetraparesis, worse in the left leg, and increased muscle strength after repeated stimuli. Deep tendon reflexes were absent at rest but present after facilitation exercises. The clinically suspected diagnosis of Lambert-Eaton myasthenic syndrome was confirmed by electrophysiologic studies with the finding of a reduced

compound muscle action potential (CMAP) amplitude in the resting abductor pollicis brevis muscle and an increment, following maximum voluntary contraction, of over 300%. Antibodies to acetylcholine receptors were negative in serum.

A chest X-ray showed an upper left lung lesion. Bronchoscopy with biopsies led to a diagnosis of small-cell anaplastic carcinoma (oat-cell carcinoma). Thoracic CT scan demonstrated a left hilar lesion with multiple homo- and contralateral mediastinal adenopathies. No distant metastasis was found on routine examination (abdominal echography, bone scintigram, brain CT scan and bilateral bone marrow biopsies).

Treatment was initiated and consisted of initial chest radiotherapy (20 G) followed by 6 cycles of cisplatin-based chemotherapy. Simultaneously, steroids (prednisone 1 mg/kg) were administered for the neurologic syndrome. Tumor response was rapid with a partial remission after irradiation and the first course of chemotherapy. Concurrently, an improvement of the weakness was observed. Repeated electrophysiologic studies showed a close correlation between the median nerve CMAP amplitude and the clinical course. After the third cycle, radiological complete remission, confirmed at the end of treatment, was obtained. Prednisone was tapered after the first month of treatment and stopped at the end of the chemotherapy, with complete recovery of the motor and the autonomic functions. However, the patient died suddenly 41 months later probably of a myocardial infarction without clinical evidence of recurrent disease. No autopsy was performed.

Physiopathology and classification of paraneoplastic neurologic syndromes

PNS may involve the central nervous system (brain and spinal cord), peripheral ganglia or the neuromuscular junction [1, 2] (Table 1). A major advance in the understanding of paraneoplastic syndromes has been the identification of various antineuronal antibodies in serum and CSF of the affected patients. These anti-

Table 1. Paraneoplastic syndromes of the nervous system.

Site	Syndrome	Associated neoplasms	Causes
Brain	Subacute cerebellar degeneration	Lung, prostate colorectal, ovary, cervix, Hodgkin's, others…	Type I anti-Purkinje cells antibody (anti-Yo)
	Encephalomyelitis – limbic encephalitis – bulbar encephalitis	Lung, germ cell, Hodgkin's, others…	Type IIa anti-neuronal antibody (Anti-Hu)
	Retinal degeneration	Lung (small cell)	Antiretinal antibodies
	Opsoclonus/ataxia	Lung, breast, neuroblastoma, retino-blastoma	Type IIb panneuronal antibody (Anti-Ri)
	Dementia	Lung	–
	Progressive multifocal leuko-encephalopathy	Leukemias, lymphomas, sarcomas	Papovavirus
	Angioendotheliosis	Lymphomas, others…	Angiogenic peptides
Spinal cord	Subacute necrotic myelopathy	Lung, kidney, Hodgkin's	?
	Subacute motor neuropathy	Lymphoma	Viral ?
	(Amyotrophic lateral sclerosis)	?	?
Peripheral nerves	Dorsal sensory neuropathy	Lung, others…	Type IIa anti-neuronal antibody (Anti-Hu)
	Sensory-motor peripheral neuropathy	Lung, gastro-intestinal, breast, others…	?
	Autonomic neuropathy	Lung (small cell)	?
Muscle/ neuro-muscular junction	Dermatomyositis, polymyositis	Lung, stomach, ovary, others…	
	Myasthenic syndrome (Lambert-Eaton Syn.)	Lung (small cell), ovary, stomach, others…	Autoimmune response against calcium channels
	Myasthenia gravis	Thymoma	Anti-acethylcholin receptors anti-body

Adapted from [1] and [2].

bodies appear to be an autoimmune response triggered by tumor antigens immunologically cross-reactive with neuronal proteins [3, 4]. Their precise role in the pathogenesis of neurologic symptoms, however, is still unknown. As shown in Table 1, the pattern of immunofluorescent staining of the brain as well as the proteins identified by Western blot analysis in serum an CSF vary according to the specific paraneoplastic syndrome and the histologic nature of the associated neoplasm. For instance, anti-neuronal nuclear antibodies, known as anti-ANNA-I or Anti-Hu have been observed in several different clinical paraneoplastic manifestations of lung cancer such as subacute sensory neuronopathy, an paraneoplastic encephalomyelitis (limbic or bulbar) [5, 6]. Pathological studies have shown common neuronal and tumoral binding as demonstrated for the anti-Hu IgG antibody; reactive neurons have been demonstrated in sections from various regions of the brain [7].

Certain clues should lead to a diagnosis of PNS. Most of these syndromes evolve subacutely and are usually severe. They are often characteristic of, but none is invariably associated with, cancer and they affect a particular portion of the nervous system with additional subtle clinical signs suggesting dysfunction outside that area.

Subacute cerebellar degeneration (SCD). SCD is the most frequently occurring PNS in the central nervous system. It is seen most often in association with lung, ovarian, and breast cancers and in Hodgkin's disease [8]. Clinical signs are subacute or progressive symmetric cerebellar syndrome with gait ataxia and eventually appendicular ataxia, dysarthria, and often nystagmus. Vertigo is common. The pathological hallmark of SCD is a severe loss of Purkinje cells. With few exceptions, inflammatory cell infiltration is not found in the cerebellar cortex but may be confined to the dentate nuclei.

Molecular analysis has shown in the serum and, at higher titer, in the cerebrospinal fluid (CSF) of patients with gynecologic cancers, the presence of a specific auto-antibody designated anti-Yo. The antibody reacts histochemically with the cytoplasm of Purkinje cells and with the tumors of patients with SCD. Ovarian and breast tumors taken from patients without SCD show no such reaction.

However, definite proof of the autoimmune origin of the disease is still a matter for discussion. Attempts to reproduce this syndrome in animals by injections of human IgG have so far failed. Immunosuppressive and plasma exchange therapy do not affect the clinical evolution. Although a decrease in the amounts of serum antibodies has been obtained, the antibody titer in the CSF is not affected. It is possible that the Purkinje cells are destroyed very early in the course of the disease, before the start of treatment.

Reaction of sera from patients with Purkinje cell extracts using the Western blot technique has identified two bands at 34 and 62 kd. Genes coding for these two proteins have been cloned [9, 10] and mapped to chromosomes X (34 kd antigen) and 16 (62 kd protein)

[11]. The function of these two proteins is still unknown but recent work suggests that they may play a role in the regulation of gene expression [12].

Female patients presenting this syndrome and a high titer of anti-Yo antibodies should be extensively investigated for gynecological or breast cancer. According to Posner, of six patients with anti-Yo-positive SCD and without evidence of tumor, gynecological cancer was established in five after abdominal surgical exploration; the sixth patient developed breast cancer a few months after the diagnosis of SCD [8].

Sensory neuronopathy. Sensory neuronopathy, also called dorsal root neuronopathy, occurs predominantly in the setting of small-cell lung carcinoma and is frequently accompanied by paraneoplastic encephalitis (see below). Patients with this syndrome exhibit progressive loss of all sensory capacity with impairment of proprioception. A distinction between paraneoplastic neuropathy and cisplatin-induced neuropathy may be difficult to determine; however, the latter mainly concerns the sensations transmitted through large fiber modalities (fine touch, vibration, position) without impairment of the small fibers (temperature, pinprick).

Encephalitis. Limbic encephalitis is characterized by progressive mental and emotional disturbances with anxiety and depression and frequent progression to dementia. Bulbar encephalitis is a progressive failure of brain stem functions, including control of the respiration.

Synchronous paraneoplastic encephalitis and neuronopathy have been observed in patients who exhibit an autoantibody termed anti-Hu. This antibody was described in 1965 and further characterized [13]. It is a polyclonal complement-fixing IgG that reacts with the nuclei of almost all neurons in the nervous system but also with all small-cell lung carcinomas (whether or not the patient clinically expresses the paraneoplastic syndrome) [8].

Opsoclonus/ataxia. Chaotic eye movement disorders (opsoclonus) with truncal or limb ataxia and other cerebellar signs have been described in patients with breast and gynecologic cancers [14]. In contrast to the syndromes associated with anti-Yo and anti-Hu, this syndrome tends to wax and wane, sometimes with spontaneous resolution of the opsoclonus. An antibody named anti-Ri-associated with this syndrome has recently been described. Although it appears to share identical histochemical properties with the anti-Hu antibody, gene cloning and protein sequencing have demonstrated that anti-Ri recognizes a different epitope [15].

Retinal degeneration. Rapid binocular loss of vision has usually been associated with small-cell lung cancer but sometimes with gynecological tumors [16]. This disorder is characterized by photosensitivity, light-induced glare, impaired visual acuity, ring scotomata and attenuated retinal arterial caliber. Patients present episodic visual obscuration and night blindness followed by a rapid and painless loss of vision. Antibodies to small-cell carcinoma antigens have been found in the serum and cerebrospinal fluid which were immunologically cross-reactive with identical retinal antigens.

Lambert-Eaton myasthenic syndrome (LEMS)

First recognized clinically in association with lung cancer in 1953 [17], LEMS has subsequently been reported in patients in whom no neoplasms were detected. In a large review of 50 LEMS patients, only one-half had no evidence of cancer, and 21 of the cancer patients suffered from small-cell lung carcinoma [18]. 1%–5% of patients with small-cell lung carcinoma (oat-cell carcinoma) present with LEMS.

Symptoms are summarized in Table 2. Their onset is usually gradual. Most patients present with slowly developing leg weakness, often associated with aching and stiff muscles exacerbated by activity or muscular cramping. Fatiguability is prominent after protracted exercise. Autonomic dysfunction is present in three-quarters of the patients, usually in the form of dry mouth, and, less frequently, blurred vision, sweating dysfunction, impotence and constipation. Involvement of cranial nerves is usually less severe and transient. Diplopia and drooping eyelids are the principle manifestations, but dysathria, dysphagia, impaired chewing and hypophonia may be present. Sensory complaints are rare and consist mainly of back pain and numbness or paresthesiae of the extremities. Respiratory disorders are infrequently reported.

Physical signs parallel the symptoms (Table 3). Although experienced by the majority of patients, muscle weakness may be difficult to demonstrate at bedside. The same is true for the increase of strenght after exercise described by some authors [18]. In contrast, a return of depressed or absent deep tendon reflexes after exercise sustained for 10 to 15 seconds is a very useful sign which is present in almost all patients. More

Table 2. Symptoms of Lambert-Eaton myasthenic syndrome.

Symptoms	Percent of patient		
	With cancer	Without cancer	All patients
Weakness	100	100	100
Lower limb	100	100	100
Upper limb	68	88	78
Muscle pain	32	40	36
Autonomic disorders	64	96	80
Cranial nerve	64	76	70
Sensory complaints	16	8	12
Respiratory	8	4	6

Adapted with permission from [18].

26

Table 3. Clinical signs of Lambert-Eaton myastenic syndrome.

Signs	Percent of patient		
	With cancer	Without cancer	All patients
Muscle weakness	88	96	92
Lower limb	88	96	92
Upper limb	72	96	82
Cranial nerves	60	64	62
Ptosis	52	56	54
Neck weakness	32	36	34
Reflexes			
Depressed/absent	96	88	92
Potentiation	80	76	78
Sensory impairment	8	0	4
Autonomic signs	12	12	12

Adapted with permission from [18].

than half of the patients present cranial involvement. The dominant sign is ptosis but weakness of neck flexion is also relatively common. Objective autonomic dysfunction such as sluggish pupillary light reflexes and an absence of sweating are infrequent.

LEMS is, in the majority of cases, a paraneoplastic syndrome even though the underlying malignancy may not be diagnosed for several months after the appearance of the neurological signs [18]. Small-cell lung cancer is the most common tumor found in association with LEMS. However, many LEMS patients, with or without cancer, may have other organ-specific autoimmune disorders. These include Hashimoto's thyroiditis, pernicious anemia, vitiligo, systemic lupus erythematosus and antibody-positive myasthenia gravis [18–20].

The muscle weakness of LEMS is due to a defect of neuromuscular transmission in the pre-synaptic region, secondary to an impaired release of acetylcholine from the motor end-plate [21]. The role of a humoral factor responsible for the syndrome was postulated when clinical and physiopathologic features were reproduced in mice injected with serum or with a purified IgG fraction from patients with LEMS [22, 23]. Moreover, clinical improvement has been noticed after plasma exchange or immunosuppressive medication [24].

Physiological studies of motor nerve terminals demonstrated that a serum component from LEMS patients was able to inactivate a substantial quantity of voltage-gated calcium channels on pre-synaptic terminals [25]. It was further shown that this inactivation was related to the destruction of the calcium channels by a complement-mediated action on IgG cross-linked receptors resembling that of the postsynaptic destruction of acetylcholine receptors observed in myasthenia gravis [26, 27]. In summary, LEMS is associated with an antibody-mediated destruction of the presynaptic voltage-gated calcium channels. Small-cell lung cancer cells express functional voltage-gated calcium channels and it is assumed that small-cell lung cancer antibodies cross-react with neuromuscular-junction voltage-gated calcium channels. However, the variety of calcium

channel subtypes and the uncertainty about which of these channels are affected by the pathologic antibodies has prevented the exact identification of the specific antigen until now.

Recently an assay for voltage-gated-calcium-channel antibody was developed using the ω-conotoxin, a specific calcium channel ligand [28, 29]. However, anticalcium channel auto-antibodies are detectable in the serum of patients with clinical and electrophysiological LEMS in a proportion ranging from 30% to 90%. For the present, the test's lack of sensitivity renders its wide clinical application unfeasible [30].

Although LEMS may strongly be suspected on clinical grounds, diagnosis is assured by electrophysiologic findings which exclude the most likely differential diagnoses of myasthenia gravis and myopathy. In brief, the resting compound muscle action potential (CMAP) amplitude is low but facilitation is the rule after rapid repetitive stimulation leading to an increase of 2 to 10 times that of the baseline value.

When LEMS is clinically suspected and confirmed by electrophysiological studies, investigations for an underlying malignant tumor must be undertaken. However, in 30% to 50% of cases, no tumor can be detected concomitantly [18]. As mentioned previously the vast majority of associated cancers are anaplastic small-cell lung carcinoma, but LEMS has been associated with other lung tumors such as adenocarcinoma. Infrequently it may be associated with extrathoracic tumors such as gastric, colic and biliary tract adenocarcinomas, and even lymphoma.

Treatment of paraneoplastic neurologic syndrome

When there is clinical suspicion of PNS at presentation, it is important to exclude any other causes – malignant or non-malignant – which could explain the neurological signs.

Detection of antineuronal antibodies must be followed by a search for the associated cancer. Investigation is directed by the clinical signs and by the type of antibody.

Although appropriate studies may detect the cancer, occasionally no tumor may be found in an antibody-positive patient. A careful follow-up must then be undertaken since neoplasm may be diagnosed up to four years after the PNS first appeared.

Because of the infrequent occurrence of PNS, information about therapy is anecdotal. There are three possible therapeutic approaches to PNS:

a) *Treatment of the underlying cancer:* Most complete recoveries from PNS have occurred when the tumor was detected at an early stage and completely removed, either by surgery or by other oncological treatment. In the case report presented above, the neurological recovery of the LEMS correlated with the rapid and complete clinical remission of the tumor. However, in Hodgkin's disease recovery of the cerebella syndrome is uncertain even after complete tumor response.

b) *Immunosuppressive therapy:* Treatment of the PNS by immunosuppressive therapy should be undertaken with caution and in association with a specific treatment of the tumor, since autoimmune mechanisms thought to be responsible for the PNS are the result of an immune response to the patient's tumor.

Immunotherapy, including plasma exchange, intravenous immunoglobulin and prednisone, has an accepted role in the treatment of LEMS [24, 31]. Some patients with opsoclonus/ataxia have also benefitted from this approach. However, as already mentioned above, the majority of patients with other PNS experienced no benefit even when there was a marked reduction of the antibody's titer.

c) *Symptomatic management:* The important neurological impairment that results from the PNS usually causes much greater patient disability than does the tumor and its treatment. Careful passive physical training during the subacute phase of the illness, and aggressive, prolonged therapy by physiotherapists is essential to enable patients to achieve optimal use of residual neurological capacities. However, improvement over time is often very limited, leading to concurrent depression. The need for social support is a major concern for patients with PNS who survive their cancers.

In the particular case of LEMS, cause of symptoms is a well understood mechanism, which allows specific symptomatic treatment. Drugs that promote the release (guanidine, aminopyridine) or prevent the breakdown (pyridostigmine) of acetylcholine and thus enhance the effector function are available in the clinic. Guanidine and aminopyridines facilitate the release of acetylcholine by prolonging duration of the action potentials. This leads to an increase in calcium uptake by the voltage gated calcium channels and consequently, acetylcholine release. However, the severe toxicities associated with guanidine (renal, hematologic, hepatic and gastro-intestinal) and with 4-aminopyridine (epileptogenic) are limiting their usefulness in practice. Clinical experience with a new agent, 3,4-diaminopyridine (DAP) has shown to be effective in increasing strength and improving autonomic symptoms in patients with LEMS. DAP is at least as potent as 4-aminopyridine and less toxic. Supplemental of pyridostigmine (acetylcholine esterase inhibitor) which prevent the breakdown of acetylcholine, may be used to enhance the effects of DAP. Unlike guanidine and 4-aminopyridine, DAP is generally well tolerated. Mild and dose-related side effects are usual in many patients and include perioral paresthesias, epigastric distress and insomnia. In patients taking large dose of DAP (>100 mg/day), seizure have been observed [32].

References

1. Bunn PA Jr, Ridgway EC. Paraneoplastic syndromes: Neurologic manifestation of malignancy. In DeVitta V, Hellmann S, Rosenberg SA (eds): Cancer, Principles and Practive of Oncology. Philadelphia: J.B. Lippincott Company 1993; 2026–71.
2. Greenlee JE, Brashear HR. Remote effects of carcinoma. In Johnson RT, Griffin JW (eds): Current Therapy on Neurologic Diseases. St. Louis, MO: Mosby Year Book Inc. 1993; 235–9.
3. Schuller-Petrovic S, Gebhart W, Lassmann H et al. A shared antigenic determinant between natural killer cells and nervous tissue. Nature 1983; 306: 179–81.
4. Bunn PA, Gazdar AF, Carney DN et al. Small cell lung carcinoma and natural killer cells share an antigen determinant, Leu-7. Clin Res 1984; 32: 413A.
5. Kimmel DW, O'Neill BP, Lennon VA. Subacute sensory neuronopathy associated with small cell lung carcinoma: Diagnosis aided by autoimmune serology. Mayo Clin Proc 1988; 63: 29–32.
6. Dalmau J, Furneaux HM, Gralla RJ et al. Detection of the anti-Hu antibody in the serum of patients with small cell lung cancer – a quantitative Western blot analysis. Ann Neurol 1990; 27: 544–52.
7. Dalmau J, Furneaux HM, Rosenblum MK er al. Detection of the anti-Hu antibody in specific regions of the nervous system and tumor from patients wih paraneoplastic encephalomyelitis/sensory neuronopathy. Neurology 1991; 41: 1757–64.
8. Posner JB. Pathogenesis of central nervous system paraneoplastic syndromes. Rev Neurol (Paris) 1992; 148: 502–12.
9. Dropcho EJ, Chen YT, Posner JB et al. Cloning of a brain protein identified by autoantibodies from a patient with paraneoplastic cerebellar degeneration. PNAS 1987; 84: 4552–6.
10. Sakai K, Mitchel DJ, Tsukamoto T et al. Isolation of a complementary DNA clone encoding an autoantigen recognized by an anti-neuronal cell antibody from a patient with paraneoplastic cerebellar degeneration. Ann Neurol 1990; 28: 692–8.
11. Siniscalco M, Oberle I, Melis P et al. Physical and genetic mapping of the CDR gene with particular reference to its position with respect to the FRAXA site. Am J Med Genetics 1991; 38: 357–62.
12. Fatallah-Shaykh H, Wolf S, Wong E et al. Cloning of a leucine-zipper protein recognized by the sera of patients with antibody-associated paraneoplastic cerebellar degeneration. PNAS 1991; 88: 3451–4.
13. Wilkinson PC, Zeromsky J. Immunofluorescent detection of antibodies against neurons in sensory carcinomatous neuropathy. Brain 1965; 88: 529–38.
14. Luque AF, Furneaux HM, Fergizer R et al. Anti-Ri: An antibody associated with paraneoplastic opsoclonus and breast cancer. Ann Neurol 1991; 29: 241–51.
15. Darnell RB, Posner JB. Cloning and characterization of the neuronal antigen recognized in paraneoplastic opsoclonus-myoclonus. Neurology 1991; 41 (Suppl 1): 363.
16. Jacobson DM, Thirkill CE, Tipping SJ. A clinical triad to diagnose paraneoplastic retinopathy. Ann Neurol 1990; 28: 162–7.
17. Anderson HJ, Churchill-Davidson HC, Richardson AT. Bronchial neoplasm with myasthenia: Prolonged apnoea after administration of succinylcholine. Lancet 1953; 2: 1291–3.
18. O'Neill JH, Murray NMF, Newsom-Davis J. The Lambert-Eaton myasthenic syndrome. A review of 50 cases. Brain 1988; 111: 577–96.
19. Bromberg MB, Albers JW, McCune WJ. Transient Lambert-Easton myasthenic syndrome associated with systemic lupus erythematosus. Muscle Nerve 1989; 12: 15–9.
20. Newsom-Davis J, Leys K, Vincent A et al. Immunological evi-

dence for the co-existence of the Lambert-Eaton myasthenic syndrome and myasthenia gravis in two patients. J Neurol Neurosurg Psychiatry 1991; 54: 452–3.

21. Eaton LM, Lambert EH. Electromyography and electric stimulation of nerves in diseases of motor unit: Observations on myasthenic syndrome associated with malignant tumors. JAMA 1957; 163: 1117–24.

22. Kim Yl. Passively transferred Lambert-Easton syndrome in mice receiving purified IgG. Muscle Nerve 1986; 9: 523–30.

23. Lang B, Newsom-Davis J, Wray D et al. Autoimmune aetiology for myasthenic Lambert-Eaton syndrome. Lancet 1981; 2: 224–6.

24. Newsom-Davis J, Murray NM. Plasma exchange and immunosuppressive drug treatment in the Lambert-Easton myasthenic syndrome. Neurology 1984; 34: 480–5.

25. Kim Yl, Neher E. IgG from patients with Lambert-Eaton syndrome blocks voltage-dependant calcium channels. Science 1988; 239: 405–8.

26. Fukuoka T, Engel AG, Lang B et al. Lambert-Eaton myasthenic syndrome II. Immunoelectron microscopy localization of IgG at the mouse motor end-plate. Ann Neurol 1987; 22: 200–11.

27. Nagel A, Engel AG, Lang B. Lambert-Eaton myasthenic syndrome IgG depletes presynaptic membrane active zone particles by antigenic modulation. Ann Neurol 1988; 24: 552–8.

28. Lennon VA, Lambert EH. Autoantibodies bind solubilized calcium channel-ω-conotoxin complexes from small cell lung carcinoma. A diagnostic aid for the Lambert-Eaton myasthenic syndrome. Mayo Clin Proc 1989; 64: 1498–504.

29. Sher E, Gotti C, Canal N et al. Specificity of calcium channel autoantibodies in Lambert-Eaton myasthenic syndrome. Lancet 1989; 2: 640–3.

30. Leys K, Lang B, Johnston I et al. Calcium channel autoantibodies in the Lambert-Eaton myasthenic syndrome. Ann Neuro 1991; 29: 307–14.

31. Bird SJ. Clinical and electrophysiologic improvement in Lambert-Eaton syndrome with intravenous immunoglobulin therapy. Neurology 1992; 42: 1422–3.

32. McEvoy KM. Lambert-Eaton myasthenic syndrome. In Johnson RT, Griffin JW (eds): Current Therapy on Neurologic disease. St. Louis, MO: Mosby Year Book Inc. 1993; 384–8.

R. L. Souhami (ed.) The Teaching Cases from Annals of Oncology, 29–36, 1997.
© 1997 *Kluwer Academic Publishers. Printed in the Netherlands.*

The management of bone metastases

J. Vinholes & R. Coleman

YCRC Department of Clinical Oncology, Weston Park Hospital, University of Sheffield, Sheffield, U.K.

Key words: bone metastases, hypercalcaemia, bisphosphonates

Introduction

Bone is the most common site of metastatic disease and is especially prevalent in tumours arising in the breast, prostate, lung, thyroid and kidney. Because of the frequency and relatively long course of breast cancer, bone metastases from this site are clinically the most important. The pattern of distribution of bone metastases is similar for most tumours, affecting the spine, pelvis, ribs, skull and proximal femora, and typically more than one site is involved. The prognosis depends fundamentally on the type of the primary tumour. The longest median survivals are seen in prostate [19] and thyroid cancers (more than 3 years), compared with two years for breast cancer [4] and multiple myeloma, and only a few months for melanoma and lung cancer.

Bone metastases cause considerable morbidity and the following case history illustrates many of the common skeletal problems encountered by oncologists and discusses new approaches to management.

Case history

In September 1988, a 47-year-old premenopausal caucasian woman presented with a 6-week history of an asymptomatic lump in the left breast. Initially, wide local excision was attempted. However this 2.5 cm poorly differentiated ductal carcinoma proved to be multifocal and she proceeded to a left mastectomy. No tumour was found in the axillary lymphnodes. Six months later a contralateral primary was identified. This was also treated by mastectomy. Histology showed a node-negative ductal adenocarcinoma. Adjuvant tamoxifen 20 mg/day was started, which she remained on for about 4 years. In November 1992 she presented with chest pain. A ventilation/perfusion radioisotope lung scan suggested a diagnosis of pulmonary embolus and she was commenced on warfarin.

In March 1993, she developed stiffness of the neck and slight rib discomfort. On examination no signs of local recurrence or neurological deficit were found.

Routine haematological and biochemistry tests were normal. A chest X-ray revealed a 1.5 cm solitary pulmonary nodule and destruction of the left 4th rib and an X-ray of cervical spine showed complete loss of the body of C3 (Fig. 1a).

Because of the severity of bone destruction and the risk of cord damage, the neck was immobilised with a hard cervical collar and the patient referred for surgical stabilisation of the spine (Fig. 1b). The operation was complicated by periods of profound hypotension precipitated by movement of the neck during surgery indicating the precarious state of the upper cervical cord. Post-operatively the patient had mild weakness and numbness of C5-C8 nerve roots, particularly on the right. After recovery from surgery she received external beam radiotherapy (3000 cGy in 10 fractions).

Staging investigations were completed and included an isotope bone scan which showed multiple hot spots with X-ray confirmation of bone metastases in both iliac wings, right calcaneum, right shoulder and D10. As she was still menstruating and had shown a 4-year disease-free interval on adjuvant tamoxifen, a radiation induced menopause (1200 cGy in 3 fractions) was performed and the tamoxifen stopped. After this, her pain and neurological symptoms slowly improved.

In August 1993, because of persistent pain, she commenced a new oral bisphosphonate – ibandronate (BM 21.0955) as part of a phase I/II evaluation. During the 4 months' trial her pain improved further and she had no side-effects. At the end of this period the lytic bone lesions were re-evaluated by X-rays and showed improvement with sclerosis of the majority of them (Figs. 2a and 2b).

In March 1994, she complained of pain in the ribs and discomfort in the left hip. X-rays showed radiological progression in both sites. She was commenced on Megestrol acetate 160 mg/day as second-line treatment and received palliative radiotherapy (3000 cGy in 10 fractions) to a new lesion in the mid shaft of the right femur. A few weeks later, both hips were also irradiated (2000 cGy in 5 fractions) due to increasing bone pain.

In June 1994, she was admitted with severe pain in the lower back. X-rays showed bone metastases at L3 and left sacrum and these were also irradiated (2000 cGy in 5 fractions).

One month after discharge she was readmitted with mental confusion, hallucinations, sickness, vomiting, constipation and dehydration. Corrected serum calcium was 3.99 mmol/l (normal 2.2–2.6) and creatinine 117 umol/l (normal 53–106). Rehydration with 3 l of normal saline per 24 h was given and on the next day she received an infusion of pamidronate 90 mg. Within 3 days her nausea and vomiting had improved and the calcium decreased to 3.23 mmol/l. One week after admission she was less confused and the calcium had fallen to 2.88 mmol/l, but a new pain appeared in the lower back.

In view of these skeletal complications, the systemic therapy was changed to chemotherapy with cyclophosphamide 600 mg/m^2, methotrexate 40 mg/m^2 and 5-fluorouracil 600 mg/m^2 (CMF) given intravenously every 3 weeks. Two days after receiving chemotherapy, she again became confused and hypercalcaemic (calcium 3.08 mmol/l). She was treated with a second infusion of pamidronate (60 mg) and within three days the

A

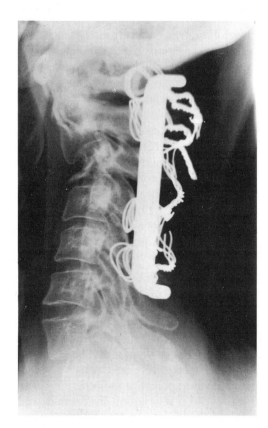

B

Fig. 1. Cervical X-ray showing complete loss of C3 body, before (A) and after (B) surgical stabilisation.

A

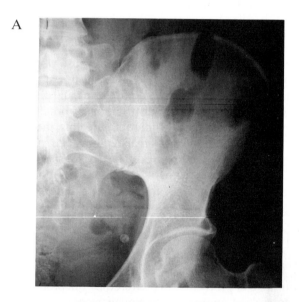

B

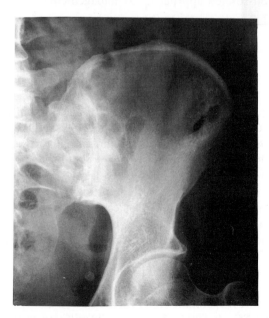

Fig. 2. Left pelvis X-ray showing a lytic bone metastasis before bisphosphonates treatment (A) with sclerosis being evident after 4 months of oral bisphosphonates (B).

calcium was again normal. One week later, a new episode of hypercalcaemia was again treated successfully with rehydration and pamidronate. Subsequently, hypercalcaemia did not recur and her pain control improved. CMF was continued for 4 courses but her general condition deteriorated and she died shortly after the 4th course, 19 months after diagnosis of bone metastases.

Discussion

Tumour cells usually disseminate to bone by blood-borne spread. This is a multi-step process determined by certain characteristics of the cancer cells, the distribution of the red bone marrow, Batson's vertebral-venous plexus which enables cells to by-pass the lungs and enter directly into the axial skeleton, and particular features of the bone microenvironment.

After reaching bone, tumour cells are attracted to the bone surface by collagen fragments and growth factors released from the bone surface. Here they produce paracrine factors which stimulate osteoclasts to resorb bone. These factors include prostaglandins, cytokines and growth factors (Fig. 3). This tumour-induced osteoclastic bone resorption is the prevailing mechanism of bone destruction by all types of malignant cells and osteoclasts have become an important therapeutic target in oncology. In addition, bone is a source of growth factors and cytokines which also stimulate tumour growth. This cancer cell-host cell interaction may be an important step in the initiation of skeletal metastases.

There are three types of bone metastases (osteolytic, osteosclerotic and mixed), each reflecting the tumour effects on bone physiology. In osteosclerotic metas-

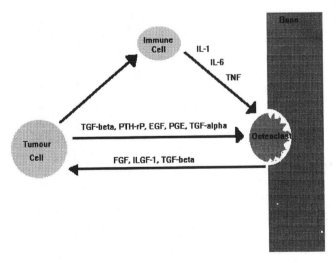

Fig. 3. Diagrammatic summary of interactions between tumour cell and bone. TGF (transforming growth factor), PTH-rP (parathyroid hormone-related protein), EGF (epidermal growth factor), FGF (fibroblast growth factor), PGE (prostaglandin E), TNF (tumour necrosis factor), ILGF-1 (insulin-like growth factor), IL-1 (interleukin 1), IL-6 (interleukin 6).

tases, bone formation predominates and excessive new bone is deposited away from sites of previous bone resorption. They are typically found in prostate cancer but also occur in breast cancer. In osteolytic metastases, which are the most common, there is uncoupling of bone resorption and formation, with loss of calcium from the skeleton and progressive destruction of bony trabeculae. This is typically found in multiple myeloma, renal cell cancer, thyroid cancer and in many patients with breast and lung cancers. A mixed appearance reflects coexistence of both processes. This is usually seen in breast cancer and occasionally in lung cancer.

Systemic anticancer treatment for bone metastases

The systemic treatment depends primarily on the type of the tumour. In breast cancer the choice is based on clinical patterns of relapse. Patients with oestrogen receptors positive tumours, a long disease-free interval (more than two years from diagnosis to relapse) and non-life threatening disease (bone metastases and/or soft tissue disease) should receive hormone therapy, while those with oestrogen receptor negative tumours, endocrine-resistant disease and those with extensive visceral disease or life-threatening disease (e.g., liver metastases with compromised hepatic function) should be treated with chemotherapy.

There are no good data to support the use of one endocrine agent over another. The claims made from time to time for both aminoglutethimide and medroxy-progesterone acetate probably reflect the imprecision of assessing response in bone rather than a specific effect on bone metastases.

Chemotherapy may be more hazardous in patients with skeletal metastases due to poor bone marrow reserve. Bone marrow infiltration by tumour and radiotherapy reduce bone marrow tolerance while immobility and generally poor performance status increase the probability of intercurrent infection.

Bone pain

Pain is the most common symptom of metastatic bone disease, affecting more than 70% of patients with bone metastases. Anti-inflammatory agents (NSAIDs) and opiates provide useful pain relief. For localised bone pain, external beam radiotherapy is the treatment of choice. More than 80% of patients show some relief, and half of them have a complete response. Most patients begin to show relief within the first two weeks, with 80% of them responding in the first month. Recurrent bone pain at the same site may be amenable to treatment but normal tissue tolerance precludes multiple retreatments.

Some studies have shown that single large fractions (between 4 and 8 cGy) are as effective as multiple fractions (usually 1 to 3 cGy in 5 to 15 fractions) [23]. A recent study has shown that 8 cGy dose is more effective than 4 cGy dose in relieving pain [14], but more data are still needed in this setting.

Bisphosphonates are a relatively new therapeutic option for bone pain. These drugs have a short plasma half-life (around two hours) and a very high affinity for bone, where they probably remain for years [10]. After binding to the hydroxyapatite bone surface, their main effect is the inhibition of osteoclast-mediated bone resorption. The antiresorptive potency varies enormously, from etidronate (~1×), through clodronate (~10×), to pamidronate (~100×). New bisphosphonates currently undergoing evaluation have even greater potency (Table 1), opening up the possibility of more reliable non-parenteral routes of administration in the future.

Bisphosphonates inhibit bone resorption in several ways; they may decrease the recruitment of osteoclasts precursors (particularly pamidronate), inhibit the attachment of osteoclasts to bone surface, and exert a direct cytotoxic effect (particularly clodronate) [9, 16].

Bisphosphonates are a useful therapy for bone pain, with relief being achieved in about half of the patients and bone healing, evidenced by sclerosis of lytic skeletal lesions, in 25% of patients [30, 3]. In addition, they induce a fall in bone resorption markers, reduce the incidence of pain requiring radiotherapy, decrease analgesic consumption, and may ameliorate mobility with improvement in the quality of life – a major goal in metastatic bone disease. The optimal dose is not yet defined, but it appears that the analgesic effect is greater with infusions of at least 60 mg of pamidronate which can be administered on a out-patient basis. Recently, it has been shown that pamidronate given as a single infusion of 120 mg alleviates pain and improves quality of life in 60% of patients with effects persisting over eight weeks, independent of the origin of the primary tumour [24].

Hypercalcaemia

Malignancy is the most frequent cause of hypercalcaemia in hospitals patients, which is the most common metabolic complication in oncology, occurring in about 5% of patients. Hypercalcaemia is most frequent in breast cancer, multiple myeloma, squamous cell lung cancer and renal cell cancer but rare in cancers arising

Table 1. Relative potency of bisphosphonates.

Relative potency	Bisphosphonates
1	Etidronate
10	Clodronate
100	Pamidronate
100–1.000	Alendronate
	Dimethyl-APD
	YM 175
1.000–10.000	Ibandronate (BM 21.0955)
	Risedronate
>10.000	CGP 42.446

from the prostate, gastrointestinal tract and female genital tract.

Calcium is present in serum in three forms: ionised (about 50%), protein-bound (40%), mainly linked to albumin, and complexed (10%) with citrate and phosphate. The ionised form is the portion tightly regulated by parathyroid hormone (PTH) and 1,25 dihydroxyvitamin D $[1,25(OH_2)]$, through a negative feedback process. The normal range of total calcium 2.2–2.6 mmol/l (8.4–10.2 mg/dl).

The pathophysiology of hypercalcaemia is now more clearly understood. The two main mechanisms are focal osteolytic destruction (osteolysis) due to bone metastases and the release of humoral factors by the tumour into the circulation. The latter may occur in the absence of bone metastases. These humoral factors have effects on bone and kidney, accelerating the rate of bone resorption and (like PTH) increasing distal renal tubular reabsorption of calcium.

In breast cancer, both osteolysis and humoral factors seem to be important, while in other solid tumours, humoral factors seem to be more relevant. In multiple myeloma, osteolytic destruction and renal impairment due to the tubular deposition of Bence-Jones protein often coexist.

There are several humoral factors, but the most important mediator is parathyroid hormone-related protein (PTH-rP) [2]. Its amino-terminal sequence is the only portion that is similar to PTH, but this is a vital part, because it is involved with the recognition of the PTH receptor [27]. Thus PTH and PTH-rP have similar biological effects.

Clinical presentation

Usually hypercalcaemia indicates progressive advanced cancer, but hyperparathyroidism should be excluded as well as the hormone flare syndrome which occasionally occurs within the first month of starting tamoxifen therapy [8]. The severity of symptoms is related to the level of serum calcium, speed of increase and individual factors (age, performance status, sites of metastases, hepatic or renal dysfunction). The initial symptoms usually appear when the serum calcium is >3 mmol/l. However, if there is a rapid increase in serum calcium, even relatively mild hypercalcaemia may cause symptoms.

Hypercalcaemia leads to a decrease in neuromuscular excitability. The initial symptoms are anorexia, fatigue, lethargy, nausea, constipation and polyuria. Without treatment hyporeflexia, mild confusion, personality changes, vomiting, dehydration, renal insufficiency, ileus and bradycardia occur. Eventually patients may develop severe confusion, arrhythmias, coma and death.

Treatment

Hypercalcaemia usually requires a change in systemic treatment where available. However, breast cancer patients have usually received previous systemic treatment and the response to second or third-line therapy is unpredictable. Even when a response is envisaged, specific measures to control hypercalcaemia are frequently needed in symptomatic patients, even though the prognosis is usually only a few months.

Dietary restriction of calcium is not useful or necessary, except in the unusual patient with lymphoma associated with high levels of 1,25 dihydroxyvitamin D. Thiazide diuretics, vitamins D and A should be stopped and patients mobilised where clinically possible.

Calcium is a potent diuretic causing loss of water and sodium, resulting in a decrease in glomerular filtration rate and further reabsorption of calcium. Therefore, the initial management is rehydration with normal saline (3–4 l/day) over the first 24–48 h, followed by 2–3 l/day for the next few days. Rehydration increases glomerular filtration and decreases proximal and distal renal tubular reabsorption of calcium, thereby increasing urinary calcium excretion. This will induce a slight fall in serum calcium (about 0.3–0.5 mmol/l) and alleviate some symptoms. However, only patients with mild hypercalcaemia become normocalcaemic and even in those, further therapy is normally required to prevent early recurrence. Rehydration needs to be carefully monitored in the elderly or in patients with significant cardiovascular disease or renal insufficiency.

Loop diuretics, although potentially able to increase urinary calcium excretion and frequently prescribed, may increase volume depletion and induce excessive urinary losses of potassium and magnesium. There is little evidence of their value in routine management.

Bisphosphonates

In the last few years, the bisphosphonates have become the drugs of choice to control malignant hypercalcaemia. Intravenous administration of these drugs is the route used in the treatment of hypercalcaemia due to the poor absorption of oral formulations and the gastrointestinal symptoms of many hypercalcaemic patients.

Pamidronate can be given safely as a single two-hour infusion in 500 ml saline, starting when a satisfactory urine output has been established [3]. Serum calcium levels fall significantly after 3 days and normocalcaemia is obtained after a median of 4 days. However, as was seen in our patient, recovery of neurological function may not occur until several days after correction of hypercalcaemia.

The bisphosphonates show a modest dose-response relationship. With pamidronate a 30 mg dose will control hypercalcaemia in approximately 70% of patients for a median of 10–14 days [4] while a 90 mg dose is effective in more than 90% [20] with a duration of about 4 weeks [25]. Recent studies have confirmed that patients with high PTH-rP levels have a reduced hypocalcaemic response to bisphosphonates [33]. Therefore, those patients with humoral hypercalcaemia and high PTH-rP levels, as well as patients with very severe hypercalcaemia (calcium $\geqslant$ 4 mmol/l), should receive 90 mg.

Recurrent hypercalcaemia can be retreated and normocalcaemia regained [12], although the response is progressively less, particularly in tumours other than breast cancer [15].

Superiority over traditional treatments such as mithramycin and calcitonin has been shown, but relatively few trials comparing bisphosphonates have been published. Pamidronate was more effective than both etidronate and clodronate in one trial [26], and superior to etidronate in another [13] while a comparison of pamidronate and clodronate at full dosage showed similar acute efficacy but a significantly longer duration of action with pamidronate [25].

Clodronate is also effective, with up to 1500 mg given as a single infusion. Its effect lasts for a median of 2 weeks [25]. Etidronate is the least effective bisphosphonate, requiring multiple infusions and pamidronate or clodronate are now preferred.

Bisphosphonates are well-tolerated drugs. They may induce a transient mild hypocalcaemia, almost always without clinical significance, and mild local phlebitis. Oral administration may cause indigestion, nausea, vomiting or diarrhoea in 5%–10% of patients. In up to 25% of patients pamidronate causes a transient pyrexia and a fall in lymphocytes [24]. This reaction is more intense within the first 48 h after the first infusion and disappears over the next few days but rigors are rare and the syndrome is normally not clinical significant. The release of cytokines from stimulated macrophages is thought to be responsible. Long-term continuous use of etidronate will cause inhibition of mineralization and hence osteomalacia and is contraindicated. At the doses currently used in clinical practice this has not been observed with the other more specific and potent bisphosphonates.

Other treatments

Calcitonin acts by both reducing tubular reabsorption of calcium and inhibiting bone resorption. It has a rapid onset of action (2–4 h), and can be given when there is renal impairment. Calcitonin is now only used for life-threatening, severe hypercalcaemia to achieve rapid partial control until the more potent bone resorption drugs begin to act [28]. Used alone, the improvement is short-lived and tachyphylaxis is common. The recommended dose of salmon calcitonin is 4–8 IU/kg every 6–8 h, by subcutaneous or intramuscular (more reliable absorption) injection.

Corticosteroids have also been frequently used, but are only of benefit in those patients with a steroid-responsive tumour (myeloma, lymphoma, occasional breast cancer). The hypocalcaemic effect normally takes at least one week to appear and except for patients with lymphoma they should not be used.

Mithramycin has a direct cytotoxic effect on osteoclasts, and is a potent bone resorption inhibitor. Toxicity and a short duration of action inhibit its usefulness.

In a randomised study, pamidronate was shown to be superior to mithramycin in achieving normocalcaemia (88% vs. 41%) [29].

Phosphate is a temporary inhibitor of bone resorption, also inducing precipitation of calcium/phosphate aggregates in soft tissues. Intravenous phosphate induces a prompt fall in serum calcium (minutes), but is associated with serious cardiovascular side-effects and now only used for severe refractory hypercalcaemia. Oral phosphate (1–3 g/day divided in three or four doses) is a weak inhibitor of bone resorption which can be used to treat mild hypercalcaemia in ambulatory patients. Induction of diarrhoea limits its usefulness and regular monitoring of serum phosphate and creatinine are necessary.

Gallium nitrate is a potent inhibitor of bone resorption, but the precise mechanism of action is not yet clear. More than 80% of patients become normocalcaemic, with the onset of action beginning after the second day of infusion and lasting for about 2 weeks. It is given after the patient is rehydrated as a continuous 5-day infusion of 200 mg/m^2/day. Renal impairment may occur and gallium is contraindicated in patients with renal insufficiency. A randomised study has shown that gallium nitrate is more effective than etidronate [32] and approval has been granted for clinical use in U.S.A.

Impending and pathological fractures

Pathological fracture is more likely if bone metastases are associated with functional pain (limb pain that worsens with use), are predominantly lytic or involve greater than half of the cross-sectional bone diameter [18]. Breast cancer is responsible for more than 50% of pathological bone fractures [1]. They occur in 15% of breast cancer patients with first relapse in bone [6] but are infrequent in prostate cancer (predominantly osteoblastic lesions) and less common in lung cancer (most patients do not live long enough to develop them). The most commonly affected site is the proximal femur, although lesions of the femoral shaft and humerus are also common. The prognosis of a pathological fracture depends on the type of tumour. For example, in a series of 80 breast cancer patients, the median survival was one year [4].

The treatment of choice for impeding fractures is prophylactic internal fixation followed by radiotherapy. Careful clinical evaluation, radiographs of the entire affected bone (it is not unusual to find other metastases in the same bone) and an isotope bone scan are required before surgery. Prophylactic treatment avoids the need for emergency surgery and the associated stress, and prevents the displacement of fracture fragments. Furthermore, it is easier to stabilise a non-broken bone and the rehabilitation is faster. If the patient is unfit for surgery, radiotherapy and non-weight bearing are indicated.

The treatment of choice for pathological fractures is primary internal stabilisation followed by radiotherapy. This will normally alleviate pain and restore mobility [11]. Radiotherapy is the primary treatment if ribs or vertebrae are affected. Systemic treatment may also be necessary.

Spinal cord and cauda equina compression

The initial symptom is pain, followed usually by motor weakness and sensory loss, and later autonomic and sphincter dysfunction. The thoracic spine is the segment most frequently involved. Cord damage may be due to mechanical damage to vertebra with fractures and collapse or compression from soft tissue extension. A recent review of magnetic resonance imaging (MRI) patterns of spinal disease revealed that bone collapse was present in only 25% of patients, while in 75% of cases there was soft tissue extension into epidural tissue [22].

Myelography has traditionally been the investigation required in this setting, but in recent years, MRI has been increasingly used. MRI does not carry the risk of rapid neurological deterioration which is seen in about 20% of patients after lumbar puncture below a complete spinal block. Furthermore, MRI is able to assess the whole spine and demonstrate paravertebral tumour extension which helps in planning local treatment.

The prognosis in this situation depends primarily on the degree of neurological dysfunction prior to therapy. There is considerable debate about the best local treatment. Surgery is preferred when the tumour origin is unknown, in the presence of spinal instability as in our patient, for previously irradiated areas, and in rapidly progressive paraplegia. High dose steroids and radiotherapy should be used in radiosensitive tumours who do not fulfil the criteria of surgical decompression. Chemotherapy may be added to local treatment in sensitive tumours such as germ-cell tumours, lymphomas, multiple myeloma and breast cancer.

Spinal instability is associated with a considerable degree of pain on movement which has a primarily mechanical origin. It is most frequently associated with breast cancer. Radiographs show destruction with vertebral collapse. Treatment is internal stabilisation with post-operative irradiation.

Prevention of skeletal complications

Several large randomised trials have been published assessing the role of bisphosphonates in preventing skeletal complications. In the first published trial, breast cancer patients were randomised to receive oral pamidronate or allocated to a control group, with systemic therapy left at the discretion of the physician. The pamidronate group showed a significant reduction in the incidence of hypercalcaemia, pain requiring radiotherapy, impending fractures and changes in systemic therapy [31].

In a double-blind controlled trial of oral clodronate

in patients with bone metastases from breast cancer, the incidence of hypercalcaemia and vertebral fractures was also reduced [9]. Recently, a randomised phase III trial was published comparing chemotherapy with chemotherapy and pamidronate 45 mg every 3 weeks. The incidence of pain requiring radiotherapy was reduced in those receiving pamidronate and the median time to disease progression in bone increased (269 days vs. 192 days, $p < 0.05$) [7].

Further studies are still needed to define more precisely the role of bisphosphonates in the prevention of skeletal complications with particular emphasis on quality of life and cost effectiveness.

Future

The bisphosphonates role in the prevention of bone metastases has been studied in animals. Effects of a risedronate injection in nude mice injected with human cancer breast cells were evaluated radiologically and histologically over six weeks. Risedronate inhibited the progression of lytic metastases and interestingly the formation of new bone metastases. In addition, it prolonged survival and decreased tumour burden in bone. The latter could be due to the establishment of a less friendly microenvironment to the bone metastases by the inhibition of bone resorption [17]. Clinical studies testing the bisphosphonates in the adjuvant setting in breast cancer are in progress.

References

1. Bross P, Reynders P, Vanderschot P. Surgical treatment of the metastatic fracture of the femur improves quality of life. Acta Orthop Belg 1993; 59 (Suppl 1): 52–6.
2. Bundred NJ, Ratcliffe WA, Walker RA et al. Parathyroid hormone-related protein and hypercalcaemia in breast cancer. BMJ 1991; 303: 1506–9.
3. Coleman R, Purohit OP. Osteoclast inhibition for the treatment of bone metastases. Cancer Treat Rev 1993; 79–103.
4. Coleman R, Rubens R. The clinical course of metastases from breast cancer. Br J Cancer 1987a; 55: 61–6.
5. Coleman R, Rubens R. Treatment of hypercalcaemia of malignancy secondary to advanced breast cancer with 3 (amino-1, 1hydroxypropyledene) bisphosphonate. Br J Cancer 1987b; 56: 465–9.
6. Coleman R. Clinical aspects of metastatic disease. In Coleman R, Rubens R (eds): Metastatic Bone Disease. The Partenon Publishing Group, Lancs 1992; 11–25.
7. Conte PF, Giannessi PG, Latreille J et al. Delayed progression of bone metastases with pamidronate therapy in breast cancer patients: A randomised, multicenter phase III trial. Ann Oncol 1994; 5 (Suppl 7): S41–S4.
8. Dauggard G. Tamoxifen and hypercalcaemia. Ann Oncol 1993; 4: 683–7.
9. Flanagan AM, Chambers TJ. Clodronate inhibits resorption through injury of osteoclast that resorbs clodronate coated bone. Bone Miner 1989; 6: 33–43.
10. Fleisch H. Pharmacokinetics of bisphosphonates. In Fleisch H (ed): Bisphosphonates in Bone Disease. Berne: Stamplfi Co. Ltd. 1993; 50–4.
11. Galasko SB. The role of the orthopaedic surgeon in the treatment of skeletal metastases. In Rubens R, Fogelman I (eds): Bone Metastases – Diagnosis and Treatment. London: Springer-Verlag 1991; 207–22.
12. Grutters JC, Hermus AR, De Muller PH, Beex LV. Long-term follow-up of breast cancer patients treated for hypercalcaemia with APD. Breast Cancer Res Treat 1993; 25 (3): 277–81.
13. Gucalp R, Ritch P, Weirnik PH et al. Comparative study of pamidronate and etidronate in the treatment of cancer-related hypercalcaemia. J Clin Oncol 1992; 10: 134–42.
14. Hoskin PJ, Price P, Easton B et al. A prospective randomised trial of 4 cGy or 8 cGy single doses in the treatment of metastatic bone pain. Radiother Oncol 1992; 23: 74–8.
15. Louviax I, Dumon JC, Body JJ. Efficacy of pamidronate for recurrences of tumor-induced hypercalcaemia according to the tumour type. Second Workshop on Bisphosphonates, 1994, Abstr 73.
16. Lowik CWGM, Van der Pluijm G, Bijvoet OLM. Migration and phenotypic transformation of osteoclast precursors into mature osteoclasts; the effects of a bisphosphonate. J Bone Miner Res 1988; 3: 185–92.
17. Mundy G. Metastatic bone disease. In Mundy G (ed): Bone Remodelling and Its Disorders. London: Martin Dunitz 1995; 104–22.
18. Mirels H. Metastatic disease in long bones. A proposed scoring system. Clin Orthop 1989; 249: 256–65.
19. Nesbit RM, Baum WC. Endocrine control of prostatic carcinoma: Clinical and statistical survey of 1818 cases. JNCI 1984; 68: 507–17.
20. Nussbaum SR, Younger J, Vanderpol CJ et al. Single-dose intravenous therapy with pamidronate for the treatment of hypercalcaemia of malignancy: Comparison of 30-, 60-, and 90-mg dosages. Am J Med 1993; 95 (3): 297–304.
21. Paterson AHG, Powels TJ, Kanis JA et al. Double-blind controlled trial of oral clodronate in patients with bone metastases with breast cancer. J Clin Oncol 1993; 11: 59–65.
22. Pigott KH, Baddely H, Matter EJ. Pattern of disease in spinal cord compression on MRI scan and implications for treatment. Clin Oncol R Coll 1994; 6 (1): 7–10.
23. Price P, Hoskin PJ, Easton D et al. Low-dose single-fraction radiotherapy in the treatment of metastatic bone pain. Radiother Oncol 1988; 12: 297–300.
24. Purohit OP, Anthony C, Owen J et al. High-dose intravenous pamidronate for metastatic bone pain. Br J Cancer 1994; 70: 554–8.
25. Purohit OP, Anthony C, Owen J et al. Randomised double-blind comparison of single infusions of pamidronate or clodronate for hypercalcaemia of malignancy. Br J Cancer 1994; 69 (Suppl XXI): 10.
26. Ralston S, Gallacher SJ, Dryburgh FJ et al. Comparison of three intravenous bisphosphonates in cancer-associated hypercalcaemia. Lancet 1989; ii: 1180–3.
27. Strewler GJ, Nissenson RA. Parathyroid hormone-related protein. In Favus MJ (ed): Primer on the Metabolic Bone Diseases and Disorders of Mineral Metabolism. New York: Raven Press 1993; 61–3.
28. Thiebaud D, Jaeger P, Burckhardt P. Fast and effective treatment of malignant hypercalcaemia with combined pamidronate and calcitonin. BMJ 1990; 292: 1549–50.
29. Thurlimann B, Waldburger R, Senn HJ et al. Plicamycin and pamidronate in symptomatic tumour-related hypercalcaemia: A prospective randomised cross-over trial. Ann Oncol 1992; 3: 619–23.
30. Tyrrell CJ on behalf of the Aredia Multinational Cooperative Group. Role of pamidronate in the management of bone metastases from breast cancer: Results of a non-comparative multicenter phase II trial. Ann Oncol 1994; 5 (Suppl 7): 37–40.
31. Van Holten-Verzantvoort ATM, Kroon HM, Bijvoet OLM et al. Palliative pamidronate treatment in patients with bone metastases from breast cancer. J Clin Oncol 1993; 11 (3): 491–8.
32. Warrell RP, Heller G, Murphy WP et al. A randomised double-

blind study of gallium nitrate compared to etidronate for acute control of hypercalcaemia. J Clin Oncol 1991; 9: 1467–75.

33. Wimalawansa SJ. Significance of plasma PTH-rP in patients with hypercalcaemia of malignancy treated with bisphosphonate. Cancer 1994; 73 (8): 223–30.

R. L. Souhami (ed.) The Teaching Cases from Annals of Oncology, 37–41, 1997.

The management of Hodgkin's disease

J. A. Radford,[1] G. R. Morgenstern[2] & D. Crowther[1]

[1] CRC Department of Medical Oncology; [2] Department of Haematology, Christie Hospital, Manchester, U.K.

Key words: Hodgkin's disease, treatment of Hodgkin's disease, treatment complications

Case history

A 27-year-old female school teacher originally present-ed in March 1987 with a six month history of painless left cervical lymphadenopathy. She had no systemic symptoms and there were no other signs of disease on clinical examination but a chest radiograph showed non-bulky mediastinal adenopathy. An abdominal CT scan was normal. Biopsy confirmed nodular sclerosing Hodgkin's disease (HD) and a staging laparotomy with splenectomy was performed. None of the lymph nodes or the spleen or the liver contained HD and it was con-cluded that the disease was confined to two sites above the diaphragm (pathological stage IIA). Mantle field radiotherapy was administered during April and May 1987 and a complete remission was obtained.

She remained well until July 1990 when, at 32 weeks of pregnancy, she presented with pruritus and weight loss. There was no palpable evidence of relapse but, following delivery at term, a CT scan was performed which showed para-aortic and bilateral iliac adeno-pathy. There was no evidence of disease within the pre-vious irradiation field. A diagnosis of relapsed HD was made and eight cycles of alternating LOPP/EVAP chemotherapy were given. Her symptoms rapidly dis-appeared and a further CT scan at the completion of chemotherapy showed complete resolution of the pre-viously noted abnormalities.

Within three months, the pruritus had returned. A repeat CT scan showed no recurrence of lymphadeno-pathy but three lung lesions (each less than 1 cm in diameter and of uncertain significance) were identified. She was treated symptomatically but the pruritus did not improve and a CT scan in February 1992 showed multiple, cavitating pulmonary lesions (largest 4 × 3 cm), several liver lesions (largest 7 × 4 cm), and para-aortic lymphadenopathy. A transbronchial lung biopsy and CT guided liver biopsy showed inflammatory changes but no other abnormalities and because of the coincidental onset of fever, opportunistic fungal infec-tion was considered. Intravenous amphotericin was commenced but her condition failed to improve and in mid-March 1992 a laparotomy was performed. Biop-sies of the liver and abdominal lymph nodes confirmed recurrence of nodular sclerosing HD and she was

transferred to the Christie Hospital for further manage-ment.

At that time she described lethargy, troublesome pruritus and heavy night sweats. Her appetite was poor and she had lost 13 kg in weight during the previous three months. Examination revealed a thin, ill-looking woman with extensive scratch marks over the trunk and limbs but there was no palpable lymphadenopathy or hepatomegaly. The blood count showed a haemoglobin of 10.6 gms/dl, a total leukocyte count of $23.2 \times 10^9/l$ (neutrophils 93%) and platelets of $423 \times 10^9/l$. The esr was 72 mm/hour and a bone marrow aspirate and trephine biopsy were clear. The serum alkaline phos-phatase (236 u/l), gamma glutamyl transferase (154 u/l) and LDH (562 u/l) were elevated but a biochemi-cal profile was otherwise normal.

Treatment with weekly VAPEC-B chemotherapy was commenced at the end of March 1992 (Fig. 1).

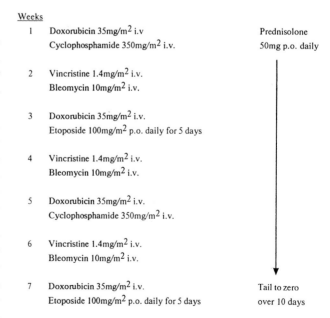

VAPEC-B : Treatment Schema

Weeks

1   Doxorubicin 35mg/m^2 i.v   Prednisolone
    Cyclophosphamide 350mg/m^2 i.v.   50mg p.o. daily

2   Vincristine 1.4mg/m^2 i.v.
    Bleomycin 10mg/m^2 i.v.

3   Doxorubicin 35mg/m^2 i.v.
    Etoposide 100mg/m^2 p.o. daily for 5 days

4   Vincristine 1.4mg/m^2 i.v.
    Bleomycin 10mg/m^2 i.v.

5   Doxorubicin 35mg/m^2 i.v.
    Cyclophosphamide 350mg/m^2 i.v.

6   Vincristine 1.4mg/m^2 i.v.
    Bleomycin 10mg/m^2 i.v.

7   Doxorubicin 35mg/m^2 i.v.   Tail to zero
    Etoposide 100mg/m^2 p.o. daily for 5 days   over 10 days

Fig. 1. VAPEC-B chemotherapy. In addition to the cytotoxic drugs and prednisolone, prophylactic co-trimoxazole 960 mg twice daily and ketoconazole 200 mg twice daily are prescribed until week 10 (when the neutropenia following week 7 has recovered and pred-nisolone has been stopped).

This resulted in the rapid resolution of symptoms and a CT scan performed at the completion of a seven week course showed partial remission of disease (largest remaining liver lesion 2×2 cm). On day 6 following the final dose of VAPEC-B (doxorubicin 35 mg/m^2 i.v. day 1 and etoposide 100 mg/m^2 orally days 1–5), filgrastim (r-HuG-CSF, Neupogen, Amgen-Roche) 300 ugs daily by subcutaneous injection was started and continued until day 15 when the total leukocyte count was 4.6×10^9/l. A single, four hour leukapheresis was performed at this time and yielded a total of 11.7×10^9 nucleated cells which were preserved in liquid nitrogen. Subsequently, she underwent a bone marrow harvest and this was also cryopreserved.

Following confirmation of satisfactory cardiac, pulmonary and renal function the patient was admitted to hospital in mid-June 1992. Cyclophosphamide 1.5 gm/m^2 i.v. with mesna and pre/post hydration was administered on days 6 to 3 inclusive with BCNU 600 mg/m^2 in 500 mls normal saline (after dissolution in ethanol) as a 1 hour infusion on day 2. The peripheral blood haemopoeitic cells were re-infused on day 0 and 24 hours later (day 1; total leukocytes 0.4×10^9/l), filgrastim 300 ugs daily by subcutaneous injection was commenced. She was severely neutropenic (neutrophils $<0.5 \times 10^9$/l) for ten days but on day 11 the total leukocyte count increased to 1.1×10^9/l (65% neutrophils) and she was allowed home on day 14 (Hb 13.6 gms/dl, total leukocytes 6.5×10^9/l, platelets 42×10^9/l). During her hospital stay she received 48 units of platelets for thrombocytopenia $<20 \times 10^9$/l and six units of red cells for anaemia but the autologous bone marrow was not used. All non-autologous blood products were irradiated before transfusion.

Three weeks after discharge the patient was re-admitted to hospital because of lethargy and low grade fever (37.8°C). The blood count was satisfactory (Hb 10.3 gms/dl, leukocytes 5.0×10^9/l, platelets 163×10^9/l) but she was hypoxic and a chest radiograph showed right lower lobe consolidation and inflammatory shadowing at the left base. Fibre-optic bronchoscopy revealed a clear bronchial tree and no bacteria, fungi or viruses were isolated from bronchial washings. Intravenous broad spectrum antibiotics and amphotericin were prescribed but the arterial hypoxia worsened and the radiographic appearances deteriorated with more extensive consolidation visible in the right lower lobe (Fig. 2a). A diagnosis of drug induced pneumonitis was proposed and oral prednisolone was started. This resulted in a rapid improvement of the hypoxaemia and within five days the radiographic abnormalities had almost completely resolved (Fig. 2b). She was discharged home on a decreasing dose schedule of prednisolone, co-trimoxazole 960 mg twice daily on three days every week, and ketoconazole 200 mg twice daily.

At present, seven month after the completion of cytotoxic treatment, the patient is well and has returned to full time work. All medication has been stopped.

There are no signs of disease and the blood count and serum biochemical profile are normal but the esr remains slightly raised at 20 mm/hr. The chest radiograph shows residual mid-zone shadowing which has remained static, but no other abnormalities.

Discussion

A patient has been described in whom HD has relapsed twice following initial radiotherapy and where the diagnosis and treatment of recurrent disease was delayed by pregnancy on one occasion and treatment for unproven fungal infection on another. Treatment of second relapse was also complicated by the development of a severe pneumonitis – probably drug induced – six weeks after receiving high dose chemotherapy. The co-existence of so many problems is unusual in HD, where the majority of patients are cured by first line therapy.

a) Management at first presentation

Hodgkin's disease is the most likely diagnosis in an otherwise asymptomatic 27-year-old patient presenting with painless cervical lymphadenopathy of several months duration and mediastinal widening on the chest radiograph. A confirmatory biopsy is mandatory and ideally this should provide a whole lymph node for histopathological examination. The biopsy specimen should be sent to the laboratoy unfixed so that material is available for cytogenetic analysis and molecular studies, in addition to more routine histology and immunohistochemistry.

Ann Arbor staging criteria [1, 2] have been used in HD for many years. However, an international committee convened in 1987 published revised criteria [3] which, although based on Ann Arbor principles, incorporate advances in imaging (in particular computerised tomography) and define what is acceptable evidence for liver or pulmonary involvement in the absence of histological confirmation. In addition, the importance of other features such as age, performance status, number of involved sites, presence of bulk disease and haematological/biochemical parameters (esr, peripheral lymphocyte count, serum LDH), all of which may provide prognostic information, is stressed. Finally, a category of complete remission, uncertain (CR(u)) is defined to take account of minor residual radiographic abnormalities following treatment, a finding which is especially common for patients who present with bulky disease [4]. The so-called Cotsworld criteria are more applicable than the Ann Arbor system to the management of HD in the 1990s and are recommended for routine use.

In the case described, staging laparotomy and splenectomy were performed to confirm the absence of sub-diaphragmatic disease in a patient with a negative abdomino-pelvic CT scan, and in whom treatment with

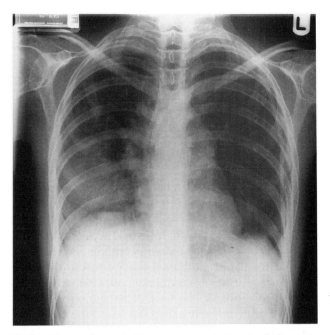

Fig. 2a. Chest radiograph (erect postero-anterior view) six weeks after high dose cyclophosphamide and BCNU showing inflammatory shadowing at the left base and right lower zone consolidation. The patient was pyrexial and hypoxaemic at this time but the bronchial tree was clear and no bacteria, fungi or viruses were isolated. A diagnosis of drug induced pneumonitis was made.

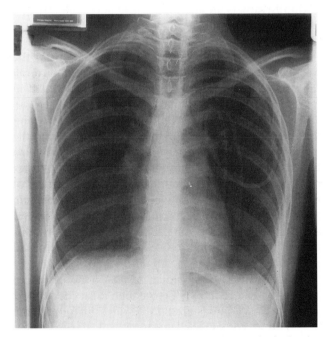

Fig. 2b. Chest radiograph (erect postero-anterior view) showing almost complete resolution of the right lower zone consolidation (Fig. 2a) after five days of oral prednisolone.

radiation alone was planned. Although this approach is reasonable, protocols incorporating pathological staging are now falling out of favour for several reasons. First, the procedure is associated with significant morbidity (infection, wound dehiscence, venous thrombosis, pulmonary embolism, cardiac arrest) [5] and is unpopular with patients. Second, there is a small but significant mortality due to fulminating pneumococcal septicaemia following splenectomy [6] and third, an in-

creased risk of secondary leukaemia has been reported in splenectomised patients eventually treated with cytotoxic chemotherapy [7].

For this reasons, clinical staging (CS) is now preferred in many centres with treatment defined by the mix of CS and other prognostic factors (such as number of involved sites, presence of B symptoms or bulk disease, esr and lymphocyte count). At this institute, the presence of mediastinal bulk (maximum horizontal transverse diameter of mediastinal tumour: internal thoracic diameter at D5/6 interspace $\geqslant 0.33$) and B symptoms have been shown to be associated with an adverse prognosis in stages I and II [8] and these features lead to initial treatment with chemotherapy. However, for patients with stage IIA disease, radiotherapy (RT) alone is appropriate first line treatment although even if pathologically staged up to 30% of cases will relapse and ultimately require chemotherapy.

Randomised trials have shown that the use of adjuvant chemotherapy after primary RT leads to a significant improvement in relapse-free survival [8, 9] for patients with stage I/II disease although overall survival is not significantly different because the majority of patients relapsing after RT alone are successfully salvaged by subsequent chemotherapy. Furthermore, the improvement in RFS is at the expense of over-treating the majority of patients who were cured by initial RT. Such a policy can only be justified if the adjuvant chemotherapy employed is subjectively well tolerated and does not, unlike MOPP derivatives, lead to a high incidence of infertility and second malignancy. The Stanford group have reported on the use of vinblastine, bleomycin and methotrexate in early stage HD [10] and other groups, including our own, are attempting to define effective chemotherapy of low toxicity in this setting.

b) Management at first relapse

Presentation of HD during pregnancy is uncommon but its management can be problematic and is normally determined by a consideration of foetal maturity and the perceived threat to the mother's immediate health. Co-operation with an experienced obstetrician is mandatory. In the first trimester of pregnancy termination may have to be recommended if disease is rapidly progressive or causing specific local problems (such as stridor or superior venal caval obstruction due to a large mediastinal mass) so that urgent treatment can be administered without fear of causing foetal damage. In the second and third trimester when organogenesis is complete it may be possible to save the foetus even if treatment is necessary for life threatening disease. In these circumstances, a local field of radiotherapy with appropriate shielding, or one or two cycles of chemotherapy can be given and may be sufficient to control the situation long enough for the foetus to reach a stage of independent viability. In the case described, disease was not life threatening and pregnancy was well advanced at the time relapse was suspected and it was possible to allow the patient to proceed to full term.

Suspected relapse must be confirmed histologically wherever possible from biopsy of an affected lymph node or other involved tissue (bone marrow, liver, lung). The differential diagnosis in these circumstances includes a second tumour (especially non-Hodgkin's lymphoma), infection or autoimmune disease, all of which would require a different approach to that adopted for relapsed HD. In addition, staging should be carried out as at first presentation in order to determine the full extent of disease and allow the effectiveness of salvage therapy to be properly measured.

At this institute the treatment of HD relapsing after previous RT is with combination chemotherapy although some clinicians would advocate additional RT for localised relapse. For many years MOPP and its derivatives (MVPP, Chlorambucil VPP) were virtually unchallenged in their role as first line regimens in HD. However, although results obtained with MOPP type therapy are considerably better than those previously seen using single agents, 30%–40% of patients treated either fail to respond or relapse after achieving a remission. In addition, MOPP/MVPP cause considerable gonadal toxicity [11] and are associated with a significant incidence of second malignancy [12].

The introduction of ABVD by Bonadonna and colleagues in the mid 1970s was an important advance. In a randomised trial involving 232 previously untreated patients, six cycles of ABVD was found to produce a significantly better complete remission rate, relapse-free survival and overall survival than six cycles of MOPP [13]. Furthermore, spermatogenesis was retained or recovered in all 24 cases treated on the ABVD arm but in only one of ten cases tested after MOPP. In a subsequent study alternating cycles of MOPP/ABVD were found superior to MOPP alone [14] and in a large, recently reported multicentre trial the advantages of ABVD either alone, or alternating with MOPP, over MOPP alone have been confirmed [15].

The concept of introducing all active drugs as early as possible into the treatment programme as proposed by Goldie and Coldman [16] was taken one step further by Klimo and Connors [17] with a so-called hybrid regimen comprising days 1–7 of MOPP and day 8 of ABV(D) (dacarbazine omitted). A direct comparison of alternating MOPP/ABVD with hybrid MOPP/ABVD by the Milan group showed no difference between the two treatment arms [18] but in a trial performed at the Christie and St Bartholomew's Hospitals, a significant advantage for a hybrid regimen over MVPP alone has been identified (progression-free survival for all patients at 5 years, 80% vs. 60%) [19].

Thus, evidence is accumulating to support a move away from MOPP-like regimens in favour of ABVD or hybrid chemotherapies. However, the long term effects of these more recently introduced treatments on gonadal, cardiac and pulmonary function and the incidence of second tumours is not yet fully defined and requires further study.

c) Management at second relapse

Diagnosis of second relapse was delayed in the case described because the pulmonary lesions when first identified by CT scan were small and of uncertain significance. In this situation lung biopsy should be performed. Later, the onset of fever and the finding of large cavitating lung lesions was interpreted as fungal infection, a complication which is more likely in the setting of neutropenia following chemotherapy. In addition, the patient had severe pruritus and focal hepatic lesions and the overall clinical picture was more in keeping with relapsed HD.

High dose chemotherapy with haemopoietic rescue should be considered for high risk patients relapsing after a doxorubicin containing combination. Such an approach is based on the knowledge that in these circumstances further conventional dose chemotherapy is unlikely to result in long term disease control in more than 30% of cases. However, the case for a high dose approach is unproven. Randomised trials are needed to compare the efficacy of conventional and high dose chemotherapy in this setting but patients are understandably reluctant to take part given that conventional therapy has previously failed to control disease. The choice of treatment for patients relapsing after initial chemotherapy is an important issue and is likely to be the subject of considerable study over the next few years.

Our policy is to first attempt cytoreduction using the weekly VAPEC-B regimen – which produces an overall response rate of 70% after six weeks of treatment in relapsed HD [20] – and then to proceed with high dose chemotherapy. Peripheral blood haemopoietic progenitors are harvested from a single apheresis during the recovery phase (augmented by r-HuG-CSF) following week 7 of VAPEC-B, and are cryopreserved until re-infusion on day 2, 48 hours after the completion of high dose cyclophosphamide/BCNU. With maximum follow-up of five years, actuarial event-free survival (time to relapse or death from any cause) using this approach is 50% at three years in our series of 30 patients.

Other centres obtain similar results to these without attempting cytoreduction before high dose chemotherapy which is administered to patients in full relapse [21]. This is not our policy for several reasons. First, non-responders to VAPEC-B fare badly after high dose treatment and these patients can therefore be spared further toxicity. Second, those that do achieve CR or PR usually have a better performance status than at the time of relapse and this may be of relevance to the subsequent tolerability of high dose therapy. Third, peripheral blood haemopoietic progenitor cells can be conveniently harvested in the recovery phase after week 7 of VAPEC-B and, finally, a short re-induction phase allows time for the patient to be scheduled into the workload of a busy transplant unit.

With regard to the choice of haemopoietic rescue after high dose chemotherapy for HD, autologous peripheral blood progenitor cells are now used routinely at this institute because compared with a time when autologous bone marrow was employed, haematological reconstitution is more rapid and total in-patient stay is shorter. Allogeneic bone marrow is not used because in many cases a suitable donor cannot be found and autologous rescue reduces the risk of graft-versus-host disease (GVHD). GVHD can still occur as a result of small numbers of allogeneic lymphocytes being transferred to a severely immunocompromised patient during routine red cell and platelet transfusion [22] and it is now our practice to irradiate all blood products required by patients with HD at any stage of their treatment.

In the first six months after high dose chemotherapy, opportunistic infection – due to continuing immunosuppression despite a normal neutrophil count – is an important cause of fever with hypoxaemia and pulmonary shadowing on the chest radiograph. Bronchoscopy with bronchial washings taken for bacteriology, a transbronchial biopsy to exclude pneumocystis and blood cultures should, if possible, be performed before the start of antibiotic therapy. Prophylaxis can significantly reduce the risk of pneumocystis infection and oral co-trimoxazole 960 mgs twice daily for three days every week is recommended [23].

In the case described, drug induced pneumonitis was the probable cause of the respiratory illness. This is a well recognised complication of treatment with BCNU and is thought to be a dose related phenomenon [24] but the patient's previous exposure to radiotherapy, bleomycin and high dose cyclophosphamide, may also be relevant. In mild to moderate cases the condition responds to corticosteroid therapy but it may progress to irreversible pulmonary fibrosis, respiratory failure and death. At this centre, the dose of BCNU has recently been reduced to 300 mgs/m^2 on account of pulmonary toxicity experienced by a minority of patients treated and etoposide 200 mgs/m^2 on days 6 to 3 has been added to the high dose regimen.

References

1. Carbone PP, Kaplan HS, Musshoff K et al. Report of the committee on Hodgkin's disease staging classification. Cancer Res 1971; 31: 1860–1.
2. Rosenberg SA, Boiron M, De Vita V et al. Report of the committee on Hodgkin's disease staging procedures. Cancer Res 1971; 31: 1862–3.
3. Lister A, Crowther D, Sutcliffe S et al. Report of a committee convened to discuss the evaluation and staging of patients with Hodgkin's disease. J Clin Oncol 1989; 7 (11): 1630–6.
4. Radford JA, Cowan RA, Flanagan M et al. The significance of residual mediastinal abnormality on the chest radiograph following treatment for Hodgkin's disease. J Clin Oncol 1988; 6: 940–6.
5. Brogadir S, Fialk MA, Coleman M et al. Morbidity of staging laparotomy in Hodgkin's disease. Am J Med 1978; 64: 429–33.
6. Weitzman S, Aisenberg AC. Fulminant sepsis after successful treatment of Hodgkin's disease. Am J Med 1977; 62: 47–50.
7. van Leeuwen FE, Somers R, Hart AAM. Splenectomy in Hodgkin's disease and second leukaemias. Lancet 1987; 8852: 210–1.
8. Anderson H, Deakin DPD, Wagstaff J et al. A randomised study of adjuvant chemotherapy after mantle radiotherapy in supradiaphragmatic Hodgkin's disease PS IA-IIB: A report from the Manchester lymphoma group. Br J Cancer 1984; 49: 695–702.
9. Hoppe RT, Coleman NC, Cox RS et al. The management of stage I-II Hodgkin's disease with irradiation alone or combined modality therapy: The Stanford experience. Blood 1982; 59: 455–65.
10. Horning SJ, Hoppe RT, Hancock SL et al. Vinblastine, bleomycin and methotrexate: An effective adjuvant in favourable Hodgkin's disease. J Clin Oncol 1988; 6 (12): 1822–31.
11. Whitehead E, Shalet SM, Blackledge G et al. The effects of Hodgkin's disease and combination chemotherapy on gonadal function in the adult male. Cancer 1982; 49: 418–22.
12. Boivin JF, Hutchison GB, Lyden M et al. Second primary cancers following treatment of Hodgkin's disease. J Nat Cancer Inst 1984; 72: 233–41.
13. Santoro A, Bonadonna G, Valagussa P et al. Long term results of combined chemotherapy-radiotherapy approach in Hodgkin's disease: Superiority of ABVD plus radiotherapy versus MOPP plus radiotherapy. J Clin Oncol 1987; 5: 27–37.
14. Bonadonna G, Valagussa P, Santoro A et al. Alternating non cross resistant combination chemotherapy or MOPP in stage IV Hodgkin's disease. A report of 8 year results. Ann Intern Med 1986; 104: 739–46.
15. Cannellos GP, Anderson JR, Propert KJ et al. Chemotherapy of advanced Hodgkin's disease with MOPP, ABVD or MOPP alternating with ABVD. N Engl J Med 1992; 327: 1478–84.
16. Goldie JH, Coldman AJ, Gudauskas GA. Rationale for the use of alternating non cross-resistant chemotherapy. Cancer Tr Rep 1982; 66: 439–49.
17. Klimo P, Connors JM. MOPP/ABV Hybrid program: Combination chemotherapy based on early introduction of seven effective drugs for advanced Hodgkin's disease. J Clin Oncol 1985; 3: 1174–82.
18. Viviani S, Bonadonna G, Santoro A et al. Alternating vs. hybrid MOPP-ABVD in Hodgkin's disease. The Milan experience. Ann Oncol 1991; 2 (suppl. 2): 55–62.
19. Radford JA, Crowther D, Rohatiner AJS et al. Results of a randomised trial comparing MVPP chemotherapy with a hybrid regimen, ChlVPP/EVA, in the initial treatment of Hodgkin's disease. J Clin Oncol 1995; 13: 2379–85.
20. Radford JA, Crowther D. Treatment of relapsed Hodgkin's disease using a weekly chemotherapy of short duration: Results of a pilot study in 20 patients. Ann Oncol 1991; 2: 505–9.
21. McMillan A, Goldstone A, Linch D et al. 100 cases of relapsed Hodgkin's disease treated with BEAM chemotherapy and ABMT in a single centre. Fourth International Conference on Malignant Lymphoma, Lugano, Switzerland 1990; abstract 20, page 28.
22. Anderson KC, Weinstein HJ. Transfusion-associated graft-versus-host disease. N Engl J Med 1990; 323 (5): 315–21.
23. Masur H. Prevention and treatment of pneumocystis pneumonia. N Engl J Med 1992; 327 (26): 1853–60.
24. Litam JP, Dail DH, Spitzer G et al. Early pulmonary toxicity after administration of high dose BCNU. Cancer Tr Rep 1981; 65 (1–2): 39–44.

R. L. Souhami (ed.) The Teaching Cases from Annals of Oncology, 43–46, 1997.
© 1997 *Kluwer Academic Publishers. Printed in the Netherlands.*

Mediastinal mass with fever and night sweats in a young farmer — potential pitfalls in the diagnostic work-up and treatment

R. A. Joss & J.-O. Gebbers

Division of Medical Oncology & Department of Pathology, Kantonsspital, Luzern, Switzerland

Key words: mediastinal mass, lymphoma diagnosis, drug-induced infertility

Case history

A 26-year-old farmer was admitted to the hospital because of a mediastinal mass.

The patient had been in good health until approximately three weeks earlier, when while serving in the army he noticed a rapid onset of swelling of his face and neck. The swelling increased and the patient became febrile up to 38.5°. He consulted his family physician who found a mediastinal mass on a chest x-ray (see Fig. 1). The patient was admitted to the hospital for investigation and treatment. He complained of fever, night-sweats, weight-loss of 5 Kg and abdominal pain when drinking beer. There was no significant past medical history.

On examination there were distended neck veins, a swollen face and conjunctival oedema. The optic fundi revealed engorged veins but normal disc margins. Superior vena cava obstruction was diagnosed. Multiple soft lymph nodes of 1 × 1 cm were found in both groins and axillae.

A full blood count and blood biochemical values were normal. The ESR was 43 mm in the first hour. A CT scan of the chest and the abdomen revealed a large mediastinal mass and multiple enlarged retroperitoneal lymph nodes (see Fig. 2). Inguinal and axillary lymph node biopsies revealed a non-specific chronic inflammatory reaction, but no neoplasm. Due to the suggestive history (fever, night-sweats, weight loss and pain on alcohol intake), the superior vena cava syndrome and

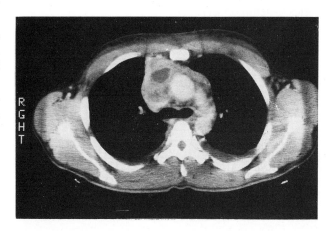

Fig. 2a. CT scan of the chest with mediastinal mass with multiple hypodense areas.

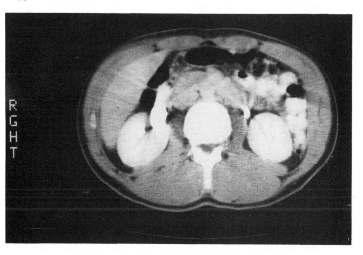

Fig. 2b. CT scan of the abdomen with enlarged retroperitoneal lymph-nodes.

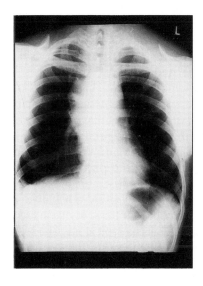

Fig. 1. Initial chest-x-ray.

the radiological diagnosis of probable retroperitoneal lymphoma, a diagnostic laparotomy was performed. The mesenteric and para-aortic lymph nodes as well as the spleen were slightly enlarged. Multiple para-aortic and mesenteric lymph nodes were biopsied. Liver biopsies were taken from the right and left lobes and a splenectomy was performed. Neither the biopsy samples nor the spleen showed evidence of lymphoma or tumour.

A mediastinoscopy was performed, which was technically very difficult. Only small fragments of the tumour mass could be biopsied. These revealed atypical tissue of medium sized, in sheets growing cells with distinct outer membranes and polymorphous nuclei (see Fig. 3a). Immunohistochemically, membrane-bound placental alkaline phosphatase (PLAP) was demonstrable in all and ferritin in the cytoplasm of some tumour cells (see Fig. 3b). Reactions for CEA, cytokeratins, S-100 protein, β-HCG, α-fetoprotein, chromogranin and desmin were all negative. The histological appearance and immuno-staining pattern is very suggestive of a germ cell tumour, since PLAP is a sensitive immunohistochemical marker of germ cell differentiation. The lack of cytokeratins and the demonstration of both PLAP and ferritin has been found in large series of seminomas [1–5].

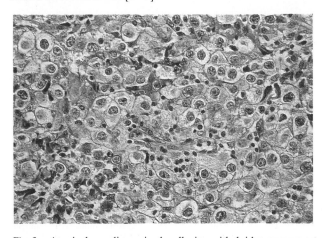

Fig. 3a. Atypical, medium sized cells in epitheloid arrangement (Hematoxylin-Eosin, ×280).

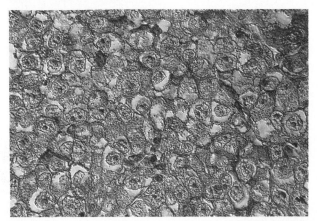

Fig. 3b. Immunohistochemical demonstration of a uniform, predominantly membrane-associated staining of placental alkaline phosphatase (Immunoalkaline phosphatase method, ×420).

The first value of serum β-HCG was 11 IE/l (normal value <5 IE/l). A subsequent level of 30 IE/l was obtained three weeks later. A diagnosis of a malignant extragonadal germ cell tumor was considered established. Results of a further investigation including an ultrasound of both testes were normal.

The patient underwent treatment with ifosfamide, etoposide and cisplatin. After the second cycle the β-HCG became normal. At this time the CT-scan revealed a small residual mass (see Fig. 4b). This mass did not change during a further three cycles of chemotherapy, when the treatment was completed (see Fig. 4c). The patient remains in unmaintained complete remission and became the father of a healthy daughter two years later.

In summary, in this young man with a mediastinal tumor mass the history and CT scan suggested disseminated lymphoma. In contrast, the significance of the slightly elevated β-HCG-level was underestimated. This led to an indirect approach to obtain a histological diagnosis with a consequent delay in establishing the final diagnosis.

Discussion

The diagnostic work-up and treatment of a cancer patient may be difficult and numerous mistakes can be made. Mistakes usually occur in one of the following categories [6]:

- During the diagnostic investigation: An indirect approach may be taken to obtain a diagnosis. There may be too much or too little investigation. Definitive histological diagnosis may be delayed.
- In planning the treatment: A curative instead of palliative intent of treatment and vice versa. An inappropriate therapy may be chosen.
- During the treatment: inadequate dose intensity, avoidable toxicity, lack of documentation of nadir counts, lack of communication between treating physicians, inappropriate treatment duration, long-treatment-free intervals in combined modality treatments, inadequate supervision of interns, residents and nurses.
- In assessing the treatment efficacy: lack of tumor parameters, misinterpretation of clinical findings.

In this patient the initial diagnostic work-up was not discussed with the oncologist. Impressed by the superior vena cava syndrome and the other symptoms suggestive of lymphoma, the physician chose an indirect approach to establish a tissue diagnosis. This led to two negative lymph node biopsies, a negative staging laparotomy and to a delay of three weeks in establishing the final diagnosis. This is a typical mistake seen in patients cared for by general internists. In a retrospective survey a delay of 8 to 10 days was observed, before a biopsy was performed, although in 67% of the patients the biopsied lesion was detected by the second day of evaluation [7]. The biopsy should usually be taken from

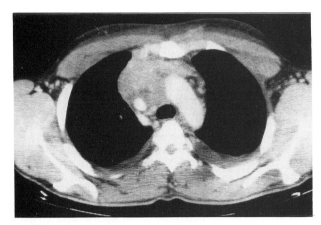

Fig. 4a. Initial CT scan.

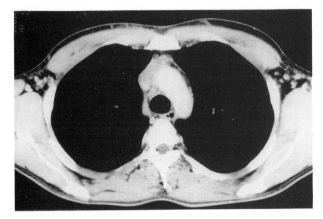

Fig. 4b. CT scan after two cycles of chemotherapy.

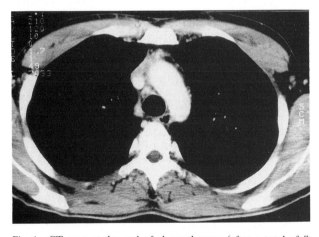

Fig. 4c. CT scan at the end of chemotherapy (after a total of fi
cycles of chemotherapy).

the site where the tumour causes its first symptoms, which is usually also the site of the largest tumour mass.

This case also illustrates the emphasis which should be placed on abnormal laboratory values when establishing a diagnosis. The β-HCG-value was initially only slightly elevated and at first was thought to be irrelevant. False positive β-HCG-levels are seen in up to 15% of patients with testicular cancer [8] and various other tumours and non-malignant diseases can cause a slightly elevated β-HCG (see Table 1) [9, 10]. Heterophilic antibodies can cause falsely elevated β-HCG

values [11]. It is therefore quite reasonable that, in the present case, the initial β-HCG value was regarded with caution. However, an abnormal value must be checked again and if still abnormal, be taken into account in the final diagnosis.

The patient initially presented with a mediastinal mass, from which only small fragments could be biopsied, revealing a malignant epithelial neoplasm. Malignant neoplasms arising in the anterior mediastinum include thymic tumours, lymphomas, germ cell tumors and thyroid neoplasms (see Table 2). Fortunately, in our patient the histological findings of an epithelial neoplasm together with an elevated and rising β-HCG level, established the diagnosis of a primary extragonadal germ cell tumour. A testicular primary was excluded by an ultrasound of the testes. Primary extragonadal germ cell tumors are uncommon neoplasms and account for approximately 1%–2% of germ cell tumors [12]. These tumors usually occur in young men, involve the midline structures and the lungs and exhibit elevated tumour markers in up to 90% of the patients. On CT scan they often exhibit low-density areas, such as were seen in our patient [13]. It is usually considered that extragonadal germ-cell tumours have a poor prognosis and that they do not respond as well to treatment as do their testicular counterparts. However, clinical symptoms often present late and therefore most patients with extragonadal germ-cell tumours exhibit a high initial tumour load [14]. These patients must therefore be treated with intensive chemotherapy regimens such as those used in patients with testicular cancer with unfavourable prognostic factors including refractory neoplasms or a high initial tumour load [15–19]. With intensive combination chemotherapies more than 60% of patients with advanced extragonadal germ cell tumours remain long-term disease-free [19, 20].

Finally, our patient illustrates another and increasingly important problem in medical oncology. With the curability of younger patients with acute leukemia, Hodgkin's disease, non-Hodgkin's lymphoma, choriocarcinoma and testicular cancer, long-term sequelae of cancer chemotherapy such as gonadal toxicity have be-

Table 1. Non-neoplastic and neoplastic diseases associated with a raised serum β-HCG value.

- inflammatory bowel disease
- peptic ulcer disease
- liver cirrhosis
- choriocarcinoma
- testicular, ovarian and extragonadal non-seminomatous germ cell tumours
- seminoma
- breast cancer
- lung cancer
- gastrointestinal cancer
- ovarian carcinoma
- uterine carcinoma
- renal cell cancer
- malignant melanoma
- lymphoproliferative diseases

Table 2. Differential diagnosis of a mass in the anterior mediastinum.

– Lymphomas	– Teratoma
– Thymic tumours or cysts	– Lipoma
Thymolipoma	– Lymphangioma
Thymoma	– Fibroma
Thymic carcinoid	– Myxoma
Thymic carcinoma	– Hemangioma
– Thyroid tumours or masses	– Chondroma
– Parathyroid tumours	– Paraganglioma from carotid
– Rhabdomycosarcoma	body
– Lung cancer	– Pericardial cysts
– Germ cell tumours	– Aneurysm

come important. The semen quality of patients with testicular germ cell tumours before chemotherapy is severely decreased in the majority of patients [20]. Chemotherapy further impairs fertility. However, in a significant number of patients recovery of spermatogenesis with subsequent fertility is possible [22, 23]. When counseling patients and their spouses several points should be addressed:

- The couple should be aware that many patients have a decreased fertility at the time of diagnosis before any treatment.
- The problem of chemotherapy-induced infertility should be discussed and options for producing a family (artificial insemination, in vitro fertilisation, adoption) should be explained.
- Widespread anxiety over an increased frequency of spontaneous abortion, genetic diseases and/or congenital anomalies in the progeny of former cancer patients should be discussed. Thus far, there is no firm evidence that any of these sequelae occur more frequently than in the general population [24].
- Finally the couple shoud understand the risk of a relapse or a second neoplasm. Thus, the timing of a pregnancy will be strongly influenced be the period of the risk for relapse. However, the partner of the patient has to be aware that he/she may eventually have to raise the child by himself/herself.

In summary the present case illustrates several important diagnostic and therapeutic problems of medical oncology. Fortunately, the errors made during the initial diagnostic work-up did not compromise the final outcome in this patient with a curable neoplasm and the patient was fortunate that his fertility was not compromised by the disease or the treatment.

References

1. Battiflora H. The biology of the keratins and their diagnostic applications. In DeLellis RA (ed): Advances in immunohistochemistry. New York: Raven Press 1988; 191–221.
2. Cohen C, Shulman G, Budgeon LR. Immunohistochemical ferritin in testicular seminoma. Cancer 1984; 54: 2190–8.
3. Jacobsen GK, Norgaard-Pedersen B. Placental alkaline phosphamtase in testicular germ cell tumors and in carcinoma-insitu of the testis. Acta Pathol Microbiol Immunol Scnad (A) 1984; 92: 323–9.
4. Manivel JC, Jessurum J, Wick MR, Dehner LP. Placental alkaline phosphatase immunoreactivity in testicular germ cell neoplasma. Am J Surg Pathol 1987; 11: 21–9.
5. Uchida T, Shimoda T, Miyata H et al. Immunoperoxidase study of alkaline phosphatase in testicular tumors. Cancer 1981; 48: 1455–62.
6. Joss R, Brand B, Kuster B et al. Häufige Fehler bei der Planung und praktischen Durchführung einer Tumortherapie. Schweiz Med Wschr 1990; 120: 1285–96.
7. Farag SS, Green MD, Morstyn G et al. Delay of internists in obtaining diagnostic biopsies in patients with suspected cancer. Ann Intern Med 1992; 116: 473–8.
8. Javadpour N. False-positive and false-negative alpha-fetoprotein and human chorionic gonadotropin assays in testicular cancer: A double blind study. Cancer 1981; 48: 2279–81.
9. Vaitukaitis JL. Human chorionic gonadotropin – a hormone secreted for many reasons. N Engl J Med 1979; 301: 324–5.
10. Klavine JV. Advances in biological markers for cancer. Am Clin Lab Sci 1983; 13: 275–80.
11. Boscato LM, Stuart MC. Heterophilic antibodies: A problem for all immunoassays. Clin Chem 1988; 34: 27–33.
12. Collins DH, Pugh RCB. Classification and frequency of testicular tumors. Br J Urol 1964; 36 (Suppl.): 1–11.
13. Lee KS, Im J-G, Han CH et al. Malignant primary germ cell tumors of the mediastinum: CT features. AJR 1989; 153: 947–51.
14. Nichols CR, Fox EP. Extragonadal and pediatric germ cell tumors. Hematology/Oncology Clinics of North America 1991; 5: 1189–209.
15. Lewi CR, Fossa SD, Mead G et al. BOP/VIP – a new platinum-intensive chemotherapy regimen for poor prognosis germ cell tumours. Ann Oncol 1991; 2: 203–11.
16. Ozols RF, Ihde DC, Linehan WM et al. A randomized trial of standard chemotherapy v a high-dose chemotherapy regimen in the treatment of poor prognosis nonseminomatous germ-cell tumors. J Clin Oncol 1988; 6: 1031–40.
17. Horwich A, Brada M, Nicholls J et al. Intensive induction chemotherapy for poor risk non-seminomatous germ cell tumours. Eur J Cancer Clin 1989; 25: 77–184.
18. Loehrer PJ, Einhorn LH, Williams SD et al. VP-16 plus ifosfamide plus cisplatin as salvage therapy in refractory germ cell cancer. J Clin Oncol 1986; 4: 528–36.
19. Bukowski RM, Wolf M, Kulander BG et al. Alternating combination chemotherapy in patients with extragonadal germ cell tumors. A Southwest Oncology Group Study. Cancer 1993; 71: 2631–8.
20. Hainsworth JD, Einhorn LH, Williams SD et al. Advanced extragonadal germ-cell tumors. Successful treatment with combination chemotherapy. Ann Intern Med 1982; 97: 7–11.
21. Myers SE, Schilsky RL. Prospects for fertility after cancer chemotherapy. Sem Oncol 1992; 19: 597–604.
22. Drasga RE, Einhorn LH, Williams SD et al. Fetility after chemotherapy for testicular cancer. J Clin Oncol 1983; 1: 179–83.
23. Nijman JM, Koops HS, Kremer J et al. Gonadal function after surgery and chemotherapy in men with stage II and III non-seminomatous testicular tumors. J Clin Oncol 1987; 5: 651–6.
24. Li FP, Fine W, Jaffe N et al. Offspring of patients treated for cancer in childhood. J Natl Cancer Inst 1979; 62: 1193–7.

R. L. Souhami (ed.) The Teaching Cases from Annals of Oncology, 47–50, 1997.

Malignant lymphoma versus sarcoma: Discordance between clinical course and immunocytochemistry
Two case reports

U. Kaiser, K.-H. Pflüger, M. Tiemann[1] & K. Havemann
Department of Haematology and Oncology, Philipps-Universität Marburg; [1]German Lymphnode Registry, Institute of Haematopathology Christian-Albrechts-Universität, Kiel, Germany

Key words: malignant lymphoma, sarcoma, immunocytochemistry

Case 1

A 56-year-old businessman was admitted for investigation of weight loss and fatigue. He had a 20-year history of recurrent gastric ulcers. Clinical examination revealed no abnormalities. Chest X-ray was normal. Haematologic values were as follows: white blood cell count (WBC) 7.0×10^9/L, haemoglobin (Hb) 127 g/dl haematocrit 0.39, platelets 150×10^9/L. Differential count was normal. LDH was 185 U/l, tumor markers CEA, CA 19-9, CA 12-5 were at normal levels. CT scan of the abdomen revealed an intra-abdominal inhomogeneous tumor of 5 cm apparently originating from the gastric antrum penetrating into the left liver and adjacent tissue. Fine needle aspiration revealed necrosis. Subsequent gastroscopy showed a rigid antral wall. Biopsies showed gastric metaplasia and gastritis. For diagnostic purposes a laparotomy was performed which showed a large gastric tumor penetrating into the liver. Multiple biopsies revealed an undifferentiated tumor consisting of large tumor cells with abundant cytoplasm and large polymorphic nuclei exhibiting bizarre nucleoli (Fig. 1). Immunohistochemistry revealed positivity of the tumor cells for vimentin and α-1-antichymotrypsin and weak positivity for epithelial membrane antigen (EMA). Markers against cytokeratin, desmin, CEA, actin, and tissue polypeptide antigen (TPA) were negative; leukocyte markers were not performed. Histological diagnosis was malignant fibrous histiocytoma.

Chemotherapy consisting of adriamycin (80 mg day 1) and DTIC (650 mg day 1 and 2) was started and followed by radiotherapy of the upper abdomen (20 Gy). After three cycles a significant tumor reduction was seen, and restaging after six cycles revealed complete remission. The patient was free of symptoms. Two years after diagnosis a routine abdominal CT scan showed a recurrent peritoneal tumor 3 cm in diameter. Because of the good response of the initial treatment, polychemotherapy consisting of adriamycin (80 mg day 1) and ifosfamide (2.5 g days 1–5) was administered. A further scan after two cycles showed marked tumor reduction.

Due to the excellent clinical response a re-evaluation of the initial biopsies by the German lymph-node registry in Kiel was requested. Immunohistochemistry revealed strong positivity of the tumor cells for the CD30 antigen using the 'Ki-1' related antibody BerH2 (Fig. 2a) and a weak reaction with anti-CD3 (for an overview of the CD system for classifying human leukocyte antigens see [1]). B-cell markers L26 and Ki-B5 were negative.

Therefore, the diagnosis had to be revised to a high-grade T-cell lymphoma, the so-called large cell anaplastic 'Ki-1' lymphoma. Subsequently the chemotherapy was switched to the lymphoma protocol CHOEP consisting of cyclophosphamide (1300 mg day 1), adriamycin (85 mg day 1), vincristine (2 mg day 1), etoposide (170 mg days 1–3) and prednisolone (100 mg days 1–5). Restaging after three cycles revealed complete remission. One year later the patient is well and still in complete remission.

Case 2

A 69-year-old woman with a history of diabetes mellitus and hypertension was admitted to the hospital complaining of left-side lower abdominal pain and constipation. Clinical examination revealed left-side abdominal tenderness on palpation. Laboratory data showed a LDH of 412 U/l and an iron deficiency anaemia. Haematologic parameters were as follows: WBC 5.3 G/l, Hb 78 g/l, hematocrit 0.25 l/l, MCH 22.6 pg, MCV 72.2 fl, platelets 308 G/l, serum iron 4.8 μmol/l and ferritin 8 μg/l. Tumor markers CEA, AFP, βHCG were within normal values. Chest X-ray was normal. Abdominal CT scan revealed a large retro-

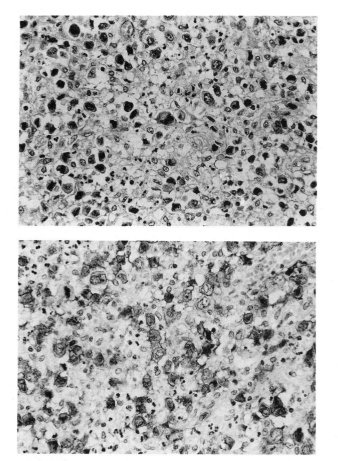

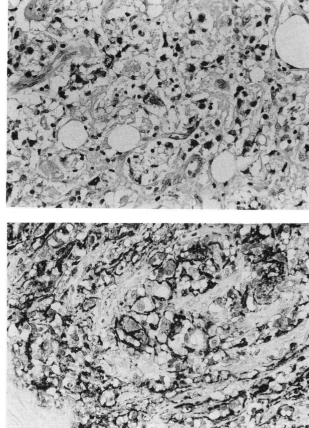

Fig. 1. Top: Tumor biopsy of case 1 consisting of atypical blasts with irregularly formed nuclei with partly gyrus-like indentations. They exhibit a dark chromatin pattern with large nucleoli. There is an epitheloid growth pattern, intermingled are macrophages and lymphocytes. H & E staining. Bottom: Immunohistochemistry of the tumor biopsy in case 1: reaction with Berh 2. Visualisation with the alkaline phosphatase anti alkaline phosphatase method (APAAP) showing cytoplasmic staring.

Fig. 2. Top: Tumor biopsy of patient 2 consisting of middle sized blasts, focally altered by artifacts. The growth pattern is follicular, intermingled are lymphocytes. H & E staining. Bottom: Immunohistochemistry of the tumor biopsy in case 2: reaction with L 26. Visualisation with the alkaline phosphatase anti alkaline phosphatase method (APAAP) showing membrane staring.

peritoneal homogeneous tumor mass reaching from the upper mesenteric artery to the aortic bifurcation. Further investigations, including bone marrow biopsy, bone scan, CT scan of the thorax, coloscopy and gastroscopy, had normal results. Laparotomy confirmed a large retroperitoneal tumor with displacement of the small bowel.

Histologic evaluation of the biopsies revealed a partly necrotic tumor with atypical spindle cells which were dense in chromatin (Fig. 2). Immunohistochemistry showed weak positivity for vimentin and actin; markers for TPA, EMA, cytokeratin, S-100, lysozyme, macrohages and leucocyte common antigen (LCA) were negative. A diagnosis of malignant mesenchymal tumor probably liposarcoma, was made.

Due to progressive abdominal pain, palliative treatment with adriamycin (80 mg day 1) and ifosfamide (2.4 g days 1 to 5) was started. After one cycle of chemotherapy LDH had returned to normal levels (246 U/l). Ultrasound control showed considerable tumor regression. After completion of three cycles the tumor mass was reduced by over 75%.

Due to the surprisingly good response, the biopsies were re-evaluated. Additional immunostaining of the initial biopsies confirmed the diagnosis of a high-grade germinal-center lymphoma, a centroblastic lymphoma of the multilobated type. On immunohistochemistry the tumor cells were negative for CD30; however, they strongly expressed CD 20 and were positive for L 26 (Fig. 2a) which detects approximately 80% of B cell lymphomas [2]. Intermingled were T cells showing positivity for CD3.

After completion of 4 cycles of chemotherapy, involved field radiation had to be postponed due to therapy-related leukopenia. Two months after completion of the chemotherapy the patient showed a rapid tumor growth and died of progressive disease in spite of palliative radiation.

Discussion

Approximately 5% of malignant specimens in pathology laboratories have to be classified as 'undifferentiated malignant neoplasm' solely on the basis of their light microscopic appearance [3]. One of the great successes in the application of immunocytochemistry to diagnostic pathology lies in the diagnosis of these cases [4]. A panel of five different antibodies has been suggested [5] as being able to lead to a definite diagnosis in 95% of anaplastic large-cell tumors.

In a study from Oxford 120 diagnostically difficult cases that were referred from re-evaluation were compared [6]. Twenty-nine of 43 cases that were previously considered to be carcinoma by routine microscopy had immunohistochemical markers for lymphoma. This led to authors to the assumption 'that lymphoma is probably underdiagnosed among routine surgical pathology samples'.

In both of the cases presented here, anaplastic tumors which had definitely been diagnosed on the basis of immunocytochemistry had to be re-evaluated because of their clinical courses. In case one an anaplastic tumor was diagnosed as being a mesenchymal tumor due to a negative reaction with epithelial markers and a positive reaction with vimentin. Vimentin, a 57 kD protein is the most widely distributed intermediate filament, being present in virtually all mesenchymal cells. However, a large array of carcinomas, lymphomas and neuroendocrine tumors has been reported to express vimentin [3]. Re-evaluation consisting of application of a wide panel of lymphocyte markers led to the diagnosis of 'Ki-1' lymphoma of T cell origin. This anaplastic large-cell lymphoma [7] is characterized by large, sometimes huge, anaplastic cells with abundant basophilic cytoplasm which tend to grow in sheets and have a histiocyte-like appearance. They typically react with the monoclonal antibody 'Ki-1' which has been assigned to the CD 30 antigen. The antibody was originally established as a marker for Sternberg-Reed cells in Hodgkin's disease [8]. Positivity for EMA [9], as in our case, as well as negativity for LCA [10], has been described in large-cell anaplastic lymphoma. Approximately 80% of large-cell anaplastic lymphomas are of T-cell origin. Due to the growth pattern with intra-sinusoidal permeation accompanied by large macrophages, the diagnosis of malignant 'histiocytosis' is often suggested [11].

In case two the diagnosis of a malignant mesenchymal tumor was made because of a weak positivity for vimentin. Malignant lymphoma was excluded because of a negative reaction with LCA. The leukocyte common antibodies are defined by a family of glycoproteins present on bone marrow – derived cells such as granulocytes, macrophages and lymphocytes. These antibodies cluster in CD 45. The antibody employed here is a cocktail of two monoclonal antibodies, PD7/26 and 2B11. With very rare exceptions, anti-LCA does not mark epithelial or mesenchymal tumors [3]. Over 90% of lymphoid malignancies are reported to react with anti-LCA [3]. However, some lymphoblastic and centroblastic lymphomas which do not stain with anti-LCA have been reported [5]. The correct diagnosis of a

centroblastic lymphoma can sometimes be established only by employing a series of lineage-specific markers. The multi-lobated centroblastic lymphoma has to be considered as a subtype of centroblastic lymphoma in which more than 10% of the blasts consist of multi-lobated nuclei with usually 3 to 4 indentations [12].

In both of the cases described here, the employment of immunocytochemistry led to diagnoses that did not correspond to clinical course. In both cases a prompt response to chemotherapy initially given for palliative reasons led us to re-evaluate the diagnosis. The diagnosis of malignant lymphoma could only be established by using a broader panel of leukocyte markers.

The differentiation between sarcoma and lymphoma may be a particularly difficult diagnostic distinction. Broad and specific markers for sarcoma do not exist. Only expression of several markers, such as S100, α-1-antichymotrypsin, and vimentin, may be of further help. When there is diagnostical doubt and LCA reactivity is negative the application of further leukocyte differentiation markers, increasingly available for use in paraffin material, should be considered.

Despite the success of immunocytochemistry in diagnostic pathology, clinicians should always have a high index of clinical suspicion when the clinical course is at variance with the histological diagnosis. It is essential to ask for re-evaluation of a pathological diagnosis based on immunohistology if the clinical course does not fit the diagnosis. A small percentage of anaplastic tumors will remain undifferentiated or can only be further distinguished by awide panel of markers.

References

1. Knapp W, Rieber P, Dörkern B et al. Towards a better definition of human leukocyte surface molecules. Immunol Today 1989; 10: 253–8.
2. Cartun RW, Coles FB, Pastuszak WT. Utilization of monoclonal antibody L26 in the identification and confirmation of B-cell lymphomas. A sensitive and specific marker applicable to formalin- and B5- fixed, paraffin-embedded tissues. Am J Pathol 1987; 129: 415–21.
3. Linder J. Immunohistochemistry in surgical pathology. Clin Lab Med 1990; 10: 59–76.
4. Mason DY, Gatter KC. The role of immunocytochemistry in diagnostic pathology. J Clin Pathol 1987; 40: 1042–54.
5. Henzen-Logmanns SC, Mullink H, Vennegoor C et al. Classification of routinely processed anaplastic large cell tumours with a small panel of antibodies. An immunohistochemical study with clinical follow-up. Histol Histopath 1987; 2: 107–18.
6. Gatter KC, Heryet A, Alcock C et al. Clinical importance of analysing malignant tumours of uncertain origin with immuno-histochemical techniques. Lancet I 1985; 1302–5.
7. Stein H, Mason DY, Gerdes J et al. The expression of the Hodgkin's disease associated antigen Ki-1 in reactive and neoplastic lymphoid tissue: Evidence that Reed-Sternberg cells and histiocytic malignancies are derived from activated lymphoid cells. Blood 1985; 66: 848–58.
8. Schwab U, Stein H, Gerdes J et al. Production of a monoclonal antibody specific for Hodgkin and Sternberg-Reed cells of Hodgkin's disease and a subset of normal lymphoid cells. Nature 1982; 299: 65–7.

50

9. Delsol G, Gatter KC, Stein H et al. Human lympoid cells may express epithelial membrane antigens: Implications for the diagnosis of human neoplasms. Lancet II 1984; 1124–9.
10. Burns BF, Dardick I. Ki1-positive non-Hodgkin lymphomas. Am J Clin Pathol 1990; 93: 327–32.
11. Suchi T, Lennert K, Tu L-Y et al. Histopathology and immunohistochemistry of peripheral T cell lymphomas: A proposal for their classification. J Clin Pathol 1987; 40: 995–1015.
12. Baroni CD, Pescarmona E, Calogero A et al. B- and T-cell non-Hodgkin's lymphomas with large multilobated cells: Morphological, phenotypic and clinical heterogeneity. Histopathology 1987; 11: 1121–32.

R. L. Souhami (ed.) The Teaching Cases from Annals of Oncology, 51–55, 1997.

The management of primary mediastinal B-cell lymphoma with sclerosis

W. Brugger, R. Engelhardt, R. Mertelsmann & L. Kanz

Albert-Ludwigs University Medical Center, Department of Hematology/Oncology, Freiburg, Germany

Key words: mediastinal large cell lymphoma, chemotherapy, high-dose chemotherapy

Introduction

Primary mediastinal large-cell lymphoma with sclerosis is a distinctive subtype of non-Hodgkin's lympoma with unique clinicopathologic aspects and aggressive behavior. The following case history illustrates the management of this disease, and discusses possible therapeutic options for patients with refractory disease or adverse prognostic factors.

Case history

A 22-year-old woman was admitted to an outside hospital, presenting with cough, chest pain and dyspnea. The physical examination showed findings of superior vena cava syndrome (SVCS) and a chest radiograph demonstrated a large mass of the anterior mediastinum with tracheobronchial compression (Fig. 1). Computer tomography (CT) revealed a bulky mediastinal mass of $14 \times 20 \times 9$ cm with displacement and compression of the trachea and the large vessels. No pleural or pericardial effusion were present or infiltration of adjacent thoracic structures. An abdominal CT-scan and a bone marrow biopsy showed no signs of disease. Lactic dehydrogenase level (LDH) was elevated at 286 U/l. A biopsy was obtained by mediastinoscopy; the tumor displayed cytomorphologic features of a large cell lymphoma with massive sclerosis and a reactive infiltrate of lymphocytes, plasma cells, eosinophils and histiocytes. Immunohistochemistry showed a positive staining of the neoplastic cells with CD45, HLA-DR, as well as the pan-B cell marker CD20. No reactivity was found for CD3, CD15, CD30 and CD43 antigens and the tumor cells were negative for cytokeratins.

Due to tracheobronchial compression, the patient required artificial ventilation following mediastinoscopy for 7 days. Immediate treatment was radiotherapy with a total dose of 20 Gy in 10 fractions. Her status improved rapidly, and she was referred to our hospital.

At our institution, she was treated wih the VACOP-B chemotherapy regimen for aggressive lymphomas. Re-

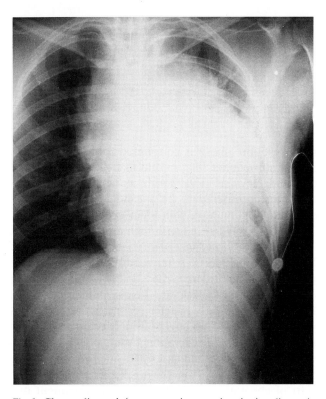

Fig. 1. Chest radiograph (erect posterior-anterior view) at diagnosis.

staging after 7 weeks on treatment resulted in a partial remission (PR) with a residual tumor mass in the anterior mediastinum (Fig. 2). Treatment was changed to a second line regimen and the patient was considered for high-dose chemotherapy with autologous peripheral blood progenitor cell (PBPC) transplantation. She received VP16, ifosfamide, and cisplatin (VIP) and PBPCs were mobilized simultaneously using G-CSF administration and collected by leukapheresis. Further restaging of the mediastinal mass after VIP chemotherapy again revealed no significant difference in the size of the tumor. A second biopsy was obtained by mini-thoracotomy. The pathologic findings included massive tumor necrosis and sclerosis but no viable tumor cells expressing the original phenotype.

Although the patient had shown a pathological com-

52

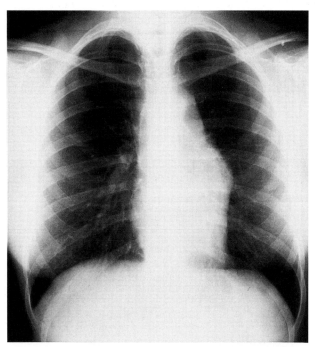

Fig. 2. Chest radiograph seven weeks after initiation of VACOP-B chemotherapy and 20 Gy emergency irradiation.

plete response she was considered to be at increased risk of subsequent relapse due to bulky disease (>10 cm) and elevated LDH levels at diagnosis. She was therefore considered to be a candidate for intensive consolidation therapy with stem cell transplantation. The patient was treated with high-dose BCNU, VP16, Ara-C and Melphalan (BEAM) chemotherapy with PBPC transplantation. After reinfusion of PBPCs, the patient received 300 µg G-CSF daily by s.c. injection in order to further accelerate hematopoietic recovery. Both neutrophil and platelet reconstitution occurred rapidly and stable. No infectious or bleeding complications occurred, and severe mucositis (WHO grade III) was the major non-hematological side effect. The patient was discharged from the hospital 15 days from the start of chemotherapy. After high dose treatment further investigation showed a residual mass in the anterior mediastinum. A positron-emission tomography (PET) scan was performed in order to differentiate between active residual tumor tissue and sclerosis. The result showed no increased metabolism due to tumor, suggesting that the residual mass consisted of inactive scar tissue or sclerosis. No further treatment has been given. The patient is well at 18 months following high dose chemotherapy and subsequent scans do not show any change in the residual mass.

Discussion

Clinical features

Patients with large-cell lymphoma of the mediastinum have some characteristic clinical features: most of them are young adults, predominantly women, with a median age of less than 30 years. They present with symptoms of a rapidly enlarging thoracic mass, often with superior venacaval compression and infiltration of adjacent structures such as lung, pleura, pericardium, and chest wall [1–4]. Due to its characteristic location in the anterior mediastinum, this lymphoma sometimes presents as an acute oncologic emergency, such as occurred in this patient. The presenting symptoms are cough, chest pain, dyspnea, or complaints from caval obstruction which occurs in 40%–50% of the patients. Few patients are asymptomatic. Fever or weight loss are present in 20% of the cases. Approximately 50% of the patients have pleural effusions, and one third demonstrate supraclavicular disease [2]. The mediastinal mass is greater than 10 cm in diameter in more than 70% of the patients, however, it is not correlated with the presence of pleural or pericardial effusions [4]. Intrathoracic extension to adjacent organs can be demonstrated in half of the patients. Despite its invasive behavior, however, the disease is confined to the mediastinum and to contiguous nodal areas in about 80%. Only 20% of all patients are clinical stages III and IV with extranodal spread being present in 10%. Bilateral renal infiltration is the most common extra-thoracic site. Other unusual sites of spread are the ovaries, the breast and the adrenal cortex [5]. Bone marrow involvement is extremely rare.

Diagnostic features

The primary mediastinal large-cell lymphoma with sclerosis is a distinct subtype of non-Hodgkin's lymphoma (NHL) which is composed of large polymorphous cells that lack of follicular pattern [6]. Sclerosis is marked in approximately 60% of the cases [3, 6, 7], which is rarely seen in other lymphomas of nodal origin, except for nodular sclerosing Hodgkin's disease. Immunohistochemistry reveals that it is a B-cell lymphoma with a uniform expression of the pan-B cell marker CD20 and the leukocyte-common antigen CD45/LCA. Light chain-restricted surface and cytoplasmic immunoglobulins, however, are usually negative [5, 8, 9]. Moreover, the tumor does not express CD3, CD5, CD10, CD15, CD30, CD45RO, and CD68. Epithelial membrane antigens (EMA) and pancytokeratins are also negative, allowing differentiation from solid tumors. Previous studies suggested that this type of lymphoma may originate in the thymus from a specific thymic B-cell population [9].

Differential diagnosis includes non-lymphoid tumors (thymoma, metastatic carcinoma, germ cell tumors) and other lymphoid malignancies, particularly nodular sclerosing Hodgkin's disease, T-lymphoblastic lymphomas as well as the Ki-1+ (CD30+) large-cell anaplastic lymphoma (Table 1). Although Hodgkin's disease may express CD20, it can be excluded from a primary B-cell lymphoma by staining for CD15, which is mostly co-expressed in Hodgkin's disease [10, 11] as well as by a negative staining for CD45. Moreover, CD30 is uniformly negative in mediastinal B-cell lymphoma with sclerosis (Table 1). Another primary lymphoma of the mediastinum which arises in boys and adolescent males is the T-lymphoblastic lymphoma, which can easily be excluded by staining for the pan-T cell marker CD3.

Table 1. Immunohistochemical characteristics of mediastinal lymphoma.

Mediastinal B-cell lymphoma with sclerosis	CD20+, CD45+, CD3−, CD15−, CD30−
Anaplastic large cell lymphoma	CD20 15%+, CD45+, CD3 75%+, CD15−, CD30+
Hodgkin's disease	CD20 20%+, CD45−, CD3 40%+, CD15+ CD30+

Management of mediastinal B-cell lymphoma with sclerosis

Several studies described this lymphoma as an aggressive disorder with a relatively poor prognosis [2, 3, 5, 12–15]. Recent studies with CHOP therapy for third-generation regimens such as MACOP-B or VACOP-B, however, reported that it is a curable disease with a 5-year failure-free survival between 40 and 60% [3–5, 14, 15]. Nevertheless, it requires prompt diagnosis and immediate treatment since it can evolve into a medical emergency.

At the present time, the patients are treated with chemotherapy regimens for aggressive NHLs, such as CHOP or VACOP-B. Achievement of a complete remission after first-line chemotherapy is essential for long-term survival, whereas primarily resistant and relapsed patients are extremely refractory to salvage therapy [13]. Moreover, the presence of bulky tumor (> 10 cm), pleural effusion or extranodal spread generally compromises survival [4, 14]. Such patients as well as patients who do not respond satisfactorily to induction chemotherapy or who relapse are poor-prognosis patients and should be considered immediately for more intensive or investigational treatment including high-dose chemotherapy with stem cell transplantation [2, 4].

Patients with localized disease without adverse prognostic factors (e.g. LDH, bulky disease, performance status, extranodal sites) [16], and no pleural effusion should be treated with either CHOP, or one of the third-generation regimens, such as VACOP-B [2, 4, 14]. However, there is at present no clear benefit of newer chemotherapy regimens over CHOP in large cell lymphomas at all sites [17, 18] suggesting that CHOP should still be considered the standard regimen for the treatment of large cell lymphoma. The role of adjuvant radiation after completion of chemotherapy remains unproven at present [2], although most centers irradiate patients after chemotherapy [14]. Using such an approach, complete response (CR) rates vary between 75 and 90% with a 3-year disease-free survival rate of approximately 70% in patients with CR [3, 14, 15]. Almost all relapses occur within the first 15 months after treatment initiation [4, 14]. The patients who are free of disease after this time period are most likely to be cured. Non-responding patients, however, do not show long-term survival [3]. Those patients and patients who relapse after having achieved an initial remission, should be considered for treatment with a salvage regimen, followed by high-dose chemotherapy with bone marrow or peripheral blood stem cell transplantation (see below).

The management for patients who present with bulky disease, pleural effusion or more than one extranodal site is somewhat different since these patients are at highest risk in terms of treatment failure or early relapse [4, 14]. Many centers would therefore recommend to treat such patients with a third-generation regimen, such as VACOP-B [19] which is also used at our own institution, but the CHOP regimen is a reasonable alternative even for less favorable tumors [2]. In any case, patients with adverse prognostic factors should be closely monitored radiologically (see below) in order to identify patients with suboptimal response at a timepoint when additional therapeutic interventions may be most effective. We undertake the first re-evaluation after 6–7 weeks of VACOP-B therapy. Patients who achieve a complete radiological response (CR) at that time can be continued with full-dose VACOP-B for 12 weeks, followed by a 36–40 Gy involved-field mediastinal irradiation. In our department, those patients who do not achieve a CR are started on second-line therapy with high-dose consolidation. Such approaches are also currently being recommended by several centers [2–4, 16, 18]. Our approach in such patients is to apply a salvage regimen using etoposide (VP16), ifosfamide and cisplatin (VIP; [20]). This regimen yields encouraging results in aggressive NHLs [21], and, moreover, the VIP regimen simultaneously mobilizes PBPCs using hematopoietic growth factors [22, 23]. Patients will then be treated with high-dose chemotherapy and autologous bone marrow or PBPC support. The reason for using PBPCs instead of autologous bone marrow is based on the finding that PBPCs induce a more rapid restoration of hematopoiesis [24] and the fact that there might be a reduced risk of tumor cell contamination in PBPC preparations [25–27]. Since the mortality rate after high-dose chemotherapy and PBPC transplantation is very low in recent series, this treatment option does not result in an increased rate of treatment-related mortality than any other third-generation regimen for aggressive NHLs [17]. Therefore, high-dose chemotherapy with PBPC transplantation should be considered in patients presenting with bulky disease, pleural effusion or more than one extranodal site as part of the front-line treatment.

The rationale for high-dose chemotherapy in high-

54

risk aggressive NHL patients in general is based on previous non-randomized trials which have indicated that this treatment option might produce superior results to conventional chemotherapy [28]. However, interim analyses of recently performed randomized trials have not yet demonstrated a significantly better survival as compared to conventional therapy [29, 30]. Until the final results of these studies are available, high-dose chemotherapy in all poor-prognosis aggressive NHL patients including this subtype of lymphoma remains to be determined.

Management of residual tumor after treatment in mediastinal B-cell lymphoma with sclerosis

Patients with bulky disease in the mediastinum frequently have residual abnormalities of uncertain significance on regular X-ray films, CT or magnetic resonance scans, independent of the subtype of the lymphoma. This situation is similar to that which can be found in nodular sclerosing Hodgkin's disease where residual masses are also frequently observed. In Hodgkin's disease, however, residual mediastinal abnormalities do not by themselves indicate persistent active disease or an increased risk of relapse [31, 32], whereas in B-cell lymphoma with sclerosis, several studies suggested that any residual tumor after treatment is associated with an increased risk of relapse [2, 4]. Therefore, a technique is needed to differentiate between active tumor tissue and fibrosis within residual radiographic masses. Gallium-67 citrate imaging has been used and shown to be a both sensitive and specific indicator of active lymphoma [33]. An alternative method to again differentiate between residual tumor and sclerosis is the positron-emission tomography (PET). This method as well as Ga-67 imaging might be particularly helpful in patients with positive-scans prior to treatment which revert to normal following completion of therapy. Persistent Ga-67 uptake after the end of treatment predicts for a poor outcome in this lymphoma [4]. At present, there are no general recommendations for the management of these patients. In addition, the role of consolidation radiotherapy in patients with residual radiographic masses after high-dose chemotherapy remains to be determined.

References

1. Levitt LJ, Aisenberg AC, Harris NL et al. Primary non-Hodgkin's lymphoma of the mediastinum. Cancer 1982; 50: 2486–92.
2. Aisenberg AC. Primary large-cell lymphoma of the mediastinum. J Clin Oncol 1993; 11: 2291–4.
3. Lazzarino M, Orland E, Paulli M et al. Primary mediastintal B-cell lymphoma with sclerosis: An aggressive tumor with distinctive clinical and pathological features. J Clin Oncol 1993; 11: 2306–13.
4. Kirn D, Mauch P, Shaffer K et al. Large-cell and immunoblastic lymphoma of the mediastinum: Prognostic and pathologic features in 57 patients. J Clin Oncol 1993; 11: 1336–43.
5. Todeschini G, Ambrosetti A, Meneghini V et al. Mediastinal large-B-cell with sclerosis: A clinical study of 21 patients. J Clin Oncol 1990; 8: 804–8.
6. Lennert K, Feller AC. Histopathology of non-Hodgkin's Lymphomas. New York: Springer-Verlag 1992; 157–61.
7. Miller JB, Variakojis D, Bitran JD et al. Diffuse histiocytic lymphoma with sclerosis: A clinicopathological entity frequently causing superior venacaval obstruction. Cancer 1981; 47: 748–56.
8. Al-Sharabati M, Chittal S, Duga-Neulet I et al. Primary anterior mediastinal B-cell lymphoma: A clinicopathological and immunohistochemical study of 16 cases. Cancer 1991; 67: 2579–87.
9. Möller P, Moldenhauer G, Momberg F et al. Mediastinal clear cell lymphoma of clear cell type is a tumor corresponding to terminal steps of B-cell differentiation. Blood 1987; 69: 1087–95.
10. Stein H, Uchanska-Ziegler B, Gerdes J et al. Hodgkin and Sternberg-Reed cells contain antigens specific to late cells of granulopoiesis. Int J Cancer 1982; 29: 283–90.
11. Zukeberg LR, Collins AB, Ferry JA et al. Coexpression of CD15 and CD20 by Reed-Sternberg cells in Hodgkin's disease. Am J Pathol 1991; 139: 475–83.
12. Trump DL, Mann RB. Diffuse large cell and undifferentiated lymphomas with prominent mediastinal involvement. A poor prognostic subset of patients with non-Hodgkin's lymphoma. Cancer 1982; 50: 277–82.
13. Haioun C, Gaulard P, Roudot-Thoraval F et al. Mediastinal diffuse large-cell lymphoma with sclerosis: A condition with a poor prognosis. Am J Clin Oncol 1989; 12: 425–9.
14. Jacobson JO, Aisenberg AC, Lamarre L et al. Mediastinal large-cell lymphoma: An uncommon subset of adult lymphoma curable with combined modality therapy. Cancer 1988; 62: 1893–8.
15. Bertini M, Orsucci L, Vitolo U et al. Stage II large B-cell lymphoma with sclerosis treated with MACOP-B. Ann Oncol 1991; 2: 733–7.
16. Shipp MA, Harrington DP. The international non-Hodgkin's lymphoma prognostic factors project: A predictive model for aggressive non-Hodgkin's lymphoma. N Engl J Med 1993; 329: 987–4
17. Fisher RI, Gaynor ER, Dahlberg S et al. Comparison of a standard regimen (CHOP) with three intensive chemotherapy regimens for advanced non-Hodgkin's lymphoma. N Engl J Med 1993; 328: 1002–6.
18. Armitage JO. Treatment of non-Hodgkin's lymphoma. N Engl J Med 1993; 328: 1023–30.
19. O'Reilly SE, Hoskins P, Klimo P et al. MACOP-B and VACOP-B in diffuse large-cell lymphomas and MOPP/ABV in Hodgkin's disease. Ann Oncol 1991; 2: 17–23.
20. Brugger W, Frisch J, Schulz G et al. Sequential administration of IL-3 and GM-CSF following standard-dose combination chemotherapy wtih etoposide, ifosfamide and cisplatin. J Clin Oncol 1992; 10: 1452–9.
21. Hickish T, Roldan A, Cunningham D et al. EPIC: An effective low toxicity regimen for relapsing lymphoma. Br J Cancer 1993; 3: 599–604.
22. Brugger W, Bross KH, Frisch J et al. Mobilization of peripheral blood progenitor cells by sequential administration of IL-3 and GM-CSF following polychemotherpay with etoposide, ifosfamide, and cisplatin. Blood 1992; 79: 1193–200.
23. Brugger W, Birken R, Bertz H et al. Peripheral blood progenitor cells mobilized by chemotherapy + G-CSF accelerate both neutrophil and platelet recovery after high-dose VP16, ifosfamide and cisplatin. Br J Haematol 1993; 84: 402–8.
24. Sheridan WP, Begley CG, Juttner C et al. Effect of peripheral-blood progenitor cells mobilised by filgrastim (G-CSF) on platelet recovery after high-dose chemotherapy. Lancet 1992; i: 640.
25. Ross AA, Cooper BW, Lazarus HM et al. Detection and viability of tumor cells in peripheral blood stem cell collections from breast cancer patients using immunocytochemical and clonogenic assay techniques. Blood 1993; 82: 2605.

26. Brugger W, Bross KJ, Glatt M et al. Mobilization of tumor cells and hematopoietic progenitor cells into peripheral blood of patients with solid tumors. Blood 1994; 83: 636–40.

27. Shpall EJ, Jones RB. Release of tumor cells from bone marrow. Blood 1994; 83: 623–5.

28. Gulati SC, Shank B, Black P et al. Autologous bone marrow transplantation for patients with poor prognosis lymphoma. J Clin Oncol 1988; 6: 1303–13.

29. Haioun C, Lepage E, Gisselbrecht C et al. Autologous bone marrow transplantation versus sequential chemotherapy in first complete remission aggressive non-Hodgkin's lymphoma: 1st Interim analysis on 370 patients (LNH87 protocol). Proc Am Soc Clin Oncol 1992; 11: 316a.

30. Gianni AG, Bregni M, Siena S et al. 5-Year update of the Milan Cancer Institute randomized trial of high-dose sequential vs. MACOP-B therapy for diffuse large-cell lymphomas. Proc Am Soc Clin Oncol 1994; 13: 373a (# 1263).

31. Jochelson MS, Mauch P, Balikian J et al. The significance of the residual mediastinal mass in the treated Hodgkin's disease. J Clin Oncol 1985; 3: 637–41.

32. Canellos GP. Residual mass in lymphoma may not be residual disease. J Clin Oncol 1988; 6: 931–3.

33. Kaplan WD, Jochelson MS, Herman TS et al. Gallium-67 imaging: A predictor of residual tumor viability and clinical outcome in patients with diffuse large-cell lymphoma. J Clin Oncol 1990; 8: 1966–73.

R. L. Souhami (ed.) The Teaching Cases from Annals of Oncology, 57–62, 1997.

The management of chronic lymphocytic leukemia — a case history

Y. Bastion, N. Dhedin, P. Felman[1] & B. Coiffier

Service d'Hématologie and [1]Laboratoire d'Hématologie, Centre Hospitalier Lyon-Sud, Pierre-Bénite, France

Key words: chronic lymphocytic leukemia, staging, prognosis, treatment, intensive treatment

Introduction

Chronic lymphocytic leukemia (CLL) is a common lymphoproliferative disease. In Western countries, CLL is the leukemia with the highest incidence among persons aged 50 to 55 years and older. Hallmarks of the disease include an absolute and sustained increase of mature-appearing lymphocytes in the blood and bone marrow. The clinical course of the disease is highly variable: some patients die within one year after diagnosis while some live as long as those in an age-matched population. This underlines the importance of prognostic factors and staging systems. Treatment strategy ranges from a watch-and-wait policy to polychemotherapy. CLL remains, however, an incurable disease and this justifies in young patients new approaches such as intensive chemoradiotherapy with autologous or allogeneic stem cell support. We report here a case history of CLL in a young patient which illustrates some of the complications of the disease and the new treatment options which are now under investigation.

Case history

A thirty-seven-year-old man presented in January 1983 with lymphocytosis. His past medical history was not significant. The initial hematological parameters were hemoglobin 145 g/L, platelet count 395×10^9/L, white blood cell count 23.3×10^9/L with 65% lymphocytes, and 32% polymorphonuclear cells. Blood cell counts performed 6 months previously showed a sustained increase of lymphocytes. Clinical examination results were normal. The bone marrow aspirate showed a lymphocytosis of 35% with mature-appearing lymphocytes, as observed in peripheral blood. Cells expressed surface membrane IgM restricted to Kappa light chain, showing clonality, CD5 antigen, and pan-B cell antigens CD19 and CD20. Binet stage A B-CLL was diagnosed.

He received no treatment until November 1983, by which time he had become asthenic, and his white blood cell count had increased to 41.2×10^9/L with 84% lymphocytes (lymphocyte count doubling time: 9 months). He was then treated with chlorambucil continuously (4 mg per day) until July 1989. The disease remained stable, with leucocytosis between 20 and 40×10^9/L. In July 1989 he presented with auto-immune hemolytic anemia with hemoglobin 64 g/L, and a positive Coombs' test result (IgG plus complement). His white blood cell count was 137×10^9/L with 95% mature-appearing lymphocytes (Fig. 1), and a platelet count of 131×10^9/L. Bone marrow aspirate showed a lymphocytosis of 80%. Clinical examination revealed a moderate splenomegaly (4 cm below left costal margin), and a superficial and deep adenomegaly (largest diameter: 2 cm). The patient responded to corticotherapy with normalization of reticulocyte count but his hemoglobin level remained at 90 g/L. Fludarabine treatment was instituted in September 1989 at the standard dose of 25 mg/m^2/d for 5 days at 4-week intervals. After 6 courses, a partial response was noted (according to the IWCLL and NCI criteria – see below), with a normal hemoglobin level, a peri-

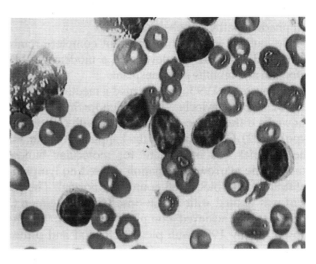

Fig. 1. Mature appearing lymphocytes from the peripheral blood (August 1989) (×1000, Wright stain).

pheral lymphocyte count of 1×10^9/L, a normal platelet count, but with a persistence of moderate deep adenomegaly and bone marrow infiltration. Six further courses of fludarabine were administered until August 1990, for a total of 12 courses.

He then presented a new episode of hemolytic anemia which did not respond to corticotherapy. The patient was splenectomized in November 1990 with a rapid normalization of hemoglobin level. Histologic examination of the spleen showed no pathological lymphoid infiltration. At that time, no superficial or deep adenomegaly was noted, and his white blood cell count was normal with normal differential. A bone marrow biopsy showed only a persistent nodular infiltration with less than 30% lymphocytes. Immunological analysis of peripheral blood mononuclear cells showed no clonal excess, and flow cytometry analysis showed that the fraction of circulating lymphocytes coexpressing CD5 and CD20 was less than 5%. However, a study of minimal residual disease by Ig gene rearrangements was not performed. The patient had no sibling donor for allogeneic transplant. The young age of the patient, and his good 'nodular' partial response, along with the usual poor prognosis of stage C CLL led us to consider the patient for intensification with autologous peripheral stem cell (PSC) support. PSC collection was performed after high-dose cyclophosphamide followed by subcutaneous granulocyte-colony stimulating factor (GM-CSF, Schering-Plough/Sandoz). He was intensively treated in March 1991 with cyclophosphamide (60 mg/kg/d for 2 days), etoposide (300 mg/m^2/d for 3 days) and fractionated total body irradiation (12 Gy in 6 fractions) followed by PSC reinfusion and received GM-CSF until neutrophil recovery. No significant toxic effects were observed. The patient had a rapid granulocyte recovery (>0.5×10^9/l at day 9 post-graft) but a delayed platelet recovery (last transfusion and platelet count >20×10^9/l at 7 months). Bone marrow biopsy performed 11 months after intensifiction showed a marked hypoplasia without evidence of lymphoid infiltration, CD5+CD20+ population remained undetectable in peripheral blood and in marrow (<1%) and no lymphadenopathy was observed.

The patient remained in apparent complete remission for 32 months. He developed a moderate CMV infection at 6 months posttransplant.

In November 1993, he presented a mediastinal mass and a supra-clavicular lymphadenopathy. Biopsies showed a diffuse large-cell lymphoma with a B phenotype (Fig. 2). Cells expressed the kappa light chain, but the material was insufficient for molecular biology study. Bone marrow examination showed no lymphoid infiltration and blood cell count was normal. The patient was treated with a high-dose CHOP regimen (3 courses) and achieved complete remission, but relapsed in July 1994 with pleural effusion and diffuse pulmonary localizations.

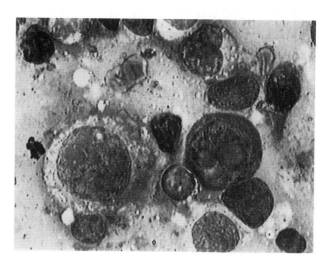

Fig. 2. Richter's syndrome: fine needle aspirates showing large lymphomatous cells (November 1993) (×1000, May-Grünewald/Giemsa stain).

Discussion points

Diagnosis, phenotypic characteristics and differential diagnosis

In typical cases, tumor cells are mature-appearing lymphocytes. Criteria for diagnosis include sustained lymphocytosis of greater than 10×10^9/L and bone marrow (BM) lymphocytosis of at least 30% in BM aspirates. In patients with 5 to 10×10^9/L lymphocytes, phenotypic analysis should be performed [1, 2].

Most CLL are B-cell malignancies. Tumor cells express surface membrane immunoglobulins, IgM, or both IgM and IgD, which are restricted to a single light chain, and antigens related to B cells such as CD19 and CD20. They also express the CD5 antigen, initially described as a pan T-cell marker but which is also present on a subset of normal B cells [2]. T CLL is a rare disorder in which cells are generally large granular lymphocytes.

CLL must be distinguished from reactive lymphocytosis, and from other B-cell malignancies. In B-prolymphocytic leukemia, the majority of tumor cells are characterized by a larger size and a prominent nucleolus, and their CD5 expression is low or absent. However, during the course of the disease, some patients with typical CLL may have an increased number of prolymphocytic cells. On the other hand, some patients have at diagnosis a significant proportion of prolymphocytic cells (10%–55%) and their disease is recognized as CLL of mixed cell type or CLL/PLL in the FAB classification [3]; this is correlated with a poor prognosis. CLL must also be distinguished from hairy cell leukemia, splenic lymphoma with circulating villous lymphocytes, and non-Hodgkin's lymphoma with a leukemic presentation: this is the case for follicular NHL, mantle cell lymphomas and lymphocytic or lymphoplasmacytic lymphoma. In the latter, lymph node biopsy may be essential, as bone marrow morphologic and immunologic features can be similar to those encountered in CLL.

Staging systems and prognosis in CLL

Two major staging systems have been proposed, and their prognostic value has been largely validated. The Rai classification, which segregates patients into five groups, was proposed in 1975 [4]. The Binet staging system defines three groups [5]. The parameters employed are roughly similar and easy to determine (Table 1). In the initial report of Binet et al. [5], median survival time was, respectively, 2, 7 and more than 10 years for patients with stages C to A disease. However, in more recent reports, the median survival for stage C patients was better, ranging from 3.5 to 4.5 years [6–9]. These reports showed that there was a lack of prognostic discrimination between Rai stages III and IV. The International Workshop on CLL (IWCLL) [1] recommended the adoption of an integrated Binet-Rai staging system in which the Binet stage was to be further defined by the addition of the appropriate Rai stage.

Along with the major prognostic factors applied in these staging systems, other parameters have been shown to have independent prognostic value, i.e., the lymphocyte count doubling time [10], the pattern of marrow infiltration (diffuse versus non-diffuse) [11], and cytogenetic analysis [12]. The influence of age at diagnosis is controversial, but prognostic factors described above are useful when applied to younger patients [13].

In 1988, Montserrat et al proposed criteria to identify patients with a 'benign' form of disease for which the term 'smouldering' CLL was proposed. The following criteria characterized this subgroup: Binet stage A disease, a non-diffuse bone marrow histology, a hemoglobin level $\geq$13 g/dL, lymphocyte value $<30 \times 10^9$/L, and a lymphocyte doubling time >12 months [10]. These patients had a life expectancy that was not different from that of the sex- and age-matched population. Slightly different criteria have been proposed by other groups to define a subset of patients with a particularly good prognosis [14, 15].

Complications developing in the course of the disease

Autoimmune manifestations are frequently observed in the course of the disease: autoimmune hemolytic anemia occurs in 10% to 25% of patients at some time and autoantibodies are generally warm reactive polyclonal IgG with activity against antigens of the rhesus system. Immune thrombocytopenia is less frequent and other autoimmune manifestations are rare (review in [16]). These manifestations often respond to corticosteroids, but this treatment is generally used concomitantly with chemotherapy.

Patients with CLL are prone to develop infections due to immunoglobulin deficiency, neutropenia and lymphoid dysfunction. The preventive use of intravenous immunoglobulins has been proposed and been shown to reduce the incidence of bacterial infections with, however, no impact on survival.

Transformation of the disease to diffuse large cell lymphoma may occur with a projected incidence of 3% to 10% [17, 18]. This event is called Richter's syndrome, and is often characterized by systemic symptoms, a rapid increase in lymphadenopathy or extranodal involvement. Prognosis is generally poor, with a median survival of 5 months despite multiagent therapy in a recent report [18]. Although this point has been controversial, the lymphomatous population generally arises from the original CLL clone, as demonstrated by Ig gene rearrangement studies [18, 19]. In rare cases, patients with typical B-CLL may develop acute lymphoblastic leukemia or myeloma or even secondary acute myeloid leukemia. Several studies have demonstrated an excess of nonhematologic neoplasms.

Table 1. Rai and Binet staging systems.

Rai staging system		Binet staging system		
Stage	Clinical features	Stage	Clinical features	% of all patients at diagnosis
0	Lymphocytosis in blood and bone marrow only	A	Hemoglobin $\geq$100 g/L; platelets $\geq$100 $\times$ 10^9/L; and <three areas[a] involved	A – 50%–60%
I	Lymphocytosis and enlarged lymph nodes			
II	Lymphocytosis plus hepatomegaly, or splenomegaly, or both	B	Hemoglobin $\geq$100 g/L; platelets $\geq$100 $\times$ 10^9/L; and $\geq$three areas involved	B – 30%
III	Lymphocytosis and anemia (hemoglobin <110 g/L)			
IV	Lymphocytosis and thrombocytopenia (platelets <100 $\times$ 10^9/L)	C	Hemoglobin <100 g/L or platelet <100 $\times$ 10^9/L, or both (independently of the areas involved)	C – 10%–20%

[a] The three areas include the cervical, axillary, and inguinal lymph nodes (whether unilateral or bilateral), the spleen, and the liver.

Table 2. Criteria of response to treatment.

Response	IWCLL criteria	NCI criteria
CR	No evidence of disease	▪ Absence of lymphadenopathy, hepatomegaly, splenomegaly or constitutional symptoms. ▪ Normal blood count: neutrophils >1.5 × 10⁹/L, platelets >100 × 10⁹/L, Hb >11 g/dL, lymphocytes <4.0 × 10⁹/L. ▪ BM biopsy normal cellularity. Lymphocytes <30%
PR	Change from stage C to stage A or B; or from stage B to A	▪ 50% reduction in blood lymphocytes and 50% reduction in lymphadenopathy and/or 50% reduction in splenomegaly and/or hepatomegaly. ▪ Neutrophils >1.5 × 10⁹/L or 50% improvement over baseline; platelets >100 × 10⁹/L or 50% improvement over baseline; Hb >11.0 g/dL (not supported by transfusion) or 50% improvement over baseline
SD	No change in the stage of the disease	▪ No CR, PR, or PD
PD	Change from stage A disease to stage B or C, or from stage B to C	▪ At least one of the following: >50% increase in the size of at least two lymph nodes or new palpable lymph nodes; ⩾50% increase of splenomegaly or hepatomegaly or appearance if they were not present; transformation to a more aggressive histology Richter or prolymphocytic leukemia: >50% increase in the absolute number of circulating lymphocytes

Standard therapy in CLL

Evaluation of treatment efficiency

Criteria of response to treatment have recently been standardized by the International Workshop on CLL [1] and the National Cancer Institute [20]; these are shown in Table 2. In fact, complete remission is rarely obtained and its assessment requires sensitive methods such as flow cytometry with the simultaneous use of CD5 and CD19 or CD20 markers, kappa-lambda clonal excess and possibly analysis of gene rearrangements by the polymerase chain reaction [1]. Progression-free survival and overall survival are major endpoints in evaluation of the impact of therapy in this disease, as in other low-grade hematologic malignancies.

Therapeutic options

There is increasing evidence that the majority of patients with stage A disease should not be treated unless their disease progresses. In a large randomized study, the survival rate of the group treated by chlorambucil was even shorter than that of the untreated group [21, 2]. The IWCLL recommended that therapy for patients with stage A disease be restricted to those with adverse prognostic factors such as lymphocyte count higher than 50 × 10⁹/L, rapid lymphocyte doubling time, diffuse bone marrow infiltration or possibly other adverse prognostic factors [1]. The optimal treatment for stages B and C patients remains controversial.

As single-agent chemotherapy, chlorambucil has been the most common treatment used in CLL and produces 40%–60% of responses in stages B and C patients. It can be used in a daily schedule (generally 0.1 mg/kg) or in an intermittent schedule with no clear advantage of either policy over the other [22, 23]. The concomitant use of corticosteroids has never been shown to improve treatment efficiency. Results obtained with other single agents are comparable or worse.

Numerous multiple drug regimens have been proposed in advanced stages such as COP (cyclophosphamide, vincristine and prednisone), MOPP, or CMP (cyclophosphamide, melphalan and prednisone) which yield results identical to those obtained with chlorambucil [24, 25]. A beneficial effect of low doses of doxorubicin ('mini-CHOP' regimen with 25 mg/m² doxorubicin) has been suggested in stage C patients, with a striking improvement in survival in a large French randomized study [6]. However, this advantage in terms of survival was not confirmed in another randomized study [26]. Other combinations with doxorubicin have been proposed, but their role needs to be clarified in randomized studies.

Chlorambucil, alone or with corticosteroids, remains the treatment of choice in elderly patients or in younger patients with an initial stage of the disease requiring treatment. In younger patients with poor prognoses polychemotherapy may be considered. However, the recent introduction of new drugs such as fludarabine could change this strategy in the future.

Although some data suggest some benefit for splenic irradiation in patients with splenomegaly [27], there is little room for radiotherapy in CLL. Irradiation of large lymph nodes may be used in patients resistant to chemotherapy. Splenectomy may be proposed in autoimmune hemolytic anemia and immune thrombocytopenia when corticosteroids are ineffective, and possibly in patients with painful splenomegaly or cytopenia secondary to hypersplenism [28].

New therapeutic options

New drugs

New nucleoside analogues have been extensively studied in recent years. A 60% response rate has been induced in previously treated CLL patients with fludarabine monophosphate [29], and in untreated patients, the CR rate reaches 75% [30]. Despite these good results, it remains unclear whether this drug can change the course of the disease. In previously treated patients, the median time to progression of responders was 21 months in a large recent study [31]. Randomized trials comparing fludarabine with CHOP are now ongoing in stages B and C patients, but results are too preliminary for conclusions. If fludarabine does improve response rates in some subsets of patients, its impact on survival remains to be demonstrated [32]. The usual schedule for fludarabine administration is 25 mg/m^2/day for 5 consecutive days every 4 weeks. Major side effects are myelosuppression and the occurrence of opportunistic infections, especially in extensively pretreated patients. The addition of prednisone does not result in a higher response rate. The combination of fludarabine with other drugs is under investigation. Although reported experience is less important, 2-chlorodeoxyadenosine seems capable of inducing similar response rates. Some patients with advanced CLL who are refractory to fludarabine therapy could benefit from treatment with 2-CDA, although this has recently been questioned [33]. Pentostatin seems to be less effective than the two previous drugs.

Fludarabine is now available in the United States for the treatment of patients with B-CLL who have not responded to, or whose disease has progressed during treatment with, at least one standard alkylating agent-containing regimen. It will soon be available in Europe.

Biologic response modifiers

Various monoclonal antibodies have been used in the treatment of CLL, with generally disappointing results. Studies with the CAMPATH-1 antibodies which are bound to the CDw52 molecule, an antigen largely expressed on T and B lymphocytes, are in progress. Some preliminary data are encouraging [34]. Treatment with Interferon-alpha offers disappointing results although it can induce a significant response rate in early stages of the disease [35]. The role of Interleukin-4, which has shown a clear in vitro activity, is under investigation.

Intensive treatment with stem cell support in young patients

Forty percent of patients with CLL are younger than 60 years at diagnosis. Some data suggest a dose-response relationship with some drugs, providing a rationale for intensive therapy followed by autologous or allogeneic hematopoietic stem cell transplant.

The use of autologous hematopoietic stem cells should theoretically require the achievement of a minimal-residual-disease state before transplantation, and in this setting, fludarabine seems to be interesting. Reduction of graft contamination by tumor cells can be achieved by marrow ex vivo treatment (mainly B-cell depletion by monoclonal antibodies) or by preferential use of peripheral blood stem cell support. In reported experience, the conditioning regimen consisted mainly of high-dose cyclophosphamide and total body irradiation. Preliminary data show that this approach is feasible in young patients with acceptable post-transplant morbidity and leads to a substantial CR rate even in patients in relapse or with advanced CLL [36–39]. However, long-term follow-up and more experience are required to evaluate the impact of this strategy on overall survival and disease-free survival.

In comparison with autologous BMT, allogeneic BMT uses a non-contaminated graft and could induce a graft-versus-leukemia effect. Data from the European and International Bone Marrow Transplant Registries with HLA-identical sibling transplants have recently been updated: fifty-four patients have been reported, of whom seven were considered to have chemosensitive disease and none of whom had achieved complete remission before transplant. The three-year leukemia-free survival is 44% despite a high transplant-related mortality [40]. As in the setting of autologous transplant, the study of post-transplant CR at the molecular level would allow better assessment of the curability of this disease. Allogeneic BMT should be considered in patients aged 50 (or 55?) years or less who have an HLA-identical sibling donor and a poor prognosis CLL. However, future studies should aim at a more precise definition of indications.

References

1. Chronic lymphocytic leukemia: Recommendations for diagnosis, staging, and response criteria. International Workshop on Chronic Lymphocytic Leukemia. Ann Intern Med 1989; 110: 236–8.
2. Dighiero G, Travade P, Chevret S et al. B-cell chronic lymphocytic leukemia: Present status and future directions. Blood 1991; 78: 1901–14.
3. Bennett JM, Catovsky D, Daniel MT et al. Proposals for the classification of chronic (mature) B and T lymphoid leukaemias. J Clin Pathol 1989; 42: 567–84.
4. Rai KR, Sawitsky A, Cronkite EP et al. Clinical staging of Chronic Lymphocytic Leukemia. Blood 1975; 46: 219–34.
5. Binet JL, Auquier A, Dighiero G et al. A new prognostic classification of Chronic Lymphocytic Leukemia derived from a multivariate survival analysis. Cancer 1981; 48: 198–206.
6. French Cooperative Group on Chronic Lymphocytic Leukemia. Long-term results of the CHOP regimen in stage C chronic lymphocytic leukaemia. Br J Haematol 1989; 73: 334–40.
7. Catovsky D, Fooks J, Richards S. Prognostic factors in chronic lymphocytic leukaemia: The importance of age, sex and response to treatment in survival. A report from the MRC CLL1 trial. Br J Haematol 1989; 72: 141–9.
8. Raphael B, Anderson J, Silber R et al. Comparison of chlorambucil and prednisone versus cyclophosphamide, vincristine and prednisone as initial treatment of chronic lymphocytic leukemia: Long-term follow-up of an Eastern Cooperative Oncology Group. Randomised clinical trial. J Clin Oncol 1991; 9: 770–6.

9. Karmiris T, Rohatiner AZS, Love S et al. The management of chronic lymphocytic leukemia at a single centre over a 24-year period: Prognostic factors for survival. Hematol Oncol 1994; 12: 29–39.

10. Montserrat E, Virolas N, Reverter JC et al. Natural history of chronic lymphocytic leukemia: On the progression and prognosis of early clinical stages. Nouv Rev Fr Hematol 1988; 30: 359–61.

11. Rozman C, Montserrat E, Rodriguez-Fernandez JM et al. Bone marrow histologic pattern. The best single prognostic parameter in chronic lymphocytic leukemia. A multivariate analysis of 329 cases. Blood 1984; 64: 642–8.

12. Juliusson G, Oscier D, Fitchett M et al. Prognostic subgroups in B cell chronic lymphocytic leukemia by specific chromosomal abnormalities. N Engl J Med 1990; 323: 720–6.

13. Montserrat E, Gomis F, Vallespi T et al. Presenting features and prognosis of chronic lymphocytic leukemia in younger adults. Blood 1991; 78: 1545–51.

14. French Cooperative Group on Chronic Lymphocytic Leukaemia. Natural history of stage A chronic lymphocytic leukaemia in untreated patients. Br J Haematol 1990; 76: 45–57.

15. Molica S. Progression and survival studies in early chronic lymphocytic leukemia. Blood 1991; 78: 895–9.

16. Kipps TJ, Carson DA. Autoantibodies in chronic lymphocytic leukemia and related systemic autoimmune diseases. Blood 1993; 81: 2475–87.

17. Armitage JO, Dick FR, Corder MP. Diffuse histiocytic lymphoma complicating chronic lymphocytic leukemia. Cancer 1978; 41: 422–7.

18. Robertson LE, Pugh W, O'Brien S et al. Richter's syndrome: A report on 39 patients. J Clin Oncol 1993; 11: 1985–9.

19. Cherepakhin V, Baird SM, Meisenholder GW et al. Common clonal origin of chronic lymphocytic leukemia and high-grade lymphoma of Richter's syndrome. Blood 1993; 82: 3141–7.

20. Cheson B, Bennett J, Rai K et al. Guidelines for clinical protocols for chronic lymphocytic leukemia: Recommendations of the NCI sponsored working group. Am J Hematol 1988; 29: 152–63.

21. French Cooperative Group on Chronic Lymphocytic Leukemia: Effects of chlorambucil and therapeutic decision in initial forms of chronic lymphocytic leukemia (stage A): Results of a randomized clinical trial in 612 patients. Blood 1990; 75: 1414–21.

22. Sawitsky A, Rai KR, Glidewell O et al. Comparison of daily versus intermittent chlorambucil and prednisone therapy in the treatment of patients with chronic lymphocytic leukemia. Blood 1977; 50: 1049–59.

23. Jaksic B, Brugiatelli M. High dose continuous chlorambucil vs intermittent chlorambucil plus predinsone for treatment of B-CLL. Nouv Rev Fr Hematol 1988; 30: 437–42.

24. Montserrat E, Alcala A, Parody R et al. Treatment of chronic lymphocytic leukemia in advanced stages: A randomized trial comparing chlorambucil plus prednisone vs cyclophosphamide, vincristine and prednisone. Cancer 1985; 56: 2369–75.

25. French Cooperative Group on Chronic Lymphocytic Leukemia. A randomized clinical trial of chlorambucil versus COP in stage B chronic lymphocytic leukemia. Blood 1990; 75: 1422–5.

26. Hansen MM, Andersen E, Christensen BE et al. CHOP regimen versus intermittent chlorambucil-prednisone in chronic lymphocytic leukemia: Preliminary results of a randomized multicenter study. Nouv Rev Fr Hematol 1988; 30: 433–6.

27. Catovsky D, Fooks J, Richards S. The UK Medical Research Council CLL trials 1 and 2. Nouv Rev Fr Hematol 1988; 30: 423–7.

28. Ferrant A, Michaux JL, Stookal G. Splenectomy in advanced chronic lymphocytic leukemia. Cancer 1986; 58: 2130–5.

29. Keating MKJ, Kantarjian H, Talpzaz M et al. Fludarabine: A new agent with major activity against chronic lymphocytic leukemia. Blood 1989; 74: 19–25.

30. Keating MJ, Kantarjian H, O'Brien S et al. Fludarabine: A new agent with marked cytoreductive activity in untreated chronic lymphocytic leukemia. J Clin Oncol 1991; 9: 44–9.

31. Keating MJ, O'Brien S, Kantarjian H et al. Long-term follow-up of patients with chronic lymphocytic leukemia treated with fludarabine as a single agent. Blood 1993; 81: 2878–84.

32. Johnson SA, Hiddemann W, Coiffier B et al. A randomised comparison between fludarabine and cyclophosphamide, adriamycin and prednisolone in the treatment of chronic lymphocytic leukaemia. First Meeting of the European Haematology Association (Brussels, 1994), Br J Haematol 1994; 87 (Suppl 1): 169 (Abstr 661).

33. O'Brien S, Kantarjian H, Estey E et al. Lack of effect of 2-chlorodeoxyadenosine therapy in patients with chronic lymphocytic leukemia refractory to fludarabine therapy. N Engl J Med 1994; 330: 319–22.

34. Dyer MSJ, Hale G, Marcus R et al. Remission induction in patients with lymphoid malignancies using unconjugated CAMPATH-1 monoclonal antibodies. Leukaemia and Lymphoma 1990; 2: 179–93.

35. Rozman C, Montserrat E, Vinolas N et al. Recombinant Alpha-2-Interferon in the treatment of B chronic lymphocytic leukemia in early stages. Blood 1988; 71: 1295–8.

36. Rabinowe SN, Soiffer RJ, Gribben JG et al. Autologous and allogeneic bone marrow transplantation for poor prognosis patients with B-cell chronic lymphocytic leukemia. Blood 1993; 82: 1366–76.

37. Khouri IF, Keating MJ, Vriesendorp HM et al. Autologous and allogeneic bone marrow transplantation for chronic lymphocytic leukemia: Preliminary results. J Clin Oncol 1994; 12: 748–58.

38. Bastion Y, Felman P, Dumontet C et al. Intensive radio-chemotherapy with peripheral blood stem cell transplantation in young patients with chronic lymphocytic leukemia. A case report. Bone Marrow Transplant 1992; 10: 467–8.

39. Michallet M, Archimbaud E, Juliusson G et al. Autologous transplants in chronic lymphocytic leukemia: Report of 11 cases. First Meeting of the European Haematology Association (Brussels, 1994). Br J Haematol 1994; 87 (Suppl 1): 172 (Abstr 671).

40. Michallet M, Archimbaud E, Bandini G et al. HLA-identical sibling bone marrow transplants for chronic lymphocytic leukemia (CLL). A collaborative study of the European Bone Marrow Transplantation Group (EBMTG) and International Bone Marrow Transplantation Registry (IBMTR). Blood 1993; (Suppl 1): 345a (Abstr 1366).

R. L. Souhami (ed.) The Teaching Cases from Annals of Oncology, 63–67, 1997.

Chylothorax in lymphoma: Mechanisms and management

A. M. O'Callaghan & G. M. Mead

C.R.C. Wessex Regional Medical Oncology Unit, Southampton, U.K.

Key words: chylothorax, non-Hodgkin's lymphoma

Introduction

Chylothorax is an uncommon and poorly described complication of non-Hodgkin's lymphoma of any histological type or grade. Though patients usually have extensive lymphoma, supra-diaphragmatic disease is not always present. This serious medical complication may not be evident at time of diagnosis. It often becomes a chronic problem, and its course does not reflect the successful treatment of the underlying lymphoma.

Here we outline the presentation, management and clinical course of four patients who had chylothoraces associated with non-Hodgkin's lymphoma and review the mechanisms by which chylothorax occurs and the available management options.

Case reports

Patient 1

A 63-year-old female presented in June 1986 with an abdominal mass. She was asymptomatic and full physical examination revealed no other abnormalities. A chest X-ray was normal. She proceeded to a laparotomy at which extensive bulky nodal enlargement was found at all sites. Histological examination of a resected lymph node showed it to be infiltrated by follicular small cleaved cell non-Hodgkin's lymphoma. A trephine biopsy showed bone marrow involvement and her disease was staged as IVA.

Treatment was commenced with chlorambucil (10 mg orally × 14 days). One week following the first course of treatment she developed rapidly progressive dyspnoea and was found to have a large right pleural effusion. The effusion was tapped and one litre of chylous fluid was obtained. Since the abdominal mass had decreased in size a second cycle of chlorambucil was commenced on day 28 and prednisolone (10 mg daily) was added.

The right sided effusion reaccumulated rapidly and repeatedly requiring five pleurocenteses, over a two week period, each yielding 1.2 to 1.5 litres of milky fluid. In view of this the chemotherapy was intensified and she received CHOP with 50% of standard adriamycin dosage [1], but this had no effect on the rate of accumulation of chyle in the pleural cavity. A lymphangiogram was performed but the lymphatic vessels were poorly visualised with none seen beyond the level of the fourth lumbar vertebra.

A thoracotomy with exploration of the thoracic duct was undertaken. The mediastinum was carefully inspected and found to be normal. The pleura was opened over the lower oesophagus and a vessel was found which was considered to be the thoracic duct; this was ligated and divided. Right pleurectomy was performed and the resected material showed inflammatory change with no evidence of lymphomatous involvement.

The patient received eight further courses of chlorambucil as treatment for her intra-abdominal disease and achieved a complete remission. She has required no further treatment and remains entirely well and free of recurrence of her chylothorax and non-Hodgkin's lymphoma at eight year follow-up.

Patient 2

A 51-year-old man presented in March 1987 with a one-year history of abdominal distension and a two-week history of increasing dyspnoea. There was no peripheral lymphadenopathy. The abdomen was distended with a large central mass and ascites. A chest X-ray confirmed the presence of a large right and a small left pleural effusion. Ultrasound examination of the abdomen showed ascites and a mid-line nodal mass (measuring 7 × 10 × 13 cm). A right pleural aspiration yielded chylous fluid but no cytological diagnosis. A diagnostic laparotomy was performed at which two litres of chylous ascites was drained and a large retroperitoneal nodal mass was biopsied. The resected node was found to be infiltrated with follicular mixed (small-cleaved and large cell) non-Hodgkin's lymphoma. A trephine biopsy showed bone marrow involvement and the patient was staged as IVA.

PACEBOM chemotherapy, an adriamycin containing alternate week schedule [2], was commenced. On this treatment his dyspnoea resolved and his abdominal distension lessened. A partial response was achieved with 12 weekly cycles, with a post chemotherapy ultrasound scan showing a residual intra-abdominal mass (measuring $6 \times 7 \times 8$ cm).

He was then given chlorambucil, 10 mg daily for 14 days every four weeks and received four cycles of this treatment, which was discontinued as his ascites was noted to be reaccumulating. During the following three months three paracenteses were necessary, yielding in total 21 litres of chylous fluid. Following this an ultrasound showed no evidence of lymphoma and his ascites did not reaccumulate.

The patient remained well for a further nine months but in December 1988 he complained of dyspnoea and was found to have recurrent pleural effusions. A large right-sided chylous effusion was aspirated on two occasions. Chlorambucil and prednisolone were given again with good result, the patient symptomatically improved and the effusions did not recur. After seven courses, this treatment was discontinued and the patient has remained in stable partial remission for three years without further recurrence of ascites or pleural effusions.

Patient 3

A 55-year-old female presented in July 1993, with a three-month history of abdominal swelling and a one-month history of increasing dyspnoea on exertion. She also reported weight loss and night sweats. On examination there were enlarged lymph nodes in both supraclavicular fossae and in the left axilla. A large left pleural effusion and ascites were present. Biopsy of the axillary node showed a follicular and diffuse large cell non-Hodgkin's lymphoma. A chest X-ray confirmed the presence of the left effusion. Abdominal CT scans showed a large para-aortic nodal mass extending superiorly into the retro-crural space and extensive ascites. A bone marrow trephine biopsy was normal and her disease was staged as IIIB.

Pleural drainage yielded 2,500 ml of chylous fluid and abdominal paracentesis yielded large amounts of chylous ascites. Chemotherapy with weekly PACE-BOM regimen was commenced [2]. Despite rapid regression of her peripheral nodal disease the patient required frequent drainage of copious amounts of pleural and peritoneal chylous fluid and accordingly her general condition deteriorated and she lost 10 kilograms in weight. On the ninth week of treatment she developed increasing dyspnoea which did not respond to pleural drainage. On clinical suspicion of pulmonary embolic disease heparinisation was undertaken but unfortunately the patient died suddenly shortly thereafter.

Post-mortem confirmed the cause of death as a massive pulmonary embolism with the probable source in the pelvic veins. There was chylous fluid in both pleural sacs and in the peritoneal cavity. Enlarged mediastinal nodes were seen which had necrotic centres, but histologically there was no evidence of lymphomatous infiltration of pleura or lung. In the abdomen enlarged lymph nodes were extensively necrotic with minimal residual lymphoma apparent on histological examination.

Patient 4

A 70-year-old male presented to his general practioner in August 1993 with a seven-month history of lower back pain, weight loss and night sweats. On examination he had firm enlarged lymph node (3×3 cm) in the left supraclavicular fossa. His chest was clinically clear. There was a deep, poorly defined mass palpable in the abdomen.

A biopsy of the supraclavicular node showed a follicular and diffuse centroblastic non-Hodgkin's lymphoma. Chest X-ray and CT scan of the chest showed a large left and small right pleural effusions which were not detected clinically or on chest X-ray two weeks previously. CT sections through the mediastinum showed a confluent nodal mass commencing at the carina and extending inferiorly into the abdomen to the level of the aortic bifurcation. A bone scan showed destruction of D11 consistent with lymphomatous involvement. His disease was staged as IVB.

Treatment was commenced with CHOP chemotherapy [1], with symptomatic improvement. Ten days later he became increasingly dyspnoeic due to enlarging left effusion and in one week, five litres of chylous fluid was removed from the left chest at repeated thoracocenteses. At this point there was a definite clinical response to chemotherapy; the abdominal mass and

Table 1. Patient characteristics.

Patient	Lymphoma	Stage	Effusion	Ascites	Treatment	Outcome
1	Low grade FSC	IVA	Right	No	Chlorambucil CHOP × 1 Surgery	CR at 8 yrs
2	Low grade FM	IVA	Bilateral R > L	Yes	PACEBOM (no MTX) Chlorambucil Radiotherapy Cyclophosphamide Etoposide	Multiple relapses Alive at 6 years
3	Intermediate DLC	IIIB	Left	Yes	PACEBOM (no MTX)	Died
4	Intermediate DLC	IVB	Bilateral L > R	No	CHOP (75%) × 6 Surgery	CR at 6 months

FSC – follicular small cleaved cell; FM – follicular mixed small and large cell; DLC – diffuse large cell; R – right; L – left; MTX – methotrexate; CR – complete remission.

peripheral lymphadenopathy were no longer palpable and the second cycle of CHOP was given. However there was no effect on the rate of reaccumulation of the pleural fluid which was draining on average one litre per day. In view of this persistent problem he was referred to the department of thoracic surgery and bilateral pleuroperitoneal shunts were inserted. He tolerated the procedure well and symptomatic improvement was dramatic. A chest X-ray showed a considerable reduction in the volume of both pleural effusions.

The patient received four further cycles of CHOP chemotherapy without complication and achieved a complete response. However chest X-ray shows persistence of small amounts of pleural fluid bilaterally.

Discussion

Chylothorax, defined as the accumulation of chyle in the pleural space, is an uncommon clinical problem. Seventy percent of cases are non-traumatic in origin with malignancy being the commonest cause. Lymphoma is the most frequently implicated malignancy and is responsible for 80% of malignancy associated chylothoraces [3].

Chyle is lymph of intestinal origin and is characteristically a thick milky or creamy liquid. The opalesence and viscosity vary according to amount and type of ingested fat. Standard analytical values show protein content of 2.2 to 6 g/dL, triglycerides greater than corresponding plasma levels and cholesterol at 65 to 220 mg/dL. Lymphocytes are the predominant cell type, and range from 0.4 to 6×10^9/L [3, 4].

Chyle is transported from the bowel mucosa by the intestinal lymphatics which coalesce to form larger lymphatic trunks which drain into the cisterna chyli. This structure is found anterior to the first two lumbar vertebrae, between the aorta and right crus of diaphragm. The thoracic duct originates at the cisterna chyli and ascends through the aortic opening of the diaphragm into the posterior mediastinum and lies to the right of midline between the aorta and the azygos vein. It crosses the midline between the sixth and fourth thoracic vertebrae, behind the oesophagus and continues posterior to the aortic arch and left subclavian vein and then arches over this structure to drain into the venous system at the confluence of the left internal jugular and subclavian veins. The pulmonary and visceral pleural lymphatics, draining non-chylous lymph from the left hemithorax, form the left bronchomediastinal trunk which joins the duct as it drains into the great veins. Lymphatic drainage of the right hemithorax is via the right bronchomediastinal trunk which delivers lymph directly to the great veins [4]. (Fig. 1).

As the thoracic duct ascends through the thorax there are many lymphatico-venous communications, and lymphatico-lymphatico anastomoses between the duct and right posterior intercostal lymphatics. These communications allow collateral flow of lymph following surgical ligation of the thoracic duct and usually provide an alternative route of flow in situations of thoracic duct obstruction [4]. If these collaterals are defective, as a result of lymphomatous infiltration or external compression by enlarged lymph nodes, there are two routes by which chyle, which should otherwise drain via the thoracic duct, may reflux into the pleural cavity. Firstly, excess pressure in the thoracic duct may cause retrograde flow of chyle from the left posterior lymphatics, via the lymphatics of parietal pleura, into the pleural cavity. Alternatively, with obstruction at a higher level, chyle may reflux via the left bronchomediastinal trunk to lymphatics of pulmonary parenchyma and visceral pleura. Chylothorax occurring as a result of duct obstruction is almost exclusively left sided. If right thoracic lymphatics are also obstructed a right chylothorax may then accumulate [5].

Thoracic duct rupture is another mechanism by which chylothorax may occur. Infiltration of the duct by lymphoma causes this usually soft and pliable structure to become increasingly rigid and thus more susceptible to rupture. This may happen with minimal and often unnoticed trauma which may be as simple as hyperextention of the vertebral column or coughing, sneezing or vomiting with resultant increasing in intra thoracic pressure [3]. Following rupture of the duct, chyle leaks first into the mediastinum and then into the pleural cavity when the parietal pleura ruptures as a result of pressure caused by the mediastinal effusion [5]. If disruption of the duct is below the level of T 5–6 a right sided effusion results (as in patient 1). If above this level the effusion is left sided [3–5].

When chylous ascites is present chylothorax is a frequent accompaniment. There is some evidence to suggest that the accumulation of pleural chyle in this situa-

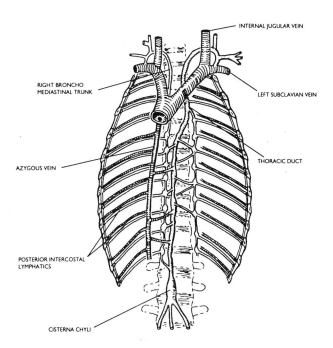

Fig. 1. The course of the thoracic duct.

tion is a result of trans-diaphragmatic movement of the chylous fluid via collateral lymphatic channels penetrating the diaphragm [6]. The initial approach to chylothorax (which is radiologically indistinguishable from pleural effusion of other aetiology) requires thoracocentesis which relieves symptoms and provides material for diagnostic purposes. Reaccumulation of chyle is almost invariable and repeated aspiration becomes necessary [7]. Continuous intercostal tube drainage allows more complete drainage of the pleural cavity but again is merely a temporary measure [3]. Attempts at pleurodesis by administration of a variety of intrapleural irritants have been ineffective, though talc pleurodesis has been reported as being successful in two cases [8, 9].

Severe nutritional depletion and immunodeficiency may result as a consequence of drainage of large amounts of chyle, which is rich in protein, fat, electrolytes, fatsoluable vitamins and lymphocytes [3]. There is much controversy as to whether there is a role for conservative management, which involves reducing thoracic duct flow in the hope that the damaged duct may heal [9, 10]. Chyle production can be reduced by dietary modification with administration of medium chain triglycerides as a source of fat, or by total bowel rest with parenteral feeding [3, 10]. This approach has little to offer in patients with lymphoma as the rupture of an abnormal/infiltrated duct is not expected to heal, and time to resolution of chylothorax may be very prolonged.

Treatment of the underlying lymphoma may reasonably be expected to improve the situation. In 1972 Lowe et al. reported two cases of chylothorax which resolved following radiotherapy to upper abdominal nodal masses [7]. However our experience is somewhat different in that all our patients were showing excellent disease regression with chemotherapy but in only one patient did the chylothorax respond to chemotherapy alone, and the time to resolution was very prolonged. In patient 1, who was being treated with an alkylating agent alone, for low grade lymphoma, the change to a more intensive combination chemotherapy regime had no therapeutic effect on the chylothorax, which was subsequently found to be caused by a ruptured thoracic duct. Patient 3, who died during her chemotherapy course, almost certainly as a complication of recurrent effusions and ascites, was found at post-mortem examination to have persistant chylous ascites and pleural fluid despite histological evidence of disease response.

Frequently surgical intervention may be required. Surgical treatment options include thoracotomy with exploration and repair or ligation of the thoracic duct, with pleurectomy as performed in patient 1 [9, 11]. This is a definitive procedure but not without potential morbidity especially in patients with widespread lymphoma who are usually receiving myelotoxic chemotherapy. Thoracoscopic techniques now offer a new method for direct approach to closure of the chylous leak allowing visualisation of the entire pleural space and ligation of a disrupted duct if visualised. This technique has not been widely employed but there are anecdotal reports documenting its successful use [11, 12].

Pleuroperitoneal shunting, as used in patient 4, has proved to an effective way to manage recurrent chylothorax [9]. This involves insertion of a device which consists of a valved pump chamber with attached fenestrated pleural and peritoneal catheters. The pump chamber is placed in a subcutaneous pocket, the pleural catheter is introduced into the pleural space by a Seldinger technique and the abdominal catheter is tunnelled subcutaneously across the costal margin and inserted into the peritoneal cavity under direct vision [9, 13]. Manual compression of the pump is required as the pleural/abdominal pressure gradient is typically negative. By manual compression of the pump chamber, at a frequency of thirty compressions per minute, for a total of 40 minutes per 24 h, 1,500 ml of fluid per day can be pumped from the pleural to the peritoneal cavity [13]. Shunt usage requires a co-operative patient with a performance status adequate to allow the required pumping [14]. The commonest complication is shunt occlusion which has been seen in 10% of usages for malignant effusion [13]. In chylothorax, there is not yet wide enough usage to ascertain occlusion rates. Replacement of a blocked shunt is easily performed.

Empirically this system works. However, the fate of the chyle pumped into the peritoneal cavity is not fully explained [9, 13]. If chylothorax occurs because the thoracic duct is incompetent, and this is the principal route of drainage of chyle into the venous system, the question arises as to whether the pump is then merely a system for circular movement of chyle [13]. As accumulation of peritoneal fluid in these patients does not occur, the abdominal lymphatics must offer an efficient alternative route of flow.

For those who have chylous ascites in addition to chylothorax, pleuroperitoneal shunting is not an option as the abdominal lymphatics are already failing to cope with the amount of chyle present in the abdominal cavity. Repeated drainage of pleural and peritoneal cavities as dictated by symptoms, along with treatment of the underlying lymphoma, are the only available management options. In a series of patients with chylous ascites, in which 10 patients had underlying lymphoma, treatment with chemotherapy for the majority gave only temporary improvement of their ascites and only two patients enjoyed long lasting benefit, being alive and ascites free at six and 14 years [15]. Of our patients, one (patient 2) required repeated paracenteses but eventually ascites resolved and has not recurred despite subsequent intra-abdominal relapses of his disease. In the other (patient 3), although disease response to chemotherapy occurred, her ascites relentlessly reaccumulated and the debility and immobility so caused undoubtedly contributed to her death from a pulmonary embolism. Irradiation can be effective but improvement tends to be partial and short-lived [15, 16].

Other interventions which have been tried with little

or no success in this clinical situation are diuretic treatment with salt restriction, dietary fat manipulation and complete bowel rest with total parenteral nutrition. The latter is a widely accepted approach for management of chylous ascites secondary to anomalies of lymphatic system which are predominantly seen in paediatric population but is not effective when malignancy is the underlying problem [15, 16]. Experiences with peritoneo-venous shunting have not been encouraging. Transient success in decreasing amount of ascites has been achieved but in the largest reported series all shunts blocked between three and six months [16]. Others report earlier blockage with shunts working effectively for only two weeks to two months post insertion [15].

In summary we report our experience in managing chylothoraces secondary to lymphoma. These tended to relentlessly reaccumulate despite excellent response of measurable lymphoma to chemotherapy. Early consideration of surgical intervention, expecially with pleuroperitoneal shunting is recommended. Management options when chylothorax is associated with chylous ascites are limited to drainage of relevant chylous collection for symptomatic benefit and appropriate treatment of the underlying disease. Chylous ascites in association with lymphoma has always proved a difficult clinical problem associated with a high mortality, and despite disease response to treatment it may persist as a significant cause of morbidity.

Acknowledgement

The authors wish to acknowledge the support of the Cancer Research Campaign.

References

1. Armitage JO, Dick FR, Corder MP et al. Predicting therapeutic outcome in patients with diffuse histiocytic lymphoma treated with cyclophosphamide, adriamycin, vincristine and prenisalone (CHOP). Cancer 1982; 50: 1695–702.
2. Sweetenham JW, Mead GM, Whitehouse JMA. Intensive weekly combination chemotherapy for patients with intermediate-grade and high-grade non-Hodgkin's lymphoma. J Clin Oncol 1991; 9: 2202–9.
3. Valentine VG, Raffin TA. The management of chylothorax. Chest 1992; 102: 586–91.
4. Seaton A, Seaton D, Leitch AG. Crofton and Douglas's Respiratory Diseases, fourth ed. Oxford, London, Edinburgh: Blackwell Scientific Publications 1989; Chapter 41: Diseases of the pleura, 1096–8.
5. Schulman A, Fataar S, Dalrymple R et al. The lymphographic anatomy of chylothorax. Br J Radiol 1978; 51: 420–7.
6. Takami A, Fujimura M, Nako S et al. A case of chylothorax resulting from malignant lymphoma – pathogenesis of chylothorax: A new concept. J Thorac 1993; 31: 112–6.
7. Lowe DK, Fletcher WS, Horowitz IJ et al. Management of chylothorax secondary to lymphoma. Surg Gynecol Obstet 1972; 135: 35–8.
8. Alder RH, Levinsky L. Persistant chylothorax. J Thorac Cardiovasc Surg 1978; 76: 859–64.
9. Milsom JW, Kron IL, Rheuban KS et al. Chylothorax: An assessment of current surgical management. J Thorac Cardiovasc Surg 1985; 89: 221–7.
10. Marts BC, Naunheim KS, Fiore AC et al. Conservative versus surgical management of chylothorax. Am J Surg 1992; 164: 532–5.
11. Ferguson MK. Thoracoscopy for empyema, bronchopleural fistula, and chylothorax. Ann Thorac Surg 1993; 56: 644–5.
12. Shirai T, Amano J, Takabe K. Thoracoscopic diagnosis and treatment of chylothorax after pneumonectomy. Ann Thorac Surg 1991; 52: 306–7.
13. Little AG, Kadowaki MH, Ferguson MK et al. Pleuro-peritoneal shunting: Alternative therapy for pleural effusions. Ann Surg 1988; 208: 443–50.
14. LoCicero J III. Thoracoscopic management of malignant pleural effusion. Ann Thorac Surg 1993; 56: 641–3.
15. Press OW, Press NO, Kaufman SD. Evaluation of management of chylous ascites. Ann Intern Med 1982; 96: 358–64.
16. Browse NL, Wilson NM, Russo F et al. Aetiology and treatment of chylous ascites. Br J Surg 1992; 79: 1145–50.

R. L. Souhami (ed.) The Teaching Cases from Annals of Oncology, 69–74, 1997.

Lymphoma of uncertain phenotype

G. B. Zulian,[1] P.-Y. Dietrich,[1] B. Conne,[2] S. Anchisi,[1] J.-C. Pache,[2] C. Rouden[2] & P. Alberto[1]
[1] Division of Oncology and [2] Institute of Pathology, Geneva University Hospital, Geneva, Switzerland

Key words: lymphoma, phenotypes, diagnosis

Case report

In February 1987, a 42-year-old caucasian man was referred to our department with symptoms of left recurrent nerve palsy and a 12-month history of lymphadenopathy involving both sides of the neck, the axillae and the anterior mediastinum. Previous neck node biopsies taken in September 1986 had shown evidence of lymphoid hyperplasia consistent with reactive lymphadenitis, and follicular and parafollicular hyperplasia was diagnosed. His past medical history included two episodes of transient transverse myelitis, in 1973 and 1980. He had suffered from nasal sinus polyposis with chronic sinusitis since infancy. Further biopsies of neck nodes were taken and showed pleomorphic malignant cells infiltrating the interfollicular areas as well as several Reed-Sternberg (RS) cells. The diagnosis of Hodgkin's disease (HD), interfollicular type, was made and confirmed by external expert review (Fig. 1a). The RS cells were CD30+ (Fig. 1b), CD15+, leukocyte common antigen (LCA)−, CD3−. In the perifollicular zone, small T lymphocytes formed rosette-like arrangements around the RS cells. The Ann Arbor clinical stage was IIA. The only blood abnormality was a monocytosis at 1.4×10^9/L ($N < 0.8 \times 10^9$). Because of the history of transverse myelitis, the patient was not considered suitable for radiotherapy and he received 3 courses of combination chemotherapy with doxorubicin, bleomycin, etoposide and prednisone, leading to partial remission, followed by 3 further courses of cyclophosphamide, vincristine, procarbazine and prednisone. A complete clinical remission was obtained in November 1987.

Ten months later, in September 1988, thrombocytopenia at 20×10^9/L was discovered in association with splenomegaly. No lymphomatous infiltration was detected in the bone marrow which showed megakaryocytic hyperplasia. A diagnosis of hypersplenism was made and a splenectomy with regional lymphadenectomy was performed. This showed interfollicular monomorphic lymphocyte infiltration of the lymph nodes and pleomorphic lymphocyte infiltration of the spleen where large numbers of epithelioid histiocytes

were found. Malignant cells present in the lymph nodes were CD3+ (Fig. 1c) and CD30−. T cell non-Hodgkin's lymphoma of the T zone (TZ) was diagnosed but no further treatment was attempted since the patient was asymptomatic and his platelet count had returned to normal immediately after surgery.

During 1989, a slight increase in the size of cervical lymph nodes (to 1–2 cm) was apparent but without any constitutional symptoms. In November 1990, erythema nodosum developed and multiple lymphadenopathy on both sides of the diaphragm as well as pulmonary infiltration were found on CT scan. Leukocytosis at 16×10^9/L and monocytosis at 5.3×10^9/L were present but there was no malignant infiltration of the bone marrow. The platelet count was 309×10^9/L. Serology for CMV, EBV, HIV 1−2 and HTLV-1 were all negative. A cervical lymph node biopsy showed a massive enlargement of the T zone filled with nucleolated lymphocytes and clusters of CD4+ and CD45 RO+ cells. Monoclonality was demonstrated by T cell receptor β chain rearrangement using Southern blotting. The patient declined further treatment.

In January 1992, massive right inguinal and left femoral lymphadenopathy appeared. Peripheral monocytosis at 5×10^9/L and a leukocytosis at 15.7×10^9/L were still present. Monocytosis was also present in the bone marrow which showed focal infiltration by CD3+ lymphocytes. Six courses of combination chemotherapy with vincristine, etoposide, mitoxantrone and prednisone resulted in a good partial remission with only 1.5 cm residual lymphadenopathies.

In March 1993 he developed abdominal pain. Lymphomatous infiltration of the gastro-intestinal mucosa was suspected, but not demonstrated despite appropriate biopsies. In the peripheral blood, however, a small band of IgG k paraproteinemia was disclosed for the first time. In April 1993, a slow clinical progression was apparent in cervical and in retroperitoneal lymph nodes. A further biopsy of neck nodes was obtained and histology confirmed TZ lymphoma but also showed persistance of follicles. Rearrangement of the T cell receptor β chain gene was again demonstrated, but germ-line configuration of the JH-Ig gene was also

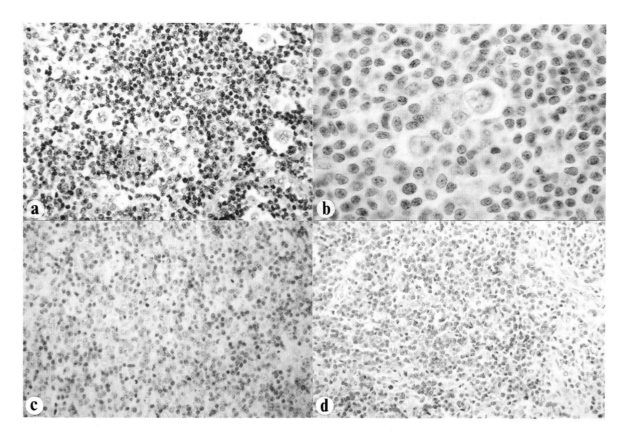

Fig. 1. Histology and immunostaining of lymph nodes removed during patient's lifetime. (a) Hodgkin's disease, interfollicular type; (b) Reed-Sternberg cells CD30+; (c) T zone lymphoma CD3+; (d) Large T cell lymphoma CD3+.

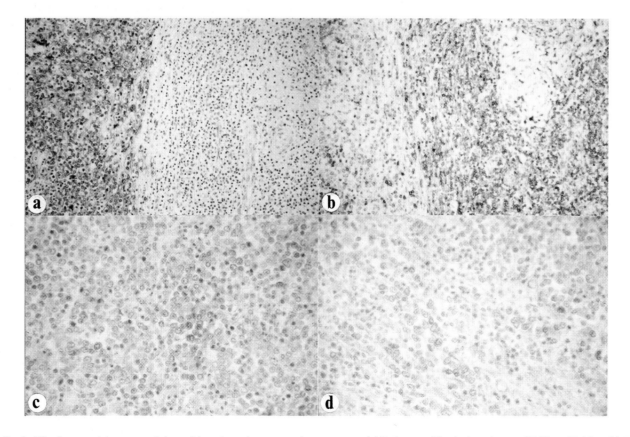

Fig. 2. Histology and immunostaining of lymph nodes removed at autopsy. (a) B immunoblastic lymphoma CD20+, CD22+; (b) T immunoblastic lymphoma CD3+; (c) Kappa light chain; (d) Lambda light chain.

shown. Bone marrow biopsy and karyotype were normal. No further treatment was offered.

In September 1993, the abdominal pain returned and diagnosis of *Helicobacter pylori* gastritis was made on endoscopy and successfully treated with a combination of bismuth, metronidazole, roxithromycine and ranitidine. In March 1994, disease progression was marked with massive lymphadenopathy and subcutaneous infiltration of the right upper anterior thoracic wall, pulmonary microdular lesions, homogeneous hepatomegaly, stomach and duodenal infiltration and bone marrow infiltration by CD3+ lymphocytes. Blood leukocytes were 25.2×10^9/L with 43% neutrophils, 1% basophils, 31% monocytes and 25% lymphocytes. Platelets were 340×10^9/L. LDH was 823 U/L, alkaline phosphatase 326 U/L (N < 370), albumin 20 g/L, β-2 microglobulin 4.6 mg/L (N < 2.5) and serum IgG k paraprotein 20.8 g/L. Axillary lymph node biopsy showed extensive and diffuse lymphomatous infiltration (Fig. 1d). Rare residual secondary follicles were still present. Several bcl-2 negative immunoblastic cells of increased size were noted. These observations were consistent with large T cell peripheral lymphoma. The patient was given 2 courses of subcutaneous cladribine (2-chloro-2′-deaoxyadenosine, 2-CDA), as part of a national study by the SAKK lymphoma group, with no response. One course of combination chemotherapy with cytarabine, etoposide, procarbazine and methylprednisolone was administered but the patient died shortly afterwards of lymphoma progression.

At autopsy, massive generalized enlargement of the lymph nodes was present as well as multiple metastases, in lungs, pleura, liver and bone marrow. Lymph node histology demonstrated diffuse lymphomatous infiltration with the co-existence of two distinct B and T immunoblastic populations. Tumour cells of B phenotype with CD20+, CD22+ cells represented most of the lymph node area (Fig. 2a) whereas T phenotype with CD3+, CD45 RO+ cells were shown in other mismatched areas (Fig. 2b). In Dubosq-Brazil fixed material, cytoplasmic κ-light chain was shown in subpopulations of B immunoblasts (Fig. 2c) while cytoplasmic λ-light chain was shown in others (Fig. 2d), thereby suggesting B cell polyclonality. T cell receptor β rearrangement was also present as well as 2 bands of IgH rearrangement, revealing 2 additional clones of B immunoblasts (Fig. 3). The final diagnosis was of T immunoblastic lymphoma developing in a TZ lymphoma with oligoclonal B immunoblastic lymphoproliferative disorder.

Discussion

Our poor understanding of the pathogenesis and natural history of some lymphomas is well illustrated by the present case. After more than a year of fluctuant lymphadenopathy, the diagnosis of interfollicular Hodg-

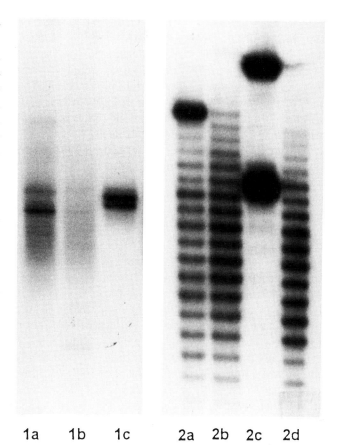

1a   1b   1c   2a 2b 2c 2d

Fig. 3. PCR analysis of lymph nodes removed at autopsy. *Panel 1.* T cell receptor β rearrangement: (1a) positive control; (1b) negative control; (1c) patient's lymph node (autopsy). *Panel 2.* IgH rearrangement: (2a) positive control; (2b) negative control; (2c) patient's lymph node (autopsy); (2d) patient's lymph node (biopsy). *Panel 1.* Determination of βTCR gene rearrangement was performed using one D oligomeric primer (Dβ1) and one J region primer (Jβ2) designed to bind the 13 J segment with varying degrees of mismatch. PCR was performed with minor modifications of the method described by Slack et al. [1]. *Panel 2.* Determination of B cell clonality was done according to Reed et al. [2] with the oligonucleotide primers shown in Table 1. PCR followed a seminested protocol using 2 sets of amplification cycles with different primers.

kin's disease (HD) was first made on the basis of both morphological Reed-Sternberg cells (RS) and immunohistochemical criteria with CD30+ and CD15+.

RS cells were described almost a century ago and, while considered pathognomonic of HD, they do not appear to be diagnostic since RS-like cells can be found in other malignant lymphomas as well as in a few benign lymphoproliferative disorders. Anaplastic large-cell lymphoma, lymphomatoid papulomatosis and mycosis fungoides are some of the lymphomas in which RS-like cells are found [3]. RS immunophenotyping may show features of more than one haemopoietic lineage with expression of B or T antigens or a monocyte-macrophage phenotype [4]. A constant expression of CD30, the Ki-1 antigen expressed on activated T and B lymphocytes, with frequent expression of CD15, a monocyte-macrophage antigen, CD25 (the IL2 receptor) and of CD40 is regarded as characteristic of the RS cell [5]. Confirmation of this multilineage expression was recently found at the gene level [6]. The relationships with the surrounding cells in the lymph node are only partially understood. Similarly, the precise role of the Epstein-Barr virus and of Herpes simplex 6 virus in pathogenesis have yet to be determined [5–8]. For the time being the nature of the RS cell, which constitutes only about 2% of the tumour tissue in HD, is still nuclear and so, therefore, is HD itself [3].

T zone (TZ) lymphoma is a term used to describe post-thymic T cell lymphoproliferative disorder which includes heterogeneous diseases with diffuse, or occasionally interfollicular, proliferation of mixed small and large atypical lymphoid cells [5]. T cell antigens are variable with CD3+/−, CD2+/−, CD5+/− and CD4>CD8. CD45RA and CD45RO may be lacking and T cell receptor genes are usually rearranged. Since RS-like cells can occassionaly be found among the neoplastic cells, the differential diagnosis between TZ lymphoma and HD can be difficult to make. In the present case, the interfollicular pattern of infiltration together with CD30+ RS cells, which was initially taken as evidence of HD, was in retrospect, most probably the presentation of TZ lymphoma. The follow-up history of this case with several relapsing episodes and final transformation into high-grade T cell lymphoma adds weight to this hypothesis. In addition, β T cell receptor rearrangement was retrospectively demonstrated on fixed material taken from the TZ lymphoma. While this further supports the diagnosis of TZ lymphoma, such rearrangement might also be found in RS cells present in HD [3].

As in other lymphoproliferative disorders of low grade malignancy, HD can transform into diffuse high-grade B cell lymphoma. However, this usually occurs with the lymphocytic predominance subtype HD (LPHD), now considered to be a B cell lymphoproliferative disorder rather than true HD. In the present case, lymphocytes were clearly of T lineage (CD3+, CD4+) and the initial morphology was not reminiscent of LPHD. HD may also be complicated by secondary B cell high grade lymphomas with an estimated risk of 6% at 15 years [11–13]. These secondary tumours may be related to treatment. Besides chemotherapy and radiotherapy, staging splenectomy increases the risk of developing secondary solid tumours and acute non-lymphoblastic leukaemias but not the risk of secondary lymphoproliferative disorders [14–15]. In the case reported here, splenectomy was done because of hypersplenism and the diagnosis of TZ lymphoma was incidental. Both the short interval between HD and TZ lymphoma and the intrinsic characteristics of the latter make unlikely any causative effects of either the treatment for HD or the splenectomy in the occurrence of TZ lymphoma.

The patient also received two courses of the adenosine analogue 2-chloro-2′-deoxyadenosine (cladribine, 2-CDA). Whereas skin infiltration and lymph node size in the upper part of the body regressed during this therapy, dramatic progression of the lymphadenopathy occurred in all other areas. Such dissociated responses have been previously described in lymphoproliferative disorders, sometimes in association with transformation to a higher grade of malignancy. Recently, beside its activity in lymphoproliferative disorders, cladribine has been identified as a potential inducer of lymphoma transformation to a higher grade of malignancy [16]. This agent could therefore have played a role in the terminal phase of the evolution of this protean lymphoproliferative disorder.

Several aspects of this complex case are illuminated by recent progress in understanding normal B cell development [17]. B and T lymphocytes recognize antigens, through their cell surface receptors, i.e. immunoglobulin (Ig) and T cell receptor (TCR), respectively. After specific recognition of the antigen, B cells bearing surface Ig differentiate either into plasma cells, secreting soluble Ig of the same specificity, or into memory B cells. In the case of a subsequent stimulation by an identical antigen, circulating B cells migrate across high endothelial venules to secondary lymphoid organs. They enter the T cell-rich para-cortical region where complex interactions between T and B cells occur. After this specific contact, B cells proliferate and then migrate into the follicle germinal center where two essential processes occur. Variable (V) region Ig genes undergo somatic mutation to optimize Ig affinity to antigens, and B cells with high-affinity receptors for antigen switch from IgM to another Ig class. T cells are crucially implicated in several steps of this B cell maturation, particularly in the interfollicular region where an effective dialogue between B and T cells occurs.

Recent data support the view that some lymphomas developed through steps similar to those by which their normal counterpart develops [5]. In addition to molecular events, the chronic stimulation of lymphocytes by a given antigen might contribute to tumor development as in the case of *H. pylori* infection [18]. In addition, primary low-grade B cell gastric lymphoma may indeed regress after eradication of *H. pylori* with antibiotics [19]. During the course of his disease, our patient presented several attacks of abdominal pain that were eventually attributed to *H. pylori* infection and that resolved after antibiotic treatment. In vitro, low-grade B cell gastric lymphomas proliferate in response to stimulating strains of *H. pylori* but exclusively in the presence of *H. pylori*-specific T cells and their products. Such data suggest that progression of B cell lymphoma might be modulated by T cells.

Other experimental data indicate that some B cell lymphomas may develop under antigenic pressure or after antigen stimulation. For example, only restricted germline V_κ genes are detected in the clonal expansion of lymphocytes in chronic lymphocytic leukaemia [20]. In addition, somatic mutation in Ig V gene hotspots occur in normal B cells in the germinal center of lymphoid follicles in order to increase antigen affinity. B cell lymphoproliferative disorders, such as multiple myeloma, macroglobulinemia or follicular lymphoma undergo antigenic selection and continue to show somatic mutations in their clinical course. In contrast, such mutations are rare in hairy cell leukaemia, pro-lymphocytic leukaemia, or mantle cell lymphoma, suggesting that these tumours are derived from more naïve cells. In the course of many follicular lymphomas, several clones may progressively emerge indicating that antigen selection is a critical event in the pathogenesis of human lymphomas [21]. Moreover, different clones may also coexist in the same tumour and can be detected by molecular analysis as shown in Fig. 3 in the case reported here [22].

The last biopsy of the present case provided evidence of the coexistence of at least two B cell clones and one T cell clone. The late development of this B cell lymphoma can be taken as an illustration of the constant and continuous dialogue between B and T cells. At the time of initial presentation, malignant cells were mainly located in the interfollicular zone where most of the intimate contact between B and T cells occurs and this led to the initial diagnosis of interfollicular HD after transition from benign follicular hyperplasia. This evolution appears to mimick what is observed during normal B cell ontogeny. TZ and finally T cell immunoblastic lymphoma subsequently developed within the same interfollicular region (Fig. 1c, d).

Conclusion

This case illustrates the gaps in our understanding of the precise origin and nature of some lymphomas based on current knowledge. Nevertheless, both the prognosis and the treatment are highly dependent upon morphological and immunohistochemical criteria. It is to be hoped that the wider use of molecular biology and other new techniques will improve the classification of tumours presenting with atypical lymphoproliferative disorders like the one reported here. More precise classification will help to clarify our ideas about treatment. The normal immune system may serve as a model for the characterization of the many steps leading to a so-called benign lymphoproliferation towards malignancy. The recently published R.E.A.L. classification of lymphoid neoplasms, which took years to be realized and which should in future prove to be a valuable tool, does not, however, take into account these subtle biological interactions [5].

Acknowledgements

The authors would like to thank Anne-Marie Kurt, M.D. and Mireille Redard for their excellent technical assistance in providing the illustrations.

References

1. Slack DN, McCarthy KP, Wiedermann, Sloane JP. Evaluation of sensitivity specifity, and reproducibility of an optimized method for detecting clonal rearrangements of immunoglobulin and T-cell receptor genes in formalin-fixed, paraffin-embedded sections. Diagn Mol Pathol 1993; 2: 223–32.
2. Reed T, Reid A, Wallberg K et al. Determination of B-cell clonality in paraffin-embedded lymph nodes using the polymerase chain reaction. Diagn Mol Pathol 1993; 2: 42–9.
3. Haluska FG, Brufsky AM, Canellos GP. The cellular biology of the Reed-Sternberg cell. Blood 1994; 84: 1005–19.
4. Agnarsson BA, Kadin ME. The immunophenotype of Reed-Sternberg cells: A study of 50 cases of Hodgkin's disease using fixed frozen tissue. Cancer 1989; 63: 2083–7.
5. Harris NL, Jaffe ES, Stein H et al. A revised European-American classification of lymphoid neoplasms: A proposal from the International Lymphoma Study Group. Blood 1994; 84: 1361–92.
6. Trümper LH, Brady G, Bagg A et al. Single-cell analysis of Hodgkin's and Reed-Sternberg cells: Molecular heterogeneity of gene expression and p53 mutations. Blood 1993; 81: 3097–115.
7. Weiss LM, Movahed LA, Warnke RA et al. Detection of Epstein-Barr viral genome in Reed-Sternberg cells of Hodgkin's disease. N Engl J Med 1989; 320: 502–6.
8. Anagnostopoulos I, Herbst H, Niedobitek G et al. Demonstration of monoclonal EBV genome in Hodgkin's disease and KI-1 positive large-cell lymphoma by combined southern blot and in situ hybridization. Blood 1989; 74: 810–6.
9. Torelli G, Marasca R, Luppi M et al. Human herpesvirus-6 in human lymphomas: Identification of specific sequences in Hodgkin's lymphomas by polymerase chain reaction. Blood 1991; 77: 2251–8.
10. Kapp U, Wolf J, Hummel M et al. Hodgkin's lymphoma-derived tissue serially transplanted into severe combined immunodeficiency mice. Blood 1993; 82: 1247–56.
11. Tucker M, Coleman CN, Cox RS et al. Risk of second cancers after treatment for Hodgkin's disease. N Engl J Med 1988; 318: 76–81.
12. Van Leeuwen FE, Somers R, Taal BG et al. Increased risk of lung cancer, non-Hodgkin's lymphoma and leukemia following Hodgkin's disease. J Clin Oncol 1989; 7: 1046–58.
13. Swerdlow AJ, Douglas AJ, Vaughan Hudson G et al. Risk of second primary cancer after Hodgkin's disease in patients in the British National Lymphoma Investigation: Relationships to host factors, histology and stage of Hodgkin's disease and splenectomy. Br J Cancer 1993; 68: 1006–11.
14. Dietrich P-Y, Henry-Amar M, Cosset J-M et al. Second primary cancers in patients continuously disease-free from Hodgkin's disease: A protective role for the spleen? Blood 1994; 84: 1209–15.
15. Kaldor JM, Day NE, Aileen-Clarke E et al. Leukemia following Hodgkin's disease. N Engl J Med 1990; 322: 7–13.
16. Emanuele S, Saven A, Kosty M et al. 2-Chlorodeoxyadenosine activity in patients with untreated low-grade lymphoma. Proc ASCO 1994; 13: 306 (Abstr 1002).
17. Clarke EA, Ledbetter JA. How B and T cells talk to each other. Nature 1994; 367: 425–8.
18. Parsonnet J, Hansen S, Rodriguez L et al. *Helicobacter pylori* infection and gastric lymphoma. N Engl J Med 1994; 330: 1267–71.
19. Wotherspoon AC, Doglioni C, Diss TC et al. Regression of primary low-grade B-cell gastric lymphoma of mucosa-associated lymphoid tissue type after eradication of *Helicobacter pylori*. Lancet 1993; 342: 575–7.
20. Kipps PJ, Fong S, Tomhave E et al. High frequency expression of conserved kappa light chain variable region gene in chronic lymphocytic leukemia. Proc Natl Acad Sci USA 1987; 84: 2916.

74

21. Zelenetz AD, Chen TT, Levi R. Clonal expansion in follicular lymphoma occurs subsequent to antigenic selection. J Exp Med 1992; 176: 1137–48.

22. Wagner SD, Martinelli V, Luzzatto L. Similar patterns of variable kappa gene usage but different degrees of somatic mutations in hairy cell leukemia, prolymphocytic leukemia, Waldenström's macroglobulinemia and myeloma. Blood 1994; 83: 3647–53.

R. L. Souhami (ed.) The Teaching Cases from Annals of Oncology, 75–80, 1997.
© 1997 Kluwer Academic Publishers. Printed in the Netherlands.

Langerhans' cell histiocytosis: A case history

J. L. Craze & J. Pritchard

Hospital For Sick Children, Great Ormond Street, London, U.K.

Key words: Langerhans' cell histiocytosis, diagnosis, prognosis, treatment

Introduction

Langerhans' cell histiocytosis (LCH) is a rare condition of uncertain aetiology characterised by the infiltration of certain organs by cells of Langerhans' cell phenotype ('LCH cells'), together with inflammatory cells. Tissue damage and fibrosis may ensue, perhaps mediated by cytokines produced by the 'LCH cells' or inflammatory cells (or both) and sometimes leading to long term sequelae after the disease has 'burnt out'. LCH may present to a variety of specialists since many different organs can be involved but the oncologist has traditionally played a major part in management because cytotoxic agents are used for many patients with the disorder. However LCH is not at the present time regarded as a true malignancy.

The disease may present at any time from infancy to old age, but the peak incidence is 1–3 years, with a male predominance (1.5:1). Prevalence is difficult to ascertain since many mild cases may not be recognised but is probably in the order of $3-4/10^6$ total population. There is a wide clinical spectrum ranging from a single bony lesion, which is usually self-limiting, to multisystem disease with organ failure and a high mortality rate. We present a patient who, like the majority, lies between these two extremes.

Case history

The patient presented in 1977, aged 3 years, with spontaneous bilateral pneumothoraces, one of which required drainage (Fig. 1a). He was treated for presumptive staphylococcal pneumonia and made a complete recovery but two months later presented with another left-sided pneumothorax (Fig. 1b). He had lost 3 kg in weight and a more careful history revealed longstanding polyuria and polydipsia.

On examination he was below the third centile for weight, and on the third centile for height. He had no rash or lymphadenopathy. Once the pneumothorax had resolved he had no residual abnormal signs in the chest. There was no hepatosplenomegaly and examination of the central nervous system was normal.

Chest X-ray showed a honeycomb appearance of both lungs with possible confluent fibrosis of the right lower lobe (Fig. 1b). The appearances were consistent with 'Histiocytosis X' (the old name for LCH), tuberous sclerosis or cystic fibrosis. Full blood count and liver function tests were normal. Bone marrow aspirate showed a normal marrow, and skeletal survey showed no lytic lesions. Results of a water deprivation test were consistent with partial diabetes insipidus which improved with DDAVP. CT scan of the brain showed no

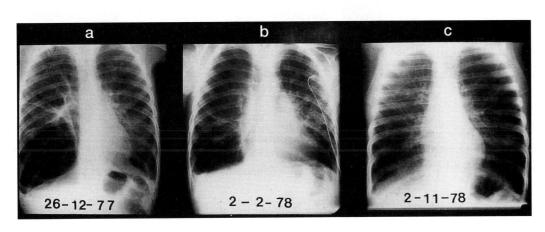

Fig. 1. (a) Chest X-ray at first presentation; (b) chest X-ray showing second left pneumothorax; (c) chest X-ray on completion of treatment, residual fibrosis.

evidence of a hypothalamic or other intracranial lesion. The diagnosis of 'Histiocytosis' was confirmed by lung biopsy.

He commenced oral prednisolone 2 mg/kg/day and weekly intravenous vinblastine beginning at 0.15 mg/kg and increasing slowly to 0.4 mg/kg. Diabetes insipidus was controlled by DDAVP 5 μg twice daily intranasally. Eleven days later he developed a right pneumothorax and talc pleurodesis was performed. Thereafter his condition stabilised, then gradually improved. Four months later he was able to run and ride a bike again. His appetite, weight gain and general well-being also improved, though his chest X-ray showed residual fibrosis (Fig. 1c). The vinblastine was discontinued after six months and the steroids gradually withdrawn over the following month.

Apart from one further small left pneumothorax in 1981 he remained generally well over the next few years with an exercise tolerance virtually identical to his peers. From the age of 9 years however, there was increasing concern about his poor growth: his height falling progressively below the third centile. Nutritional supplements failed to produce an improvement. He was teased at school about his small stature, which distressed him considerably. He perceived his exercise tolerance as diminishing and avoided sport apart from swimming, although there was little objective evidence of altered exercise tolerance.

It was felt that pituitary dysfunction was the most likely cause of his poor growth and weight gain because there was no clinical evidence of either active generalized or gastrointestinal LCH. At 12 years 3 months his hypothalamic-pituitary axis was formally assessed. His height velocity was 4.5 cm/year, (tenth centile for age) and he was prepubertal. Combined pituitary function testing (insulin tolerance test, LHRH/TRH stimulation test) gave results within normal limits and he therefore commenced oxandrelone to encourage pubertal development. Ten months later his growth velocity had increased to 10.2 cm/year (greater than 97th centile) and he was entering puberty. The oxandrelone was then stopped.

Since then he has remained in reasonable health and is considered to have 'burnt out' his disease. Since 1989 he has suffered intermittent lower back pain. Clinical examination and X-rays show a scoliosis, commencing at the eleventh thoracic vertebra with a compensating lower lumbar curve, thought to have developed as a consequence of his pulmonary fibrosis. (Figs. 2a and b) Chest X-ray now shows diffuse 'honeycombing' typical of pulmonary fibrosis (Fig. 3b) and lung function testing shows a restrictive defect with diminished Car-

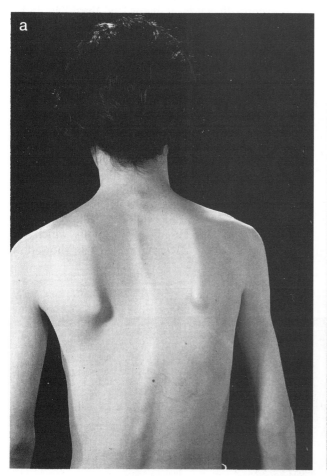 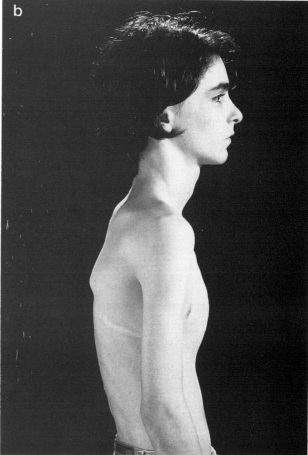

Fig. 2. (a and b) The patient aged 17 years, demonstrating scoliosis and chest deformity.

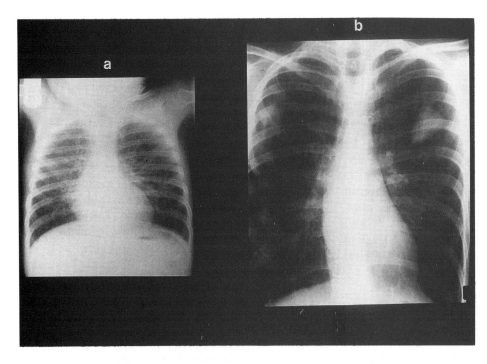

Fig. 3. (a) Chest X-ray aged 15 years; (b) chest X-ray aged 19 years, pulmonary fibrosis.

bon Monoxide transfer (TLCO) consistent with this diagnosis.

Now aged 21 years, the patient works full time but has limited exercise tolerance. He has recurrent back pain for which he receives physiotherapy, and remains on intranasal DDAVP. His adult height is 162 cm (third centile), weight 42.2 kg (third centile).

This patient therefore ran a course commonly seen in LCH of a chronic illness ultimately remitting but leaving several sequaelae, and long term suboptimal health.

Discussion

Background

In 1953, Lichtenstein proposed the unifying concept of 'Histiocytosis X' to include the syndromes previously recognised as 'eosinophilic granuloma', 'Hand Schuller Christian disease' and 'Letterer-Siwe disease' [1]. Since the recognition by Nezelof in 1973 of the central appearance of the Langerhans' cell in the lesions, the term Langerhans' cell histiocytosis (LCH) has been preferred [2].

Clinical and tissue diagnosis

Diagnosis of LCH with its variable presentation and course can be difficult, not least because it is often not suspected. Clinical suspicion arising because of a typical lesion at a typical site (see below) should lead to evaluation of other possible disease sites. Virtually any organ can be affected, including many where Langerhans' cells are not normally found. Organs most often affected are bone, skin, lymph nodes, bone marrow, liver and spleen, lungs, central nervous system and GI tract. Investigation of a patient suspected of having LCH should therefore include skeletal survey (radionucleide bone scan is less helpful than plain X-rays) full blood count and film, liver function tests and early morning urine osmolality proceeding to water deprivation test if indicated. Other tests e.g. lung function tests, bone marrow aspiration should only be added if clinically indicated [3]. The definitive diagnosis should then be established by biopsy of a suitable and accessible lesion – usually a bony lesion, skin rash or lymph node.

Histology of a typical LCH lesion shows an infiltrate of histiocytes together with varying proportions of macrophages, lymphocytes, eosinophils and giant cells with occasional neutrophils and plasma cells. The 'LCH cells' express the phenotype of normal Langerhans' cells which are dendritic antigen-presenting cells derived from bone marrow. The 'LCH cell' is thought to be less capable of antigen presentation than its normal counterpart and is presumed to be a Langerhans' cell 'frozen' in an early stage of activation. Both contain characteristic Birbeck granules which are tennis racket-shaped intracytoplasmic organelles. The cells can also be identified by a number of surface antigens of which the CD1a glycoprotein is the most specific. Immunophenotypic markers include S-100 protein, ATP-ase, αD-mannosidase, peanut agglutinin (PNA), interferon γ receptor and placental alkaline phosphatase (PLAP). The last three molecules appear on 'LCH cells' but not normal Langerhans' cells [4].

In 1987 the Histiocyte Society established 'confidence levels' for diagnosing LCH [5]. The appearance of conventional histological characteristics allows a 'presumptive diagnosis' to be made. If stains for at least two of S-100 protein, ATP-ase, αD-mannosidase or PNA are positive the term 'diagnosis' is used. The highest level of significance is attached to either the presence of Birbeck granules on electron microscopy or positivity for CD1a antigen which allows a 'definitive diagnosis' to be made. When the patient described here was diagnosed in 1977 we relied on histology alone, the other diagnostic 'tools' becoming available more recently (and unfortunately not amenable to use retrospectively on old samples).

Clinical manifestations

Approximately 25% of patients have single system disease, usally skin or bone. This hardly ever progresses to multisystem disease. The commonest presentation in young infants is of severe multisystem disease, often with fever, failure to thrive, hepatosplenomegaly and organ failure. The third and largest group is those with grumbling, fluctuating and ultimately remitting multisystem disease.

Specific organ involvement

Bony lesions most commonly arise in the skull and may present as symptomless skull deficits, painful lesions, scalp lumps due to overlying soft tissue swelling or proptosis due to a lesion in the retro-orbital region. Pathological fractures may occur through lesions in long bones. Bony lesions may rarely cause neurological complications by compression, e.g. of the optic nerve or spinal cord. The lesions are typically lytic on X-ray, sometimes with periosteal reaction. Aspiration of material from bony lesions to establish a diagnosis often precipitates resolution of the lesion.

Skin involvement is most common in babies. Brownish-red maculopapules, very similar to seborrheic eczema are seen, distributed most often on the scalp (resembling severe cradle cap), postauricular areas, midline of the trunk, axillary and groin creases and nappy area. Persistently discharging ears are a common presenting symptom and reflect involvement of skin within the ear canal or occasionally extension of bony disease into the ear canal. Super-infection is often present.

Lymph node enlargement is not as common as one might expect. Any regional nodes can be involved, particularly the cervical nodes; size varies but occasionally nodes are massive. Chronically discharging nodes can pose problems. Bone marrow involvement is also of variable severity: bone marrow failure may occur, usually in sick young infants with severe disease. 'Anaemia of chronic disease' is much commoner than marrow involvement per se.

Hepatomegaly is common and histologically periportal infiltration by LCH cells can be demonstrated. Obstructive jaundice and hepatic failure are fortunately rare. Splenomegaly, if massive, may cause pancytopenia. Again it is the young infants who are most likely to have symptomatic hepato-splenic involvement.

Shortness of breath suggests lung involvement. Radiologically a 'honeycomb appearance' is seen due to fibrosis and cyst formation: pulmonary function testing demonstrates a restrictive defect. Spontaneous pneumothorax can occur due to cyst rupture.

The usual manifestation of central nervous system involvement is diabetes insipidus (DI) which develops in 15% to 40% of LCH patients and may be present at the time of first presentation [6]. MRI scanning shows loss of the bright posterior pituitary signal and thickening of the pituitary stalk. Anterior pituitary hormone deficiencies may also occur, particularly growth hormone deficiency. Aside from pituitary involvement, CNS disease is rare, perhaps as low as 1%–4%, but can be severely disabling. It may commence many years after initial diagnosis, with cerebellar symptoms being the most common [7]. To date, 'LCH cells' have only rarely been demonstrated in the CNS. The mouth is the only part of the GI tract to be frequently involved. The mucosa may become thickened and ulcerated, and teeth may become loosened and 'float'. Premature eruption of milk teeth is characteristic of LCH, though its significance is often overlooked at the time. Involvement of the rest of the GI tract is less commonly diagnosed, but is one cause of failure to thrive in these patients. Colonic/rectal involvement manifests as diarrhoea often with blood and mucus [8].

Prognosis

Prognosis is extremely variable. Single system disease almost always resolves completely without long term sequelae hence it is important to avoid potentially toxic treatment in this group [9]. Survival in young infants with multisystem disease and organ failure is relatively poor, mortality rate in most studies being in the region of 30%–50%, irrespective of treatment and not apparently improving over the years [9–11]. In most patients with multisystem disease without organ dysfunction the active phase of disease eventually burns itself out. Around 50% of these children, however, develop long term sequelae due to residual fibrosis or gliosis and scarring in affected organs [6, 9, 10]. Long-term morbidity results and these patients require indefinite follow up.

Treatment

The variable outcome and lack of clear understanding of the pathogenesis of the disease have hampered efforts to establish better, more specific treatment. Over the years various modalities have been tried including antibiotics, steroids, radiotherapy and cytotoxic drugs. We shall outline some of the local treatments available for single lesions and then discuss systemic therapy for multisystem disease.

Treatment for single system disease

The main objective is to use a conservative treatment approach whilst awaiting spontaneous resolution of the lesion. Bony lesions often resolve after diagnostic biopsy especially if the lesion is also curetted. Asymptomatic bony lesions should be left alone: intervention is only required if the lesion is painful, disfiguring or likely to encroach on an adjacent vital structure. Injection of intralesional steroid has been found to be very effective, and can be repeated at intervals if necessary [12, 13]. In the past radiotherapy has been used for bony lesions but is now usually avoided because of the effects on bone growth in children and concern about radiation-induced neoplasia. It is still occasionally used when vital structures, e.g. the optic nerve are threatened but curettage or intralesional steroid injection are impractical.

Skin disease often responds well to topical corticosteroids. More severe disease can be treated with topical 20% mustine paint [14] (under dermatological supervision). In a few patients PUVA phototherapy has been shown to be effective [15]. Good aural toilet and topical treatment with steroid or combined antibiotic-steroid drops is usually effective for discharging ears. Curettage of the mouth if there are severe mucosal lesions can produce dramatic results, and may markedly improve oral intake and nutritional status in younger children. DI can be controlled with oral or intranasal DDAVP.

Management of patients with LCH may thus require the assistance of many different specialists. For the patient with multisystem disease one role of the oncologist, in addition to supervising systemic treatment, is to coordinate input from various colleagues to treat troublesome lesions as detailed above. For paediatric patients the oncologist is also involved in more general issues such as monitoring growth, behaviour, development and occasionally special educational needs of the more severely affected children.

Therapy for multisystem disease

Although cytotoxic agents have been used in the past, recognition that the disorder, though clonal [16, 17], is probably not neoplastic, and that multisystem disease may sometimes also regress spontaneously has led to adoption of a more conservative approach in some centres [12]. Observation alone is used for those without organ failure or severe pain or constitutional disturbance (fever, failure to thrive etc.). The presence of these features, or disease progression, is an indication for treatment. In a recent study [9] treatment, only when indicated on these criteria, was instituted with a short pulse of prednisolone (60 mg/m^2/day). Further progression was treated with either vincristine, vinblastine or etoposide (VP16). This strategy produced an overall survival (in 44 patients, 8 of whom received no treatment) of 82%; and 64% survival in those with organ dysfunction. However, 66% of survivors suffered long-term sequelae, 36% developing DI.

Other studies also show that VP16 is an effective single agent, but this is tempered by concern over its apparent ability to induce acute non-lymphoblastic leukaemia [18, 19].

A more aggresssive first line treatment approach has been advocated by other centres. A recent Italian multicentre study divided patients into two risk groups on the basis of presence or absence of organ dysfunction [11]. The good risk group received sequential vinblastine, doxorubicin and VP16 and the poor risk group combination chemotherapy with cyclophosphamide, doxorubicin and prednisolone. Again VP16 was the most effective single agent but outcome in the poor risk group remained poor – only 18% achieved remission and mortality rate was nearly 50%.

A large Austrian/German multicentre trial stratified patients into 3 risk groups and after the same inital treatment (prednisolone, vinblastine and VP16) one year of 'stratified' maintainance treatment was given [20]. Those with multiple bony lesions alone received 6-mercaptopurine, vinblastine and prednisolone; those with multisystem disease without organ dysfunction received additional vinblastine and those with organ dysfunction received additional vinblastine and VP16. Response rates were high (89%, 91% and 67%, respectively) and maintained. Median time to response was 4 months. In addition a low rate of long term sequelae was noted (20%; with only 10% having DI).

These two studies raise the possibility that achieving a more rapid response by more intensive (multidrug) therapy may lead to a decrease in long term morbidity.

The physician, whilst wishing to avoid overtreating those who may spontaneously improve, may also wish to achieve a rapid response and perhaps reduce the risk of long term problems in a patient with progressive, or very symptomatic, LCH by using one of a number of regimens that have not been directly compared. There is therefore a great need to establish which treatment is the most effective but least toxic, and for this reason the Histiocyte Society launched the international LCH-1 trial in 1991.

Newly diagnosed, previously untreated patients with multisystem disease aged less than 18 years and with a 'definitive diagnosis' on standard criteria are eligible for randomisation. All patients receive an initial pulse of high dose methylprednisolone for 3 days followed by randomisation to 24 weeks' treatment with either weekly vinblastine (6 mg/m^2/day) or 3 weekly VP16 (150 mg/m^2/dose for 3 days). Failure to respond is an indication to change to the opposite arm of the trial. Preliminary results [21] suggest that approximately 50% of patients show disease regression within 6 to 12 weeks, with those responding within 6 weeks more likely to show a sustained response. Non-responders who have switched to the other arm of the trial seem not to benefit – only 5 of 24 showing a response after the change. The trial is still continuing and it is hoped to accrue a large number of patients and delineate the optimal treatment for those with moderately severe disease. However, it seems that there is still a residuum of difficult-to-treat patients.

Possible alternative therapies

The existence of a poor risk group plus advances in the understanding of the nature of LCH – for example, the role of cytokines – provides a continuing stimulus to look for other effective agents. Cyclosporin A has been suggested as an immunomodulatory agent: it has been used in a few patients with some effect [22] and warrants further larger studies. Thymic extract and interferon α have both been tried but there is no good evidence that either is useful. The recognition of CD1a surface antigen raises the attractive possibility of using monoclonal antibody against the antigen. It has been shown that radiolabelled antibody localises to disease sites [23]; a pilot study of the use of the antibody as a therapeutic agent has just commenced.

For the poor risk group of patients with organ failure investigation of potentially more toxic treatment seems justified. Since the cells in LCH lesions – including 'LCH cells' – are bone marrow derived, bone marrow transplantation may be effective. A few patients have been treated with megachemotherapy followed by autologous or allogeneic bone marrow rescue: 4 out of 6 published cases survive [24]. In the recently opened LCH-1S trial of the Histiocyte Society the benefits of marrow ablative therapy and autograft will be compared to the effects of antithymocyte globulin and cyclosporin A in patients who have failed to show a response on LCH-1.

The future

Current treatment strategies have been based on an oncological approach since, in the 1960's and 1970's, LCH was thought to be a malignant disease. The demonstration of clonality of 'LCH cells' seems to support this view but, in fact, the aetiology and pathogenesis are still uncertain. Further basic research is needed to help elucidate the nature of LCH and hence suggest treatment approaches. The reader wishing to learn more about current research is referred to 'The Proceedings of the Nikolas Symposia on the Histiocytoses 1989–1993 (Br J Cancer 1994; Suppl XXIII).

Note added in proof
Since this article was prepared the LCH-1 trial has closed. Plans are under way for the new LCH-2 trial for the treatment of multisystem LCH.

References

1. Lichtenstein L. Histiocytosis X. Integration of esoinophilic granuloma of bone, 'Letterer-Siwe disease', and 'Schuller-Christian disease' as related manifestations of a single nosologic entity. AMA Arch Pathol 1953; 56: 84–102.
2. Nezelof C, Basset F, Rousseau MF. Histiocytosis X; histogenic argument for a Langerhans' cell origin. Biomedicine 1973; 18: 365–71.
3. Clinical Writing Group of the Histiocyte Society: Broadbent V, Gadner H, Komp DM et al. Histiocytosis syndromes in children: II. Approach to the clinical and laboratory evaluation of children with Langerhans' cell histiocytosis. Med Pediatr Oncol 1989; 17: 492–5.
4. Pritchard J, Malone M. Histiocyte disorders: 1878–1886. In
5. Peckham M, Pinedo HM, Veronesi U (eds): Oxford Textbook of Oncology. Oxford: Oxford University Press 1995.
5. Writing Group of the Histiocyte Society: Chu T, D'Angio GJ, Favara B et al. Histiocytosis syndromes in children. Lancet 1987; 1: 208–9.
6. Dunger DB, Broadbent V, Yeoman L et al. The frequency and natural history of diabetes insipidus in children with Langerhans' cell histiocytosis. N Engl J Med 1989; 321: 1157–62.
7. Grois N, Tsunematsu Y, Barkovich AJ et al. Central nervous system disease in Langerhans' cell histiocytosis. Br J Cancer 1994; 70 (Suppl XXIII): S24–8.
8. Egeler RM, Schipper ME, Heymans HSA. Gastrointestinal involvement in Langerhans' cell histiocytosis (Histiocytosis X): A clinical report of three cases. Eur J Pediatr 1990; 149: 325–9.
9. McLelland J, Broadbent V, Yeomans E et al. Langerhans' cell histiocytosis: The case for conservative treatment. Arch Dis Child 1990; 65: 301–3.
10. Komp DM, El Mahdi A, Starling KA et al. Quality of survival in Histiocytosis X: A Southwest Oncology Group Study. Med Pediatr Oncol 1980; 8: 35–40.
11. Ceci A, De Terlizzi M, Colella R et al. Langerhans' cell histiocytosis in childhood: Results from the Italian cooperative AIEOP-CNR-H.X '83 study. Med Pediatr Oncol 1993; 21: 259–64.
12. Broadbent V, Pritchard J. Histiocytosis X – current controversies. Arch Dis Child 1985; 60: 605–7.
13. Egeler RM, Thompson RC, Voute PA et al. Intralesional infiltration of corticosteroids in localized Langerhans' cell histiocytosis. J Pediatr Orthop 1993; 12: 811–4.
14. Sheehan MP, Atherton DJ, Broadbent V et al. Topical nitrogen mustard: An effective treatment for cutaneous Langerhans' cell histiocytosis. J Pediatr 1991; 119: 317–21.
15. Neumann C, Kolde G, Bonsmann G. Histiocytosis X in an elderly patient. Ultrastructure and immunochemistry after PUVA photochemotherapy. Br J Dermat 1988; 119: 385–91.
16. Willman CL, Busque L, Griffith BB et al. Langerhans' cell histiocytosis (Histiocytosis X): A clonal proliferative disease. N Engl J Med 1994; 331: 154–60.
17. Yu RC, Chu C, Buluwela L et al. Clonal proliferation of Langerhans' cells in Langerhans' cell histiocytosis. Lancet 1994; 343: 767–8.
18. Ceci A, De Terlizzi M, Collela R et al. Etoposide in recurrent Langerhans' cell histiocytosis: An Italian cooperative study. Cancer 1988; 62: 2528–31.
19. Broadbent V, Pritchard J, Yeomans E. Etoposide (VP16) in the treatment of multisystem Langerhans' cell histiocytosis (Histiocytosis X). Med Pediatr Oncol 1989; 17: 97–100.
20. Gadner H, Heitger A, Grois N et al. A treatment strategy for disseminated Langerhans' cell histiocytosis. Med Pediatr Oncol 1994; 23: 72–80.
21. Ladisch S, Gadner H. Treatment of Langerhans' cell histiocytosis – evolution and current approaches. Br J Cancer 1994; 70 (Suppl XXIII): S41–6.
22. Mahmoud HH, Wang WC, Murphy SB. Cyclosporin therapy for advanced Langerhans' cell histiocytosis. Blood 1991; 77: 721–5.
23. Kelly KM, Beverley PC, Chu AC et al. Successful in vivo localization of Langerhans' cell histiocytosis with use of a monoclonal antibody, NA1/34. J Pediatr 1994; 125: 717–22.
24. Morgan G. Myeloablative therapy and bone marrow transplantation for Langerhans' cell histiocytosis. Br J Cancer 1994; 70 (Suppl XXIII): S52–3.

R. L. Souhami (ed.) The Teaching Cases from Annals of Oncology, 81–84, 1997.

Second cancers complicating Hodgkin's disease

E. O'Reilly & J. Crown

St. Vincent's Hospital, Dublin, Ireland

Key words: Hodgkin's disease, leukaemia, second cancers

Case #1

A 58-year-old man presented with a two-month history of exertional shortness of breath, left-sided pleuritic chest pain, cough and decreased energy. He had smoked cigarettes for forty years.

Seventeen years prior to the current admission, he had been diagnosed with stage IA, lymphocyte-depleted Hodgkin's disease. He was treated with 35 Gy of mantle radiotherapy, and five cycles of MOPP (mustine, vincristine, procarbazine, and prednisolone) chemotherapy. He had been in complete remission since. Physical examination was remarkable for finger clubbing and for a left pleural effusion. Chest radiograph confirmed the effusion, and in addition showed a left hilar mass. Bronchial and mediastinal biopsies revealed the presence of an adenocarcinoma. Cytology of the pleural fluid was also positive for malignant cells.

The patient was thus diagnosed with stage IIIB non-small-cell lung cancer. A left chest drain was inserted, and the patients underwent a successful pleurodesis. He started chemotherapy with cisplatin and etoposide, but developed progressive cancer and died within three months of diagnosis.

Case #2

A 64-year-old man presented with widespread lymph node enlargement. Biopsy revealed a diagnosis of diffuse mixed small-cleaved and large-cell lymphoma.

He had been diagnosed with stage II lymphocyte-depleted Hodgkin's disease 19 years previously. He was treated, following staging laparotomy, with mantle radiotherapy, but developed a recurrence of Hodgkin's disease three years later and was then treated with MOPP chemotherapy. He had been in remission since that time.

On the current admission, the original biopsy was reviewed, and it was confirmed that these were two separate malignancies. He was treated with cyclophosphamide, doxorubicin, prednisolone and vincristine for six cycles, and obtained a complete remission which ended in relapse after one year. The patient was treated palliatively with COP chemotherapy, but died six months later.

Discussion

Hodgkin's disease is one of the few cancers in which the cure rate is so high that late complications of therapy have emerged as a major problem for long-term survivors. The introduction of effective radiotherapy regimens in the late 1950s [1] and of MOPP (mechlorethamine, vincristine, prednisolone, procarbazine) chemotherapy and its variants in the mid 1960s extended the prospect of remission and possible cure to patients with all stages of this formerly lethal disease [2]. As more patients with Hodgkin's disease achieved prolonged survival, it became apparent that a greater than expected number were developing second malignancies, which included leukaemia, non-Hodgkin's lymphoma (NHL) and solid tumours [3–6].

Acute leukaemia has been reported to occur in from 2%–10% of long-term HD survivors who were treated with chemotherapy. Early reports suggested that combined radio-chemotherapy might pose an increased risk [6, 7] but these have not been uniformly confirmed [8]. Some, but not all, studies have incriminated splenectomy as co-factor [6–9]. The actual drugs used may also be of relevance, with a particularly high risk reported for nitrosoureas, mechlorethamine, chlorambucil and procarbazine [4, 10, 11]. Somewhat surprisingly, vinblastine, but not mechlorethamine, was reported to increase the leukaemia risk in one large international study [11]. However, the ABVD (doxorubicin, bleomycin, DTIC, vinblastine) regimen has been reported to be substantially less leukaemogenic than MOPP [7], as has an alternating program of MOPP and ABVD [12].

The amount of alkylating agent exposure appears to be important, with patients who had been treated with repeated chemotherapy treatment programs for relapsed disease reportedly having a substantially higher risk (up to 40 times higher) than those who received a single regimen [13]. Prolonged schedules of maintenance chemotherapy might also increase the risk [4].

Treatment-related acute leukaemia is generally myeloid and is frequently preceded by a phase of myelodysplasia. Cytogenetic studies may reveal deletions involving chromosomes 5 and 7. The disease is more resistant to therapy than is de novo acute myeloblastic leukaemia [14].

The increased incidence of solid tumours in long-term survivors of Hodgkin's disease is also very likely to be therapy-related. Unlike leukaemia, where the risk remains elevated throughout the first 10 years following chemotherapy, and then falls off [15], the risk of solid tumours continues to rise, with no apparent plateau in incidence emerging within 10 years. Importantly, while the relative risk (RR) for solid tumours is substantially smaller than it is for leukaemia, the absolute risk is higher. Several reports have suggested that radiotherapy was primarily responsible for the increased incidence of solid tumours. Tucker et al. [16] reported that the relative risk for the development of a solid tumour in patients who survived Hodgkin's disease was 1.1 for patients who received chemotherapy only, 2.8 for patients who received single modality radiotherapy, and 4.4 for patients who received definitive radiotherapy plus adjuvant chemotherapy. Other studies have also suggested that there is an increased incidence of solid tumours in patients treated with radiotherapy, without any significant incidence in patients who received chemotherapy alone [9, 12, 17]. Doria et al. [18] reported that patients who received definitive chemotherapy with adjuvant radiotherapy for newly diagnosed HD had a modest increase in the incidence of second solid cancers, whereas an identical program administered as salvage therapy to patients whose disease had relapsed following definitive radiotherapy, resulted in a 41% incidence of these tumours. Our first case describes a patient who developed lung cancer after successful treatment of Hodgkin's disease seventeen years previously. Abrahemsen et al. [9] reported that the lung cancer risk was elevated in patients who received single modality radiotherapy, and that the risk of this and other solid tumours was increased following combined modality treatment. In this study, there was no increase in the incidence of solid tumours following single modality chemotherapy.

In recent years several studies have yielded conflicting data concerning a possible role for chemotherapy in the causation of solid tumours. The report of the British National Lymphoma Investigation confirmed the known excess incidence of solid tumours following radiotherapy, but also showed an increased risk after chemotherapy [19]. Other recent reports have also suggested that the solid tumour risk was increased by chemotherapy [20, 21].

One possible explanation for the apparent discordance between these more recent studies and the earlier reports is the duration of follow-up. Radiotherapy is an older treatment, and thus radiotherapy-treated cohorts have tended to have longer follow-up, possibly biasing the results to suggest that solid tumours are more common following this form of treatment. However, even in studies with prolonged follow-up, an increased incidence of solid tumours in patients who received chemotherapy as a single modality is not uniformly reported. Van Leeuwen recently reported the combined experience of two large cancer centers in The Netherlands, which included 1939 patients. The follow-up in this study extended for 20 years (median 9.2). These investigators found no impact of chemotherapy on the occurrence of solid tumours [12]. An analysis of the single institution data from Milan with nine-year follow-up also failed to detect an increase in solid tumours following chemotherapy, as did the data from the International Hodgkin's Disease Database. In this latter study, increased age at treatment was an independent risk factor for the development of second cancers [6, 7].

Beatty et al. [22] studied the incidence of second malignancies in survivors of paediatric Hodgkin's disease. They found that the overall cancer incidence was increased in these patients. This was most evident in those who were older at the time of treatment, in females and in patients treated for relapsed disease. However, the higher overall cancer incidence was not associated with a particular treatment.

As our second case illustrates, the incidence of non-Hodgkin's lymphoma is also increased in survivors of Hodgkin's disease. The disease occurs in patients who were treated with chemotherapy, radiotherapy and combined modality treatment. While some studies suggest that the incidence may be higher with one or other of these treatment approaches, it is possible that disease-related rather than treatment-related variables may be the main causative factors [6, 12].

The occurrence of these second malignancies has two main implications for oncologists. Firstly, physicians should be aware that long-term survivors of Hodgkin's disease are at an increased risk for the development of new cancers, and require life-long monitoring. Some authorities for example recommend that women who have undergone mantle radiotherapy during their teenage years and twenties (a group who appear to have a particularly high risk of developing breast cancer) should have regular screening mammography performed [12]. Particular attention should also be paid to smoking cessation.

These findings could also influence the choice of therapy for patients with early Hodgkin's disease. If, in theory, both of the main modalities of treatment produced equivalent anti-tumour results in this setting, then the occurrence of late complications, especially cancers, might be an important factor in determining which one to use. The increasing suspicion that second solid tumours might be increased in chemotherapy-treated patients tends to undermine one argument which has been advanced in favour of the substitution of chemotherapy for radiotherapy. It must, however, be remembered that the literature concerning chemotherapy-induced cancers and leukaemias, is derived virtually entirely from reports of MOPP-like regimens, and that most of the published evidence suggests that the ABVD combination is substantially less leukaemogenic than MOPP and its variants. It may also be less carcinogenic [7]. Definitive confirmation of this latter impression would be important, since ABVD was shown to be superior to MOPP in a prospective randomized trial, and is increasingly prescribed [23]. The same caution regarding duration of follow-up will have to be exercised in the analysis of the data from these studies. Attempts have also been made to develop other non-alkylating agent-containing regimens [24, 25]; however, the epipodophyllotoxins [10, 26] and the anthracyclines [27] may also be leukaemogenic. Finally, the increasing use of high-dose regimens with autologous marrow or peripheral blood progenitor cell autografts in the therapy of patients with poor risk disease may introduce another substantial risk factor for the development of secondary leukaemia [28].

In summary, the risk of developing a second cancer is increased substantially in long-term survivors of Hodgkin's disease. The incidence of acute leukaemia is considerably increased in those who were treated with chemotherapy. The risk of developing a solid tumour is increased following radiotherapy, and is also, probably higher in patients who have received chemotherapy. Improvements in therapy, primarily the widespread substitution of ABVD for MOPP-like regimens will probably reduce the incidence of leukaemia post-chemotherapy, and speculatively, may also influence the frequency of solid tumours as well, although the latter will require confirmation.

Table 1. Risk factors for acute leukaemia in long-term survivors of Hodgkin's disease.

Alkylating agent chemotherapy, especially mechlorethamide
Prolonged chlorambucil maintenance
Multiple chemotherapy regimens
Older age at treatment
? Splenectomy
? Combined modality
? Salvage chemotherapy following radiotherapy
? Vinblastine

Table 2. Risk factors for solid tumours in long-term survivors of Hodgkin's disease.

Radiotherapy
Chemotherapy
Older age at treatment

References

1. Kaplan HS. Long-term results of palliative and radical radiotherapy of Hodgkin's disease. Cancer Res 1966; 26: 1250–2.
2. DeVita VT, Serpick A. Combination chemotherapy in the treatment of advanced Hodgkin's disease. Ann Intern Med 1970; 73: 891–5.
3. Coltman CA, Dixon DO. Second malignancies complicating Hodgkin's disease: A Southwest Oncology Group 10-year follow-up. Cancer Treat Rep 1982; 66: 1023–33.
4. Glicksman AS, Pajak TF, Gottlieb A et al. Second malignant neoplasms in patients successfully treated for Hodgkin's disease: A Cancer and Leukaemia Group B study. Cancer Treat Rep 1982; 66: 1035–44.
5. Cunningham J, Mauch P, Rosenthal DS, Canellos GP. Long-term complications of MOPP chemotherapy in patients with Hodgkin's disease. Cancer Treat Rep 1982; 66: 1015–22.
6. Henry-Amar M. Second cancer after treatment for Hodgkin's disease: A report from the International Database on Hodgkin's Disease. Ann Oncol 1992; 3 (Suppl 4): S117–S28.
7. Valagussa P, Santoro A, Fossati-Bellani F et al. Second acute leukemia and other malignancies following treatment for Hodgkin's disease. J Clin Oncol 1986; 4: 830–7.
8. Kaldor JM, Day NE, Clarke A et al. Leukaemia following Hodgkin's disease. N Engl J Med 1990; 322: 7–13.
9. Abrahemsen JF, Andersen A, Hannisdal E et al. Second malignancies after treatment of Hodgkin's disease: The influence of treatment, follow-up time and age. J Clin Oncol 1993; 11: 255–61.
10. Van Leeuwen F, Chorus AMJ, van den Belt-Dusebout AW et al. Leukaemia risk following Hodgkin's disease: Relation to cumulative dose of alkylating agents, treatment with teniposide combinations, number of episodes of chemotherapy and bone marrow damage. J Clin Oncol 1994; 12: 1063–73.
11. Boivin JF, Hutcison GB, Zauber AG et al. Incidence of second cancers in patients treated with Hodgkin's disease. J Natl Cancer Inst 1995; 87: 732–41.
12. Van Leeuwen F, Klokman WJ, Hagenbeek A et al. Second cancer risk following Hodgkin's disease: A 20 year follow-up study. J Clin Oncol 1994; 12: 312–25.
13. Devereux S, Selassie TG, Vaughan Hudson G et al. Leukaemia complicating treatment for Hodgkin's disease: The experience of the British National Lymphoma Investigation. BMJ 1990; 301: 1077–80.
14. Coltman CA, Dahlberg S. Treatment-related leukaemia. N Engl J Med 1990; 322: 52.
15. Blayney DW, Longo DL, Young RC et al. Decreasing risk of leukaemia with prolonged follow-up after chemotherapy and radiotherapy for Hodgkin's disease. N Engl J Med 1987; 316: 710–4.
16. Tucker MA, Coleman CN, Cox RS et al. Risk of second cancers after treatment for Hodgkin's disease. N Engl J Med 1988; 318: 76–81.
17. Boivin JF, O'Brien K. Solid cancer risk after treatment of Hodgkin's disease. Cancer 1988; 61: 2541–6.
18. Doria R, Holford T, Farber LR et al. Second solid malignancies after combined modality therapy for Hodgkin's disease. J Clin Oncol 1995; 13: 2016–21.
19. Swerdlow AJ, Douglas AJ, Vaughan Hudson G et al. Risk of second primary cancers after Hodgkin's disease by type of treatment: Analysis of 2846 patients in the British National Lymphoma Investigation. BMJ 1992; 304: 1137–43.
20. Boivin JF, Hutchison GB, Zauber AG et al. Incidence of second cancers in patients treated with Hodgkin's disease. J Natl Cancer Inst 1995; 87: 732–41.
21. Cimino G, Papa G, Tura S et al. Second primary cancer following Hodgkin's disease: Updated results of an Italian multicentric study. J Clin Oncol 1991; 9: 432–7.
22. Beatty O, Hudson M, Greenwald C et al. Subsequent malignancies in children and adolescents after treatment for Hodgkin's disease. J Clin Oncol 1995; 13: 603–9.
23. Canellos GP, Anderson JR, Propert KJ et al. Chemotherapy of Hodgkin's disease with MOPP, ABVD or MOPP alternating with ABVD. N Engl J Med 1992; 327: 1478–84.
24. Crown JP, Gulati S, Straus D et al. Mitosantrone, etoposide,

84

mitoguazone and vinblastine chemotherapy in relapsed and refractory lymphomas. Invest New Drugs 1991; 9: 185–6.

25. Canellos GP, Petroni GR, Barcos M et al. Etoposide, vinblastine and doxorubicin: An active regimen for the treatment of Hodgkin's disease in relapse following MOPP. J Clin Oncol 1995; 13: 2005–11.

26. Ratain MJ, Kaminer LS, Bitran JD et al. Acute non-lymphocytic leukaemia following etoposide and cisplatin combination chemotherapy for advanced non-small cell carcinoma of the lung. Blood 1987; 70: 1412–7.

27. Levine M, Bramwell V, Bowman D et al. A clinical trial of intensive CEF versus CMF in premenopausal patients with node-positive breast cancer. Proc Am Soc Clin Oncol 1995; 14: 103.

28. Darrington DL, Vose JM, Anderson JR. Incidence and characterization of secondary myelodysplastic syndrome and acute myelogenous leukaemia following high-dose chemoradiotherapy and autologous stem cell transplantation for lymphoid malignancies. J Clin Oncol 1994; 12: 2527–34.

R. L. Souhami (ed.) The Teaching Cases from Annals of Oncology, 85–89, 1997.
© 1997 Kluwer Academic Publishers. Printed in the Netherlands.

The management of ovarian cancer

A. M. Prové, L. Y. Dirix, D. Schrijvers & A. T. Van Oosterom
Department of Medical Oncology, University Hospital of Antwerp, Belgium

Key words: ovarian cancer, role of CA-125 in ovarian cancer, staging for ovarian cancer

Case history

A 52-year-old, postmenopausal woman presented to her gynecologist in October 1986 with fatigue, abdominal distention and intermittent vaginal bleeding. Pelvic examination revealed a right adnexal mass. She had no relevant medical history. After a minimal staging, including routine blood tests and a chest x-ray, she underwent an exploratory laparotomy. A right-sided ovarian tumour was found with no macroscopic evidence of disease spread beyond the ovary. Both of her ovaries and her appendix were removed. Histopathological examination led to diagnosis of a cystadenocarcinoma of the right ovary. Microscopy revealed that the tumour had invaded the peritoneal layer lining the posterior side of the uterus. Malignant cells were present in the posterior section planes. Therefore, a second laparotomy was performed and a radical hysterectomy, omentectomy and extensive tissue sampling were done. Definitive pathological staging showed carcinomatous infiltration of the dorsal peritoneal lining of the uterus and negative peritoneal washings. Thus this patient was staged as having an ovarian carcinoma FIGO stage II b (Table 1).

Subsequently she started combination chemotherapy. She received six cycles of CP-1 chemotherapy (cyclophosphamide 800 mg/m^2 and cisplatin 50 mg/m^2, q3 weeks), between December 1986 and April 1987. A postoperative abdominal CT scan and tumour marker analysis, CA-125 (13.5 U/ml, normal value <35 U/ml) were normal after her second surgery and remained so throughout the treatment period.

The regular follow-up examinations were uneventful until March 1989 when the CA-125 rose from normal to 728 U/ml over a three-month period with no major physical complaint. She was then seen at our hospital for the first time. She complained of vague pains in the right iliac fossa which had increased in intensity over the previous few months. Physical examination revealed a 4- to 5-cm tender mass situated in the right iliac fossa. On pelvic examination numerous nodules were felt at the top of the vaginal stump with a bloody discharge. Rectal examination was normal.

The sedimentation was 30 mm/hour, blood counts were normal, serum LDH was 350 U/L (normal <250). Chest x-ray was normal. A CT-scan of the pelvis confirmed the local recurrence at the vaginal stump and the mass in the right lower abdomen (Fig. 1). She was restarted on chemotherapy. The regimen consisted of carboplatin 350 mg/m^2 i.v. on day 1 and cyclophosphamide 100 mg/m^2 orally on day 2 through 6, to be repeated every 3 weeks.

Table 1. FIGO staging for ovarian cancer.

I	Tumour limited to the ovaries.
IA	Tumour limited to one ovary, capsule intact, no tumour on ovarian surface, no malignant cells in ascites or peritoneal washings.
IB	Tumour limited to both ovaries, capsule intact, no tumour on ovarian surface, no malignant cells in ascites or peritoneal washings.
IC	Tumour limited to one or both ovaries with any of the following: capsule ruptured, tumour on ovarian surface, malignant cells in ascites or peritoneal washings.
II	Tumour involves one or both ovaries with pelvic extension.
IIA	Extension and/or implants on the uterus and/or tube(s), no malignant cells in ascites or peritoneal washings.
IIB	Extension to other pelvic structures, no malignant cells in ascites or peritoneal washings.
IIC	Pelvic extension with malignant cells in ascites or peritoneal washings.
III	Tumour involving one or both ovaries with microscopically confirmed peritoneal metastasis outside the pelvis and/or regional lymph node metastasis.
IIIA	Microscopic peritoneal metastasis beyond the pelvis.
IIIB	Macroscopic peritoneal metastasis beyong the pelvis, 2 cm or less in the greatest dimension.
IIIC	Peritoneal metastasis beyond the pelvis more than 2 cm in the greatest dimension and/or regional lymph node metastasis.
IV	Distant metastasis (excludes peritoneal metastasis).

Note: Pleural effusion must have positive cytology for stage IV.
Liver capsule and peritoneal metastases are stage III.
Liver parenchymal metastasis is stage IV.

Standard chemotherapy regimens are:
CP-1: 650-1000 mg/m^2 cyclophosphamide
75–100 mg/m^2 cisplatin, q 3 weeks
CC: 600 mg/m^2 cyclophosphamide
350–450 mg/m^2 carboplatin (if normal kidney function), q 3 weeks

Calvert-formula: carboplatinum dose mg = AUC × (GFR + 25) [21].
Target-AUC (area under the curve) = 7 for untreated patients
GFR (glomerular filtration rate) (ml/mm) = (140-age) × weight in kg/72 × (serum creatinine conc) − 15% for women.

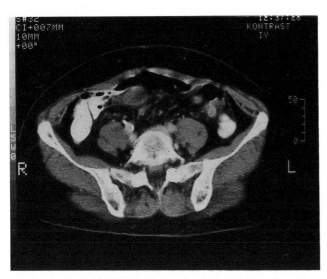

Fig. 1. Right lower abdominal mass.

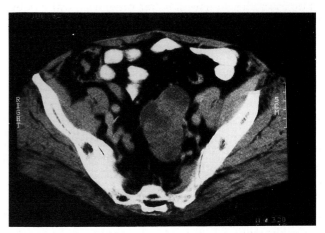

Fig. 2. Cystic mass in the central and left lower abdomen and pelvis.

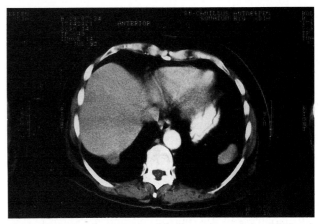

Fig. 3. Metastases between the right liver edge and the right hemi-diaphragm.

After two courses no clinical abnormalities remained and the CA-125 dropped from 2250 U/ml at the start of therapy to 19 U/ml, which is a normal value. A CT scan performed after 2 cycles was considered normal. Six cycles of this chemotherapy were given from April 1989 until August 1989. Tumour marker as well as CT scan remained normal. In August she underwent a 'second look' laparotomy. No metastatic lesions were found, and biopsies were taken at different sites. Her clinical complete response was confirmed on pathology.

She remained in remission without symptoms until June 1992. At that time her CA-125 had again risen to 100 U/l. Blood counts and biochemical values were normal. Clinical examination showed a left lower abdominal tenderness. Pelvic examination was normal. Chest x-ray was normal. CT scan revealed a cystic mass in the middle and left lower abdomen (Fig. 2) and a metastatic implant between the right liver and the diaphragm (Fig. 3).

Chemotherapy was restarted with an essentially identical regimen using carboplatin 400 mg/m^2 and cyclophosphamide 600 mg/m^2 both intravenously at day 1, every 3 to 4 weeks. After two courses CA-125 returned to normal and CT scan showed a clear partial response with diminution of the pelvic mass and disappearance of the metastatic implant. In October 1992, a re-laparotomy was performed after four cycles of chemotherapy. A solitary mesenterial metastatic lesion was discovered and a partial sigmoidal resection was performed, with reanastomosis protected by a temporary transverse colostomy. Multiple biopsies were taken. Pathological examination confirmed the presence of carcinoma in the excised nodule, but all other biopsies were negative. Two more courses of the same chemotherapy were given afterwards. In December 1992 the transverse colostomy was closed.

At present, In August 1993, nearly 7 years after initial diagnosis, after 4 surgical procedures and 3 periods of intensive chemotherapy, this patient is in perfect physical condition with no evidence of disease.

Discussion

1. Prognosis

Overall survival in patients with ovarian carcinoma changed dramatically with the introduction of cisplatin-based chemotherapy, especially for patients who present with more advanced stages of the disease. Patients with FIGO stage I or stage II (Table 1) disease have a five-year survival ranging from 50% to 85% and from 37% to 79%, respectively [1]. These differences may partially be due to variable staging criteria. In the more advanced stages the overall survival with the best treatment in the pre-cisplatin era (e.g., Hexa-CAF) was 18% at 5 years, and 9% at 10 [2]. Treatment with cisplatin-based chemotherapy (CHAP-5 or CP) appears to improve survival by more than 10%: 30% after 5 years and 21% after 10 [2, 3]. Only a minority of patients with stage IV disease will survive longer than 5 years, and this survival does not seem to be improved by the cisplatin-based regimens [3]. Well-differentiated (grade

1) tumours clearly have a better prognosis, with about 50% of stage IV patients alive at 5 years and 30% at 10. For other grades the survival rates are halved [4].

2. Surgical management in ovarian carcinoma

Surgery is still essential in the management of patients with ovarian cancer. The task of the surgeon can be diagnostic, therapeutic and/or palliative. In the early stage of the disease appropriate surgery is a critical element in the determination of prognosis and the choice of further treatment. The FIGO staging system (Table 1), currently the most widely accepted one, is based upon the results of exploratory laparotomy.

Appropriate surgical staging consists of a midline vertical incision, meticulous exploration of the entire peritoneal cavity, biopsies of the retroperitoneal lymph nodes, omentum and diaphragm, and the obtaining of peritoneal cytologic washings.

Surgery should include complete hysterectomy and removal of both the ovaries and fallopian tubes. The risk of occult tumour in the opposite ovary, as well as of developing a subsequent cancer, is substantial, and outweighs the concern of preserving hormonal function in younger women. Optimal staging allows patients to be separated into different risk and treatment categories. Many patients present with advanced rather than early-stage disease, as in the case described here.

The concept of cytoreduction or 'debulking' of ovarian cancer has been controversial. Substantial experimental and clinical evidence has emerged which show that patients with minimal residual disease live longer than those with greater residual disease. The removal of large tumour masses may enhance the response to subsequent chemotherapy. It has been demonstrated that patients whose tumours were reduced to 'optimal-disease' were more likely to achieve a clinical as well as a pathological complete response [2].

The optimal margin for providing a significant survival benefit proved to be at a cut-off point of 1 cm. The 3-year survival rate for patients with residual tumor less than 1 cm was 70% in contrast to 35% in patients with tumor residue larger than 2 cm. These differences persist even with longer follow-up [2].

Thus, at the initial laparotomy every effort should be made to reduce the tumor masses to less than 1 cm. In general, optimal primary cytoreduction will be possible in about one-third of patients, although reports range from as low as 17% to as high as 87% [2–4].

Recently the EORTC Gynecological Cancer Cooperative Group studied the effect of intervention debulking surgery on advanced ovarian cancer. After sub-optimal initial debulking all patients received 3 cycles of CP chemotherapy and those who did not have progressive disease were randomly assigned to undergo, or not to undergo, intervention debulking surgery. In this study intervention debulking surgery proved to be a safe procedure which improved progression-free and overall survivals [5].

Our patient underwent a second laparotomy immediately to complete surgical staging and clearance of residual tumour. This optimal surgery is still indicated in all stages, but even more so in the case at hand because of the relatively early stage of disease. Patients with FIGO I and II and those with well-differentiated histology, are potentially cured after optimal surgery.

A second-look operation is a laparotomy performed on a patient with no evidence of disease after completion of chemotherapy in order to determine the response to therapy. It is much like the initial staging operation performed in early-stage ovarian cancer, and includes multiple washings for cytology, a thorough exploration of the abdominal cavity, removal of any remaining internal reproductive organs, biopsy of any suspicious area, and biopsy of retroperitoneal lymph nodes. Grouping all stages together, approximately half of the patients will have tumour identified at the time of second-look surgery. The amount of tumour at the time of second-look laparotomy is a strong predictor of prognosis. Most patients with large unresectable tumour masses will die within 3 years. When only microscopic tumour can be found, which can be expected in some 20% of second-look operations, prognosis is far better, with a reported 5-year survival rate of 71% [6].

Performance of a second-look laparotomy does not per se influence patient survival. In patients with no evidence of disease and in patients with few remaining intraperitoneal tumour localisations after chemotherapy, as in this case, second-look laparotomy may become important when active second-line chemotherapy is available. This could be intraperitoneal or systemic chemotherapy (e.g., taxol, taxotere). The possible influence on patient survival in this situation remains to be established. Our patient shows the unusual pattern of relapse of ovarian carcinoma with recurrence seemingly limited to two sites, one at the site of the vaginal suture and the other a large mass. She underwent surgery on 2 separate occasions, after each episode of disease recurrence and remission induction with chemotherapy. This is a more debatable situation in which to perform surgical intervention aimed at removing all residual disease. In our opinion this remains a useful option in instances of localized recurrence with rapid normalization of both tumour markers and regression of clinical and/or radiological abnormalities after chemotherapy.

3. Adjuvant chemotherapy in ovarian carcinoma

Our patient was treated initially for stage IIb disease after extensive surgery and without clinical, biochemical or radiological signs suggestive or residual disease. In this case chemotherapy was given in the adjuvant setting, which is quite different from the more frequently encountered condition of stage III or IV disease. What evidence, if any, is there of benefit from treatment with chemotherapy for stage I and II disease?

Few randomised trials have addressed the role of

adjuvant treatment in early-stage ovarian cancer. A study from the Gynecologic Oncology Group (GOG), showed no survival benefit in stage Ia and Ib well- or moderately-differentiated ovarian carcinoma from adjuvant treatment with melphalan (0.2 mg/kg/d for 5 days, q 4 to 6 weeks, for up to 12 cycles) versus no treatment. In a second GOG trial, patients with poorly differentiated stage I tumours and with stage II disease received adjuvant treatment with either melphalan or a single intraperitoneal dose of ^{32}P (15 mCi). Although the trial sizes were too small for definite conclusions to be drawn, the outcome for the 2 treatment groups appeared similar with regard to 5-year disease free (80%) and overall survival (81% vs. 78%) [7]. Initial surgical staging can identify those patients who can be followed without adjuvant treatment. The remaining group will benefit from adjuvant therapy.

Cisplatin is considered the most active single agent in ovarian cancer, and in combination therapy response rates reach 80%. It is possible that cisplatin-based adjuvant therapy will show greater efficacy in preventing relapses than has been shown in the old trials with less aggressive chemotherapy [8]. Our patient received six cycles of cisplatin and cyclophosphamide. The dose of cisplatin was somewhat low as will be discussed later.

4. Chemotherapy in metastatic disease

Ovarian cancer is most frequently diagnosed at an advanced stage, when resection alone is no longer curative. Chemotherapy has become the major treatment modality in this stage of disease. Active single agents in advanced ovarian cancer include cisplatin, carboplatin, and the alkylating agents melphalan, chlorambucil, cyclophosphamide and ifosfamide. Other active drugs such as adriamycin and hexamethylmelamine have been used in combination regimens.

Following cytoreductive surgery, the standard chemotherapeutic approach until recently consisted of the administration of six cycles of chemotherapy with cisplatin and cyclophosphamide. Addition of adriamycin or hexamethylmelamine (CAP, CHAP-5) to the CP regimen does not appear to improve relapse-free or overall survival [2, 3, 8–10]. Carboplatin, a second generation platinum analogue that shows far less non-haematological toxicities, especially neuro- and nephrotoxicity, is reported to be equally effective with regard to disease-free and overall survival at a dose of 400 mg/m^2 when compared with 100 mg/m^2 cisplatin [11–14]. Since the most effective dose of cisplatin remains unclear, the commonly used dose is 75 mg/m^2 in combination with alkylating agents, probably chosen as a compromise between efficacy and toxicity. A dose-response relation has been established for cisplatin in ovarian carcinoma, when 50 mg/m^2 is compared with 100 mg/m^2 in combination with cyclophosphamide 750 mg/m^2 [15]. However, toxic effects were significantly greater in the high-dose group, especially neuro-

toxicity and ototoxicity, alopecia, vomiting and anaemia [15].

Carboplatin is more myelosuppressive, which leads more often to dose reductions when used in combination with alkylating agents. Fixed-dose schedules may lead to underdosing because of interpersonal variations in renal clearance. It is therefore possible that despite its better toxicity profile, the overall long-term results with carboplatin can be inferior to those with cisplatin [12, 16, 17].

The optimal duration of chemotherapy remains to be established. However, it appears that there is no advantage to treatment with more than six cycles of intensive chemotherapy. Patients who do not achieve a pathological complete remission after six cycles of combination chemotherapy are unlikely to do so after an additional five or six cycles of the same regimen.

5. Salvage therapy for advanced ovarian carcinoma

The patient described here was retreated with a platinum-based chemotherapy at both relapses (one after 24 months, and the second other after a further 34 months), and showed complete response after completion of each treatment. Is it logical to retreat patients repeatedly with cisplatin or carboplatin? Selection of salvage therapy is primarily based upon the nature of the response to induction chemotherapy. The longer the disease-free interval following cisplatin-based chemotherapy, the greater the likelihood of a second response to a platinum drug [16]. The choice of platinum drug is based upon the toxicity of the previous platinum-based therapy.

When response to platinum-based chemotherapy is of very short duration, or when there is no response, patients are considered to be primarily platinum-resistant, and prognosis is much worse than in the present case. When used in this clinical setting the response rates of second-line treatment with either ifosfamide or hexamethylmelamine are as low as 10% to 20% [16, 18, 19]. Changing from one platinum compound to another when there is progressive disease during, or shortly after, treatment with a platinum-based chemotherapy is nearly always unsuccessful. Cross-resistance between platinum drugs is so rare in ovarian cancer that it is unexploitable clinically and of no practical value [20]. Because of these poor results of current salvage chemotherapy, there is no place for surgical debulking in advanced drug-resistant ovarian cancer.

It can, however, be considered, as in our patient, in a case with a limited number of disease sites and a second good response to chemotherapy. Hopes have been raised with respect to several new drugs. Of these the taxanes, taxol and taxotere, look most promising in early phase II studies including pretreated and cisplatin resistant patients [21, 22].

These data, when confirmed in more mature studies, suggest the possibility of more active regimens in first-line treatment and the availability of active schedules in patients with tumours refractory to a platinum-alkylator combination. Under such circumstances the role of second-look laparotomy in patients treated with a first-line combination, and achieving tumour marker normalisation, may need reconsideration. Indeed repeated cytoreduction may become an important tool in the management of advanced-stage ovarian cancer.

6. The role of CA-125 in the follow-up of ovarian cancer patients

In our patient an elevated CA-125 at routine follow-up visit predicted recurrence of the disease at both relapses, without major physical complaints. Elevated serum levels of CA-125 are present in the serum of over 80% of ovarian cancer patients [23]. However, elevated levels are also present in approximately 6% of patients with benign disease as well as in approximately 1% of apparently healthy individuals. The sensitivity of CA-125 in detecting ovarian carcinoma in its earliest stages is not known. Jacobs, in a review of literature, reported that only 50% of clinically detectable stage I ovarian cancers had elevated levels of CA-125 [24].

Van der Burg et al. [25] showed in a prospective study the value of serum CA-125, which in combination with a gynecological and general physical examination, detected progression of disease in 92% of the patients. The additional contribution of second-look surgery, chest x-ray and routine laboratory tests to the diagnosis of relapse, was minimal. There are arguments suggesting a particular prognostic value of the half-life of CA-125 following treatment. A T $\frac{1}{2}$ <20 days during induction chemotherapy corresponded to progression rate and progression-free survival. Median time to progression was 11 months for patients with T $\frac{1}{2}$ >20 days versus 43 months with a T $\frac{1}{2}$ <20 days.

References

1. Rubin SC. Surgery for ovarian cancer. Hematol/Oncol Clin North America 1992; 6: 851–65.
2. Neijt JP, ten Bokkel Huinink WW, van der Burg MEL et al. Long term survival in ovarian cancer. Mature data from the Netherlands Joint Study Group for Ovarian cancer. Eur J Cancer 1991; 27: 1367–72.
3. Neijt JP, ten Bokkel Huinink WW, van der Burg MEL et al. Randomized trial comparing two combination chemotherapy regimens (CHAP-5 vs CP) in advanced ovarian carcinoma. J Clin Oncol 1987; 8: 1157–68.
4. Redman JR, Petroni GR, Saigo PE et al. Prognostic factors in ovarian carcinoma. J Clin Oncol 1986; 4: 515–23.
5. Van der Burg MEL, Van Lent M, Kobierska N et al. Intervention debulking surgery (IDS) does improve survival in advanced epithelial ovarian cancer (EOC); An EORTC Gynecological Cancer Coöperative Group (GCCG) Study. ASCO Proceedings 1993; 12: abstract 818.
6. Copeland LJ, Gershenson DM, Wharton JT et al. Microscopic disease at second-look laparotomy in advanced ovarian cancer. Cancer 1985; 55: 472–8.
7. Young RC, Walton LA, Ellenberg SS et al. Adjuvant therapy in stage I and stage II epithelial ovarian cancer: Results of two prospective randomized trials. New Engl J Med 1990; 322: 1021–7.
8. Advanced Ovarian Cancer Trialists Group. Chemotherapy in advanced ovarian cancer: An overview of randomized clinical trials. BMJ 1991; 303: 884–93.
9. Conte PF, Bruzzone M, Chiara S et al. A randomized trial comparing cisplatin plus cyclophosphamide versus cisplatin, doxorubicin, and cyclophosphamide in advanced ovarian cancer. Gynecol Oncology 1986; 4: 965–71.
10. Omura GA, Bundy BN, Berek JS et al. Randomized trial of cyclophosphamide plus cisplatin with or without doxorubicin in ovarian carcinoma: A gynecologic oncology group study. J Clin Oncol 1989; 7: 457–65.
11. ten Bokkel Huinink WW, Dalesio O, Rodenhuis S et al. Replacement of cisplatin with carboplatin in combination chemotherapy against ovarian cancer: Long-term treatment results of a study of the Gynaecological Cancer Coöperative Group of the EORTC and experience at the Netherlands Cancer Institute. Semin Oncol 1992; 19 (Suppl 2): 99–101.
12. McGuire WP, Abeloff MD. Carboplatin substitution for cisplatin in the treatment of ovarian carcinoma – A word of caution. J Natl Cancer Inst 1989; 81: 1438–9.
13. Mangioni C, Bolis G, Pecorelli S et al. Randomized trial in advanced ovarian cancer comparing cisplatin and carboplatin. J Natl Cancer Inst 1989; 81: 1464–71.
14. Edmonson JH, McCormack GM, Wieand HS et al. Cyclophosphamide-cisplatin versus cyclophosphamide-carboplatin in stage III-IV ovarian carcinoma: A comparison of equally myelosuppressive regimens. J Natl Cancer Inst 1989; 81: 1500–4.
15. Kaye SB, Lewis CR, Paul J et al. Randomized study of two doses of cisplatin with cyclophosphamide in epithelial ovarian cancer. Lancet 1992; 340: 329–33.
16. Markman L, Rothman R, Hakes T et al. Second-line platinum therapy in patients with ovarian cancer previously treated with cisplatin. J Clin Oncol 1991; 9: 389–93.
17. Calvert AH, Newell DR, Gumbrell LA et al. Carboplatin dosage: Prospective evaluation of a simple formula based on renal function. J Clin Oncol 1989; 7: 1748–56.
18. Sutton GP, Blessing JA, Homesley HD et al. Phase II trial of ifosfamide and mesna in advanced ovarian carcinoma: A Gynecologic Oncology Group Study. J Clin Oncol 1989; 7: 1672–6.
19. Manetta A, MacNeil C, Lyter JA et al. Hexamethylmelamine as a single second line agent in ovarian cancer. Gynecol Oncol 1990; 36: 93–6.
20. Gore ME, Fryatt I, Wiltshaw T et al. Cisplatin/carboplatin cross-resistance in ovarian cancer. Br J Cancer 1989; 60: 767–9.
21. McGuire WP, Rowinsky EK, Rosenshein NB et al. Taxol: A unique antineoplastic agent with significant activity in advanced ovarian epithelial neoplasms. Ann Intern Med 1989; 111: 273–9.
22. Piccart MJ, Gore M, Ten Bokkel Huinink W et al. Taxotere (RP 56976, NSC 628503): An active new drug for the treatment of advanced ovarian cancer. ASCO Proc 1993; 12: abstr. 820.
23. Bast RC, Klug TL, St. John E et al. A radioimmunoassay using a monoclonal antibody to monitor the course of epithelial ovarian cancer. N Eng J Med 1983; 309: 883–7.
24. Jacobs I, Bast RC Jr. Clinical review: The CA 125 tumour-associated antigen: A review of the literature. Human Reproduct 1989; 4 (1): 1–12.
25. van der Burg MEL, Lammes FB, Verweij J. The role of CA 125 in the early diagnosis of progressive disease in ovarian cancer. Ann Oncol 1990; 1: 301–2.

R. L. Souhami (ed.) The Teaching Cases from Annals of Oncology, 91–94, 1997.
© 1997 *Kluwer Academic Publishers. Printed in the Netherlands.*

The endodermal sinus tumour and clear cell ovarian cancer

M. E. R. O'Brien, T. Perren, S. Tan, C. Fisher & E. Wiltshaw
The Gynaecological Oncology Unit, Royal Marsden Hospital, London, U.K.

Key words: clear cell, endodermal sinus, markers, alpha-feto protein, ovarian cancer

Introduction

Clear cell ovarian cancer was originally called 'meso-nephroid' on the basis of its morphological appearance and resemblance to renal cell carcinoma. At the time it was thought to be derived from mesonephric nests, but since then the group referred to as 'mesonephroid' has become divided into 2 distinct entities: a group of tumours of mullerian origin referred to as clear cell epithelial ovarian cancer (CCC) which occur in the >30 age group and a group of tumours of germ cell origin – endodermal sinus tumours (EST) – which occur in the <30 age group (Table 1). The prognosis in clear cell ovarian tumours is generally thought to be poor but recently this bad prognosis has been described as limited to early stage disease. Stage for stage patients with advanced disease do no worse than other patients with ovarian cancer [1]. The prognosis on the other hand in EST is good overall and in the early stages of disease most patients are cured.

Pathologically the clear cell entity is characterised by clear cells and 'hobnail' cells (where the cytoplasm collapses around the nucleus) and the sheets of cells have a distinct pattern of either solid, tubulocystic, papillary or mixed pattern. The EST have a more primitive appearance and can contain Schiller-Duval bodies. In CCC immunohistochemically the Leu-M1 antigen is positive while staining for alpha-fetoprotein (AFP) is negative and the serum AFP is not raised. EST on the other hand show the opposite with a negative Leu-M1 antigen, a positive AFP and a raised serum AFP. However none of these markers are infallible. In this report we describe 3 cases of pure clear cell ovarian cancer with raised serum AFP.

Case 1

A 51-year-old woman presented with a large mass arising from the pelvis. At laporotomy, a multilocular right ovarian cyst was found which was equivalent in size to a 36 week pregnancy. There was no evidence of tumour penetrating the capsule and no evidence of peritoneal spread. The patient did not consent to complete surgery and therefore only a right salphingo-ophorectomy was performed. The tumour was completely removed and there was no obvious residual disease, however the cyst had been punctured pre-operatively and therefore the disease was staged as stage Ic. Pre-operative tumour markers showed a normal beta human chorionic gonadotrophin (HCG) but an AFP of 374 kU/litre and CA 125 of 57.

History review at the above hospital showed an adenocarcinoma with clear cell morphology (focally papillary and tubulocystic). Both Leu M1 and AFP were positive. Further staging investigations including abdominopelvic CT scan were normal apart from the unexpected finding of a liver haemangioma confirmed by a labelled red blood cell scan with tomography. Full blood count, biochemistry and liver function tests were normal.

Table 1. Differential diagnosis – Clear Cell Carcinoma (CCC) versus Endodermal Sinus Tumour (EST).

	CCC	EST
Origin	Mullerian	Germ cell
Age	>30	<30
Path	Clear and hobnail	More primitive appearance
	Solid, tubulocystic or papillary pattern	Schiller-Duval bodies PAS+
Immuno	Leu-M1 +, AFP−	Leu-M1 −, AFP+
Serum	AFP−	AFP+

Repeat markers after surgery fell progressively (Fig. 1). One year later, a total abdominal hysterectomy and left salphingoophorectomy were carried out. Multiple biopsies and peritoneal washings were taken, none of which showed any evidence of malignancy. The patient has been subsequently followed up by serial CT scans and markers and remains in remission at reporting.

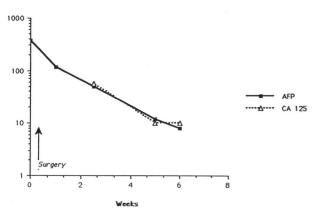

Fig. 1. Case 1 clear cell carcinoma with raised AFP and CA 125.

Case 2

A 64-year-old woman became aware of increasing abdominal girth. At laporotomy there was ascites, the pelvis was found to be full of friable tumour which completely replaced the omentum and there were parietal and visceral peritoneal secondaries of tumour under the right hemi-diaphragm but the liver appeared normal on inspection. A left salphingoophorectomy only was performed leaving residual disease > 5 cms. Histology showed a clear cell adenocarcinoma with representation of the 3 described morphological patterns in varying proportions – tubulocystic, papillary and solid areas. She was referred to the Royal Marsden where she was found to be breathless on exertion and clinically and recurrence of ascites with a palpable central abdominal mass.

She had normal liver function tests and a staging CT scan showed ascites, a large fixed mass in the pelvis, omental disease and a large solid deposit in the lower part of the paracolic gutter. There were small metastases on the inferior surface on the right diaphragm. No parenchymal liver deposits were seen but there were enlarged paracardiac lymph nodes within the chest and a splenic deposit. Review of histology confirmed a clear cell carcinoma with a solid and papillary pattern with immunohistochemistry negative for AFP and positive for Leu M1. At presentation liver function tests were normal but the serum AFP was 4359 kU/l, HCG = 7 UI/l and CA 125 = 1170 IU/l.

The patient was therefore treated as having a stage IV epithelial ovarian cancer and received high dose carboplatin. She achieved a surgical and pathological complete remission confirmed at laporotomy.

Six months later, she relapsed in the pelvis with a CT scan abnormality and rising serum CA 125 and AFP (Fig. 2A and B). She received a combination of cisplatin, bleomycin and vinblastine and had a further remission. This was of short duration and the patient died of relapsed disease on 6.10.90.

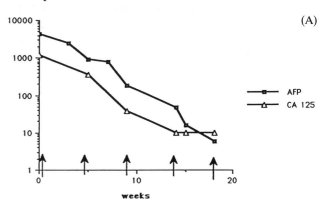

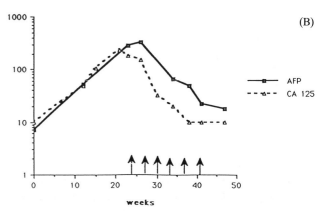

Fig. 2. (A) Case 2 clear cell carcinoma with raised AFP and CA 125 at presentation and during initial treatment – arrows indicate treatment with cisplatin. (B) Case 2 clear cell carcinoma at relapse and retreatment – arrows indicate treatment with cisplatin, vinblastine and bleomycin.

Case 3

In December 1989 a 36-year-old woman from Nigeria had a tumour removed from the right ovary. There was widespread bulky residual disease and the histology was reported as 'metastatic papillary adenocarcinoma'. She came to Britain for further management and presented with fever, ascites and a palpable abdominal mass. Her blood film confirmed malaria, she had normal liver function tests, and a CT scan of her abdomen and pelvis showed a normal liver and bulky disease extending to the right diaphragm, anterior abdominal wall and to each side of the pelvis.

The limited pathological material from Nigeria was reviewed and reported as clear cell carcinoma of the ovary but there was no tissue available for immunohistochemistry. Serum AFP was 12,941 kU/l, HCG 2 IU/l, and CA 125 52 IU/l. She had received one course of carboplatin (AUC 8) and her AFP on the 1.2.90 was 8706 kU/l. In view of her young age and the very high AFP it was thought more likely that this lady had a germ cell tumour rather than a clear cell carcinoma. Thus after a second course of carboplatin the chemotherapy was changed to a combination of carboplatin, etoposide and bleomycin frequently used for endodermal sinus tumours. Chemotherapy was given twice and she went into complete remission. The patient then developed hepatitis B and thus never had any more cytotoxic drugs. One year later there was no evidence of recurrent disease and AFP was normal (Fig. 3).

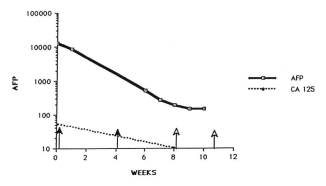

Fig. 3. Case 3 clear cell carcinoma with raised AFP and CA 125 – arrows indicate treatment with carboplatin and then cisplatin, vinblastine and bleomycin.

Discussion

There have been many studies of tumour markers carried out in patients with epithelial ovarian cancer. The best marker to date is CA 125 which is currently used in diagnosis, as a measure of bulk of residual disease and as a marker of response to treatment when raised. Carcinoembryonic antigen (CEA) is raised in 40% of patients with ovarian cancer but is not used in routine practice due to its lack of sensitivity [2]. HCG has been the most effective tumour marker for patients with trophoblastic disease [3]. It has been described in tissue culture from epithelial ovarian cancer cells [4] but has not been detected in serum of these patients.

AFP has been isolated from the tumours and plasma of patients with primary hepatocellular carcinomas, endodermal sinus tumour, embryonal carcinoma of the ovary and testicular cancers. Other tumour sites associated with raised AFP are lung, GIT, pancreas, kidney etc. Donaldson et al. have reported raised AFP in 30% of gynaecological malignancies including patients with ovarian epithelial tumours as well as invasive carcinoma of the cervix and endometrium, however these patients and their histologies are not described in detail [5]. There are case reports in the literature of raised AFP in endometrial adenocarcimoma [6], mixed mesodermal tumour of the ovary [7] and single cases of a mucinous cystadenocarcinoma [8] and a serous papillary cystadenocarcinoma [9]. However there are no reports of this association with clear cell ovarian cancer.

Other causes for raised AFP were considered in the cases described here particularily in case 3. Below 1000 kU/l there is diagnostic difficulty as these levels can be found in patients with severe viral hepatitis and active cirrhosis. However both these conditions are associated with abnormal liver function tests and the level in case 3 was over 12000 kU/l. Levels above 1000 kU/l in a patient with liver disease are highly suggestive of hepatocellular carcinoma. The patient described in case report 3 had no evidence of any liver disease on CT scanning and our diagnosis was substantiated by the response to chemotherapy since hepatocellular carcinoma is in general insensitive to chemotherapy.

There are morphological similarities between clear cell ovarian cancer and endodermal sinus tumours apart from the clinical characteristics (Table 1). Immunohistochemical markers are of value in differentiating these 2 tumours and the detection of a raised serum AFP is again helpful. These cases we described show the fallibility of these criteria: the original report of the Leu M1 marker showed 94% positivity in clear cell carcinoma and 29% with endodermal sinus tumours, while AFP staining was positive in 86% of the endodermal sinus tumours and 18% of the clear cell tumours [10]. The patient in case 1 clinically presented as an ovarian cancer of the clear cell type both morphologically and immunohistochemically with a positive Leu M1. However in addition she had a raised serum AFP and evidence of AFP production from the tumour by immunohistochemistry. In case 2, again a case of clinical and morphological clear cell cancer with positive Leu M1 immunohistochemistry but AFP was negative on immunohistology despite the high serum level. There was no other obvious cause for a raised AFP in particular there was no detectable liver metastases, however micrometastases may have been present. The immunohistochemistry was repeated with positive controls but was consistently negative on the piece of tissue sampled. It is possible that the AFP secreting cells were in pockets and were missed in sampling.

The patient described in case 3 is more complicated as this patient had some clinical features suggestive of an EST with young age, raised markers and good response to chemotherapy; however morphologically her tumour looked like a clear cell ovarian cancer. A possible explanation for this patient is that this was a clear cell ovarian cancer presenting in a young patient with a coincidental raised AFP due to liver involvement with preclinical malaria or hepatitis B. The liver function tests were initially normal and remained so and the liver had a normal appearance on imaging. In addition the excellent response to chemotherapy and continuing remission in this patient is more in keeping with an EST. From our series of clear cell carcinomas we have tested stored sera for AFP in 5 other patients who presented to this hospital recently having not received any previous treatment except surgery. One patient had stage I disease with no residual disease after surgery (CA 125 = 35) and the other 4 had disease staged II to

94

IV, all with normal serum levels of AFP (CA 125 <20, 38, 127, 230 respectively).

Of all primary ovarian cancers, 89%–92% are of the epithelial type and 8% are tumours of sex cord stromal or germ cell origin. Within the epithelial group 42% are serous cystadenocarcinomas, 12% mucinous, 15% endometrioid, 17% undifferentiated and 6% are clear cell [11]. It has been suggested that clear cell ovarian cancer represents a variant of endometrioid ovarian cancer rather than a distinct entity [12] but there are distinct morphological histochemical and ultrastructural differences between these two tumour types [13]. Clear cell ovarian cancer is associated with endometriosis in 25%–30% of cases, but this is not of prognostic significance [14]. It is thought to have a bad prognosis but in a retrospective clinicopathological study of 86 patients with clear cell ovarian cancer in our hospital, stage for stage patients with advanced disease (II-IV) did no worse than other subtypes of epithelial tumours but patients with stage I disease did significantly worse at both 5 ($p < 0.05$) and 10 years ($p < 0.02$). Young age (<60 years), advanced stage and the presence of vascular invasion were independently poor prognostic factors [1]. Therefore we recommend that stage II-IV clear cell ovarian cancer be treated in standard protocols with other subgroups of epithelial ovarian cancers. In view of the aggressive nature of stage I disease some form of adjuvant therapy should be offered and as the numbers will be too small for a meaningful randomised study, at least if patients were treated in a standard fashion we would be able to report our experience and hopefully improve outcome.

We feel it is important to recognise the subgroup of clear cell carcinoma with raised AFP for a number of reasons: first to check carefully the diagnosis and thereby confirm that the treatment is appropriate and a curable tumour is not being undertreated. Secondly, AFP is a useful marker when raised in following the response to treatment in these patients. Finally the presence of these oncofetal markers may teach us more about the origin and the biology of these tumours.

Acknowledgement

MO'B was supported by the Cancer Research Campaign.

References

1. O'Brien MER, Schoefield J, Tan S et al. Clear cell epithelial ovarian cancer (mesonephroid) – bad prognosis only in early stages. Gynecol Oncol 1993; 49: 250–4.
2. Van Nagell JR, Donaldson ES, Gay EC et al. Carcinoembryonic antigen in ovarian epithelial cystadenocarcinomas: The prognostic value of tumour and serial plasma determinations. Cancer 1978; 41: 2335–40.
3. Vaitukaitis J, Braunstein G, Ross G. A radioimmunoassay which specifically measures human chorionic gonadotrophin in the presence of human luteinizing hormone. Am J Obstet Gynecol 1972; 113: 751–8.
4. McManus L, Naughton M, Martinez HA. Human chorionic gonadotrophin in human neoplastic cells. Cancer Res 1976; 36: 3476–81.
5. Donaldson ES, Van Nagell JR, Gay EC et al. Alpha-fetoprotein as a biochemical marker in patients with gynecological malignancies. Gynecol Oncol 1979; 7(1): 18–24.
6. Majsukuma K, Tsukamoto N. Alpha-fetoprotein producing endometrial adenocarcinoma: Report of a case. Gynecol Oncol 1988; 29: 370–7.
7. Blumenfeld A, Kerner H, Thaler et al. Increased alpha-fetoprotein levels in mixed mesodermal tumor of the ovary. Gynecol Obstet Invest 1984; 17: 169–73.
8. Konishi I, Fujii S, Kataoka N et al. Ovarian mucinous cystadenocarcinoma producing alpha-fetoprotein. Int J Gynecol Path 1988; 7: 182–9.
9. Higuchi Y, Kouno T, Teshima H et al. Serous papillary cystadenocarcinoma associated with alpha-fetoprotein production. Arch Pathol Lab Med 1984; 108: 710–2.
10. Zirker TA, Silva EG, Morris M et al. Immunohistochemical differentiation of clear-cell carcinoma of the female genital tract and endodermal sinus tumor with the use of alpha-fetoprotein and Leu-M1. Am J Clin Pathol 1989; 91: 511–4.
11. Young RC, Knapp RC, Perez CA. Cancer of the ovary. In: De Vita VT (ed): Cancer. Principles and Practice of Oncology. 1st Ed. J. B. Lippincott Company: Philadelphia 1982; 884–913.
12. Shevchuk M, Winkler-Monsanto B, Fenoglio C et al. Clear cell carcinoma of the ovary: A clinicopathologic study with review of the literature. Cancer 1981; 47: 1344–51.
13. Rogers LW, Julian CG, Woodruff JD. Mesonephroid carcinoma of the ovary: A study of 95 cases from the Emil Novak Ovarian Tumor Registry. Gynecol Oncol 1972; 1: 76–89.
14. Scully RE, Barlos JF. 'Mesonephroma' of the ovary: Tumor of mullerian nature related to endometrioid carcinoma. Cancer 1967; 20: 1405–17.

R. L. Souhami (ed.) The Teaching Cases from Annals of Oncology, 95–98, 1997.

The management of granulosa cell tumor of the ovary — a case history

C. A. H. H. V. M. Verhagen,[1] Q. G. C. M. van Hoesel,[1] C. P. T. Schijf[2] & P. H. M. De Mulder[1]

[1]Department of Medical Oncology; [2]Department of Gynaecology and Obstetrics, University Hospital St. Radboud, Nijmegen, The Netherlands

Key words: corticosteroids, granulosa cell tumor, treatment

Introduction

Granulosa cell tumors comprise 3% to 10% of all malignant ovarian tumors. They are diagnosed at all ages, but usually occur after the menopause [1]. The most common presenting symptom is abnormal uterine bleeding due to hormonal activity of the tumor. Complete surgical removal is the management of choice for these tumors. The stage at the initial operation appears to be the most important prognostic factor for cancer-related survival. The management of metastatic disease or inoperable loco-regional relapse has yet to be defined for this uncommon ovarian tumor. The following case history illustrates a number of management problems in a patient with granulosa cell tumor of the ovary. Therapeutic options for the different stages of the disease will be discussed.

Case history

A 59-year-old woman presented with a history of abdominal discomfort and dysuria of six months' duration, with additional symptoms of dyspareunia and anal tenesmus. There was no history of vaginal discharge or bleeding. She was multiparous and had been post-menopausal for eight years. On examination the only abnormal finding was a mobile mass in her lower abdomen. Laboratory investigations including full blood count, plasma electrolytes, serum creatinine and liver function tests all showed normal results apart from an elevated lactate dehydrogenase of 369 U/L (normal ≤ 250) and 17-beta-estradiol of 250 pmol/L (postmenopausal woman normal ≤60). A cervical smear showed no abnormalities except for an absence of atrophy of epithelial cells. The chest X-ray picture was normal. Intravenous pyelography showed an impression on the bladder but no urethral obstruction and ultra-sound confirmed a solid mass originating in the right ovary.

An exploratory laparotomy was performed. Apart from adhesions of the enlarged right ovary to the small intestine, no abnormalities were found. After washout of the peritoneal cavity an infracolic omentectomy and total hysterectomy was performed with bilateral salpingo-oophorectomy including the adhesent part of the small intestine. Histological examination showed a granulosa-cell tumor of the right ovary confined within the capsule (FIGO stage IA) and a carcinoma in situ of the endometrium of the uterus. The patient's postoperative recovery was uneventful and her serum beta-estradiol level returned to normal postmenopausal levels.

During follow-up the patient complained of disabling flushes which were treated successfully with conjugated estrogen 1.25 mg daily.

After two years the patient again experienced abdominal pain. On examination no tumor was found but ultra-sonography revealed an abdominal mass. Determination of her estradiol levels was not helpful due to the estrogen medication. Laparotomy was performed and in addition to extensive adhesions, two peritoneal lesions of 1.0 and 4.0 cm diameter were found. Both lesions proved to be granulosa cell tumor and could be completely resected. No adjuvant therapy was given.

Six months later a routinely performed CT scan of the abdomen showed a local recurrence and liver metastases. The endogenous 17-beta-estradiol level (after cessation of the estrogen medication) was elevated to 180 pmol/L. Palliative poly-chemotherapy was started with PVB courses; cisplatin (20 mg/m^2 day 1–5), vinblastine (0.15 mg/kg days 1 and 2) and bleomycin (30 mg/24-hour infusion on day 2 and 15 mg short infusion day 15) every four weeks. After two courses there was a reduction in tumor size. After four courses early signs of bleomycin lung toxicity were detected on the chest X-ray and bleomycin was discontinued. After six courses the patient developed polyneuropathy and chemotherapy was stopped. A partial response was obtained with normalization of estradiol levels and elevation of luteinizing hormone (LH), follicle-stimulating hormone (FSH) levels to postmenopausal values.

One and a half years later, four years after the initial presentation, abdominal pains recurred due to growth of the liver metastases. Elevation of her serum estradiol levels (156 pmol/L) had preceded clinical manifestations four months earlier. Chemotherapy was re-instituted with carboplatin (day 1, 340 mg adjusted to creatinine clearance of 50 ml/min) and etoposide (120 mg/m^2 days 1–3) every three weeks. Again a partial response was seen after four courses, with normalization of estradiol to postmenopausal levels. No further tumor regression could be achieved and treatment was stopped after the sixth course. The response lasted only six months. A third attempt with polychemotherapy (carboplatin and etoposide) was less successful and stabilization of the tumor was the best response achieved with a total dose of six courses.

No further treatment was given and slow progression of the tumor advanced to end-stage disease one year later. At that time the patient was completely bed-ridden, complained of abdominal pain, loss of appetite, night-sweats and tumor-related fever. The enlarged liver extended into the pelvis and the patient became dependent on blood transfusions at 10-day intervals. Palliative therapy with dexamethasone orally 3 mg daily was started, with considerable benefit. Her subjective symptoms disappeared and the massive liver mass shrank to only a small palpable rim just below the right costal margin. The patient became transfusion-independent and was able to resume her normal daily activities. This unexpected objective response on dexamethasone lasted for one year. Fifteen months later, eight years after her initial diagnosis, the patient died of progressive disease.

Discussion points

1. Presenting symptoms, diagnosis and prognosis of granulosa-cell ovarian tumor

A minority of granulosa cell stromal tumors occur in children before their fifth year and may present with sexual pseudo-precocity. The majority of the tumors occur after the menopause (55%) or during reproductive life (40%) [2]. A higher incidence has been reported after ovarian stimulation with clomiphene citrate and/or gonadotrophins in patients with primary and secondary infertility [3]. Abnormal uterine bleeding due to hormonal activity of the tumor is a presenting symptom in more than one-half of the adult victims. The endometrium may show cystic hyperplasia (60%) and adenocarcinoma is reported in 3% to 13% of cases [4, 5]. Abdominal discomfort and distension is noted in one-third of the patients, of whom 8% may present with acute symptoms due to torsion or rupture of the ovarian tumor [4, 6]. Virilization is a rare complication of androgen production by the tumor.

Granulosa-cell tumors are diagnosed at an early stage more often than other ovarian tumors due to their hormonal activity; they account for 70% of all feminizing ovarian tumors. Precocity in young girls, estrogen-stimulated vaginal smears and cervical mucus or endometrial hyperplasia may alert the gynaecologist to the possible existence of a granulosa cell tumor. Laboratory tests may show an elevated estrogen level and low FSH and LH levels in menopausal women, but one-third of these tumors are not steroid-producing and investigations will be hampered by premenopausal status or the use of exogenous estrogens. Inhibin, a polypeptide produced by granulosa cells, is stimulated by FSH and itself inhibits the release of FSH from the pituitary gland. Elevated levels of inhibin may also act as a marker for this tumor [7], but not specifically, as other ovarian cancers may also be associated with elevated levels of inhibin [8]. Histology is therefore necessary to prove the nature of the tumor. Thecomas must be differentiated from granulosa cell tumors and mixed granulosa–theca cell tumors. Pure thecomas are benign tumors of stromal origin, and only rarely do they recur after complete surgical removal [5]. Mixed tumors and pure granulosa-cell tumors are both malignant and have the same, less favourable prognosis. The tumors may show different histological patterns, but the pattern does not correlate with survival [9].

Advanced clinical stage (FIGO II–IV), presence of tumor rupture, large tumor (>5 cm) and high number of mitotic figures are all associated with poor prognosis [4–6, 9, 10]. The majority of patients (78%–92%) present with FIGO stage I with five-year survival rates of 92%–98% and at 10 years of 86%–92%. The five-year survival of FIGO stage II is reported to be 57%–76%, and at 10 years 30%–61%. Survival in FIGO stages III and IV at 5 and 10 years is 11%–22% and 6%, respectively, but the total number of patients with advanced disease is very low in most series. The overall survival with granulosa cell tumor is more favourable than with epithelial cell cancer of the ovary. This may be at least partially due to the earlier stage at diagnosis of granulosa cell cancer, as stage for stage survivals are comparable for the two tumor types. Tumor relapses occur on an average six years after initial diagnosis, but late recurrences of more than 20 years have been reported [2].

2. Initial management according to FIGO stage of granulosa-cell tumor of the ovary

The initial treatment for granulosa-cell tumor of the ovary should be a bilateral oophorectomy with hysterectomy and removal of as much metastatic disease as possible. Incomplete surgical removal is associated with a poorer overall prognosis [5, 11, 12].

There is no general consensus concerning the advisability of a conservative unilateral oophorectomy in younger patients with limited disease and a strong wish for preservation of fertility. The available retrospective studies are inconclusive. Conservative surgery was acceptable to Malkasian [2] only for patients with

FIGO stage IA disease. In contrast, Kietlinska [11] has pointed out that although the five-year survival in stage I disease is not compromised by conservative surgery, longer follow-up revealed that it carries a much less favourable prognosis than the one following radical surgery. Conservative surgery must also deal with the possibility of associated endometrial cancer and the occasional bilateral occurrence of the tumor. Although bilateral tumors are uncommon, with a reported incidence usually of 2%–5% of cases [4–6, 9], a much higher incidence was noted by Ohel (26%) [10]. Unilateral oophorectomy should be preceded by dilatation and curettage of the uterus, and biopsy of the remaining ovary has been advocated.

Radical surgery is therefore probably preferable in terms of overall prognosis, and the loss of child-bearing potential must be weighed carefully against the increased chance of an incurable relapse after conservative surgery. Initial-presentation FIGO stage IV is very rare for granulosa-cell tumor and experience with management is sparse. The role of primary or secondary debulking in these patients is unclear. Palliative chemotherapy with cisplatin containing regimens may be advisable [13].

3. Adjuvant therapy in the management of granulosa-cell tumor of the ovary

The majority of patients present with FIGO stage IA or IB disease, and surgery alone will be adequate primary therapy. Local recurrence and metastases occur especially in the higher stages. Compared with epithelial cancer of the ovary the role of adjuvant therapy in granulosa cell tumor FIGO stage IC and higher is less well understood. Prospective randomized studies are impracticable because of the low incidence of the tumor and the long interval during which relapses may occur. Results of treatment are derived from small nonrandomized studies with short follow-up often not permitting meaningful conclusions.

Many retrospective series report the use of adjuvant radiotherapy. Adjuvant radiotherapy seemed to be associated with a better prognosis after long-term follow-up in the study of Kietlinska [11]. However, existing data are too incomplete for meaningful comparison of survival by stage of disease or other important prognostic factors. Retrospective analysis by Evans [5], Ohel [10] and Stenwig [4] did not document a possible positive effect of radiotherapy. At present there are no firm scientific arguments for adjuvant radiotherapy.

Colombo presented the results of cisplatin-containing polychemotherapy in 11 patients with advanced or recurrent disease [13]. In six patients (four with FIGO stage III and two with stage IV) adjuvant therapy was given after primary surgical debulking. In all five patients in whom surgery had been optimal, a surgically verified complete remission was subsequently obtained, while a patient who had sub-optimal surgery showed progression during polychemotherapy. During follow-up lasting 6–36 months no signs of relapse have been noted. In addition to this small study, only anecdotal reports of adjuvant chemotherapy have been presented in the literature [14, 15]. Chemotherapy seems to be indicated for patients with FIGO stage IC–III tumors after surgical debulking, but the exact role of adjuvant chemotherapy in the management of granulosa cell tumor of the ovary remains speculative.

4. Follow-up after initial therapy of granulosa-cell tumor of the ovary

Because of the possibility of late recurrence even more than twenty years after initial treatment, follow-up for granulosa tumor of the ovary should be life-long [2, 11].

History, physical examination and biochemical markers will be included in the follow-up examination. Serum estradiol levels may be a marker in those patients in whom elevated levels were found before initial therapy. Serum inhibin, although not specific for granulosa-cell cancer alone [8], may be an alternative and sensitive marker for primary as well as recurrent disease and is less hampered by endogenous or exogenous estrogen. Elevation of the markers may precede clinical manifestations of recurrent disease by as long as 20 months [7].

The role of routine radiological diagnosis is not clear. Recurrence may occur intra-abdominally as in epithelial ovarian cancer. The first sites of metastases outside the peritoneal cavity are lungs, liver and even the brain, spread hematogenously. Although there are many recurrences within the first five years after initial therapy, the median interval is six years. The best approach is to perform radiological investigation in patients in whom there is suspicion of relapse, based on the symptoms, physical examination or laboratory results.

In addition to associated endometrial cancer, there is evidence of an increased incidence of breast cancer in patients with granulosa-cell tumor of the ovary [2, 10]. Incidences of 3.7% to 20% have been reported. Periodic examination of the breasts and mammography have been advocated.

5. Management of inoperable advanced or relapsed granulosa-cell tumor of the ovary

There is no consistently effective management in advanced or relapsed granulosa cell cancer of the ovary. Published experience with these patients is anecdotal. Although no cure is achieved, there have been reports of complete responses of long duration achieved by surgery, radiotherapy and chemotherapy, both alone and in combination.

Repeated surgical removal after recurrence has been reported to be successful in limited disease. Combination therapy of surgical debulking and radiotherapy or radiotherapy alone has been used [4, 5, 11, 12, 16]. The combination of surgery and radiotherapy was superior in the opinion of Kietlinska [11], but comparative data are lacking.

Chemotherapy has been used in patients with large residual disease, metastases and inoperable recurrences. A twenty to twenty-five percent objective response rate has been reported in small groups of patients on monotherapy with melphalan and cyclophosphamide [16]. Anecdotal successes with L-phenylalanine mustard, adriamycin and actinomycin D have been published [14, 17, 18]. Combination chemotherapy with vincristine, adriamycin and cyclophosphamide (VAC), cisplatin, adriamycin and cyclofosfamide (PAC) or actinomycin D, 5-FU and cyclophosphamide (AcFuCy) has been used, yielding similar results [19, 20]. Colombo presented a successful combination with cisplatin, vinblastine and bleomycin (PVB) [13]. Five of six patients with residual disease after primary debulking surgery derived complete responses and four of five patients with recurrent disease responded, but two toxic deaths occurred. In his study only patients with residual disease <2 cm had a complete response with chemotherapy and longer-lasting responses. Until now reported studies have been too small to serve as a basis for conclusions regarding optimal combination chemotherapy or the number of courses to be given. Moreover, nothing is known of the possible activity of newer drugs such as taxol in granulosa cell tumor of the ovary.

In this case history an unexpected response occurred on dexamethasone. Until now no such response has been reported in the literature. Clarification of the implications of this observation await publication of the experiences of others.

Conclusion

Many questions about the management of granulosa-cell tumor of the ovary remain unanswered. Its low incidence and long relapse interval preclude a rapid comprehension of the biology of the tumor and definition of the best treatment option in advanced or metastatic disease. The cornerstone of treatment remains surgery. In all studies patients with early-stage disease and optimal debulking proved to have the best prognoses even in recurrent disease. Patients with stage IC disease or worse may benefit from adjuvant therapy especially after optimal surgery, but there have been no well-designed studies to determine the role of radiotherapy or chemotherapy. Theoretically chemotherapy has the advantage of treating distant metastases as well, which do occur in granulosa cell tumors. Recurrent disease may respond to radiotherapy or chemotherapy, but the best results have been obtained after optimal surgery. Nevertheless individual patients may benefit from one treatment modality subsequent to the other after a long period has elapsed.

References

1. Young RH, Scully RE. Ovarian sex cord-stromal tumours: Recent advances and current status. Clin Obstet Gynecol 1984; 11: 93–134.
2. Malkasian GD. Tumors of granulosa-theca derivation. In Williams CJ (ed.): Textbook of Uncommon Cancers of the Mayo Foundation. Chichester: Wiley 1988; 3–13.
3. Willemsen W, Kruitwagen R, Bastiaans B et al. Ovarian stimulation and granulosa-cell tumour. Lancet 1993; 341: 986–8.
4. Stenwig JT, Hazekamp JT, Beecham JB. Granulosa cell tumors of the ovary. A clinicopathological study of 118 cases with long-term follow-up. Gynecol Oncol 1979; 7: 136–52.
5. Evans AT, Gaffey TA, Malkasian GD, Annegers JF. Clinicopathological review of 118 granulosa and 82 theca cell tumors. Obstet Gynecol 1980; 55: 231–8.
6. Malström H, Högberg T, Risberg B, Simonsen E. Granulosa cell tumors of the ovary: Prognostic factors and outcome. Gynecol Oncol 1994; 52: 50–5.
7. Lappöhn RE, Burger HG, Bouma J et al. Inhibin as a marker for granulosa-cell tumors. N Engl J Med 1989; 321: 790–3.
8. Cooke I, O'Brien M, Charnock FM et al. Inhibin as a marker for ovarian cancer. Br J Cancer 1995; 71: 1046–50.
9. Björkholm E, Silfverswärd C. Prognostic factors in granulosa-cell tumors. Gynecol Oncol 1981; 11: 261–74.
10. Ohel G, Kaneti H, Schenker JG. Granulosa cell tumors in Israel: A study of 172 cases. Gynecol Oncol 1983; 15: 278–86.
11. Kietlinska Z, Pietrzak K, Drabik M. The management of granulosa-cell tumors of the ovary based on long-term follow-up. Eur J Gynaecol Oncol 1993; 14 (Suppl): 118–27.
12. Pankratz E, Boyes DA, White GW et al. Granulosa-cell tumors a clinical review of 61 cases. Obstet Gynecol 1978; 52: 718–23.
13. Colombo N, Sessa C, Landoni F et al. Cisplatin, vinblastine and bleomycin combination chemotherapy in metastatic granulosa-cell tumor of the ovary. Obstet Gynecol 1986; 67: 265–8.
14. Camlibel FT, Caputo TA. Chemotherapy of granulosa-cell tumors. Am J Obstet Gynecol 1983; 115: 763–5.
15. Jacobs AJ, Deppe G, Cohen CJ. Combination chemotherapy of ovarian granulosa-cell tumor with cis-platinum and doxorubicin. Gynecol Oncol 1982; 14: 294–7.
16. Malkasian GD, Webb MJ, Jorgensen EO. Observations on chemotherapy of granulosa-cell carcinomas and malignant ovarian teratomas. Obstet Gynecol 1974; 44: 885–8.
17. Lusch CJ, Mercurio TM, Runyon W. Delayed recurrence and chemotherapy of a granulosa cell tumor. Obstet Gynecol 1978; 51: 505–7.
18. Disaia PJ, Saltz A, Kagan AR et al. A temporary response of recurrent granulosa-cell tumor to adriamycin. Obstet Gynecol 1978; 52: 355–8.
19. Slayton RE. Management of germ-cell and stromal tumors of the ovary. Semin Oncol 1984; 11: 299–313.
20. Slayton RE, Johnson G, Brady L et al. Actinomycin D, 5-fluorouracil and cyclophosphamide (AcFuCy) chemotherapy for ovarian stromal tumors; a gynecologic oncology group study. Proc Am Soc Clin Oncol 1980; 21: 430.

R. L. Souhami (ed.) The Teaching Cases from Annals of Oncology, 99–104, 1997.

The management of non-seminomatous germ cell tumours (GCT)

L. Paz-Ares,[1] P. Lianes[2] & H. Cortes-Funes

Servicio de Oncologia Medica, Hospital Universitario 'Doce de Octubre', Madrid, Spain; [1]CRC Department of Medical Oncology, University of Glasgow, Glasgow, UK; [2]Laboratory of Molecular Immunopathology, Memorial Sloan Kettering Cancer Center, New York, NY, USA

Key words: germ cell tumours, non-seminomatous tumours, cisplatin, chemotherapy, management

Case history

In April 1992, a 40-year-old TV assistant presented to his general practitioner with a two-day history of swelling of the left testicle. He had had no previous local injury or systemic symptoms apart from possible mild fever. Clinical examination revealed tenderness, swelling and increased temperature of the left gonad, but no separate mass. His family and past medical histories were unremarkable. He was on no medication.

A suspected diagnosis of acute epididymo-orchitis was made and a 10-day course of antibiotics and analgesics was prescribed. As only a slight improvement was noted 14 days later, further investigations were performed, including alpha-fetoprotein (AFP), beta subunit of the chorionic gonadotropin (B-HCG), chest X-ray and testicular ultrasound. The ultrasound revealed a solid mass in the left testis and both tumour markers were elevated (AFP: 150 IU/ml; B-HCG: 25 IU/ml). A high inguinal orchidectomy was performed, and the patient was discharged 5 days following the procedure. The testis contained a 4.5-cm tumour which did not extend to the epididymis or involve the tunica vaginalis. The histology was reported as embryonal carcinoma with areas of mature teratoma. There were no other germ cell elements, and no vascular or lymphatic invasion (Fig. 1).

On referral to the medical oncology department, the patient was asymptomatic and physical examination results were normal. A CT scan of chest, abdomen and pelvis showed no abnormal findings, and serum markers progressively normalized (B-HCG on day 7, and AFP on day 17 postoperatively). No further therapy was advised but close follow-up was arranged. The first four scheduled monthly examinations (physical exam, serum markers and chest X-rays) yielded normal results, as did a CT scan in the second month post-orchidectomy. This was reported as showing non-significant para-aortic lymph node enlargement <1.5 cm, without changes since the previous study. Five months after orchidectomy, relapse was detected by increased AFP

(106 IU/ml) and the appearance of two intraabdominal masses, one behind the left kidney hilum of 4 cm diameter and the other, in the left paraaortic area, of 2.5 cm (Fig. 2A).

Chemotherapy was started, and the patient received 3 courses of BEP (bleomycin 30 U i.v. in continuous infusion, days 1–5, etoposide 100 mg/m² i.v., days 1–5, and cisplatin 20 mg/m² i.v., days 1–5, every 3 weeks) and one course of EP (the same regimen without bleomycin). Tolerance of chemotherapy was good, but grade II nausea/vomiting, universal alopecia and grade II tinnitus developed. AFP normalized after the second course of chemotherapy, but a CT scan after the third cycle showed persistent abnormalities in the sites of previous disease, although of reduced size. A further CT scan 5 weeks following the fourth course persisted unchanged (Fig. 2B), and the patient was sent back to the urologist for surgical removal of the residual masses. A unilateral retroperitoneal lymphadenectomy was carried out and histology showed mature teratoma in both macroscopically enlarged nodes (Fig. 3).

Following the operation, the patient was followed closely for one year and then at decreasing intervals.

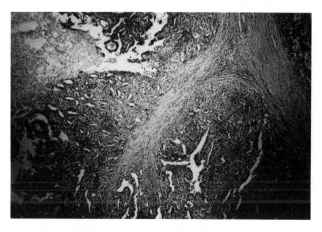

Fig. 1. Histological section of the primary tumour showing a predominance of undifferentiated germ cells (embryonal carcinoma). No vascular or lymphatic invasion is apparent.

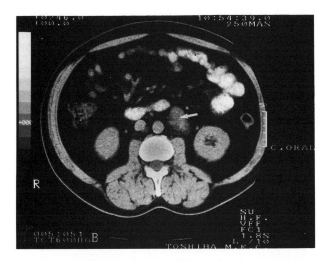

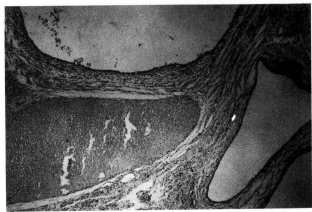

Fig. 3. Histological section of one of the post-chemotherapy lymph nodes showing mature teratoma.

Discussion

Although germ cell tumours (GCT) are not common (1%–1,5% of all cancers in males), they have a fundamental role in oncology for several reasons; (a), they usually arise in young individuals; (b), the availability of two serum markers (AFP, B-HCG) often allows more detailed assessment of the course of the disease; and (c), a high cure rate is achievable even in advanced stages. GCT have therefore been regarded as a model of a curable neoplasm [1].

The natural history of testicular tumours is of local growth involving the testicular layers, early spread to retroperitoneal lymph nodes, and thence to supradiaphragmatic regions, and vascular invasion with visceral metastases, particularly the lungs. Treatment varies for each patient, depending on the stage, histology and other prognostic factors (AFP and B-HCG levels, burden of disease, visceral involvement, etc.) [2], as well as patient characteristics. The case history presented here is not typical because most non-seminomatous GCT (NSGCT) patients are rendered continuously disease-free with first treatment. This case illustrates some important aspects of the current management of this disease.

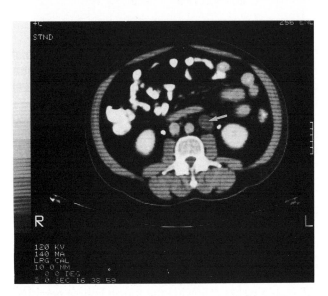

Fig. 2. Abdominal CT scans at the time of relapse (A) and 5 weeks following chemotherapy (B). Although the initial metastases decreased in size, a persistent residual mass is easily detectable behind the left kidney hilum (arrowed).

I. Diagnosis and staging

The characteristic presentation of a testicular GCT is as a hard and painless mass. About 15%–20% of patients complain of local pain with or without local inflammatory components. This may lead to the misdiagnosis of epididymo-orchitis and thus delay diagnosis. Therefore, in the presence of an asymptomatic testicular mass or with atypical evolution of an orchitis, as in our case history, testicular ultrasound is essential. Determination of AFP and B-HCG in this context is often helpful, but negative values do not negate the diagnosis. Delayed diagnosis is common, but is more often due to patient delay in seeking medical evaluation than to physician misdiagnosis. Several studies have

There has been no evidence of recurrence in the last 5 years. On the other hand, he complained of tinnitus, which improved initially during the first 6 months following chemotherapy but has persisted unchanged since then. After lymphadenectomy, he lacked anterograde ejaculation for 2–3 months. Although he subsequently recovered semen emission, the patient complained of persistent decreased sexual appetite and potency. Endocrine investigations showed normal testosterone levels with moderate increases in those of FSH (20–25 IU/ml) and LH (16–20 IU/ml) and subfertility in semen analysis (4–6×10^6 sperms/ml). He has been attending sessions of group psychotherapy without significant improvement. In addition, he developed hypercholesterolemia and hypertriglyceridemia in the second year post-treatment. With a low-fat diet and treatment with clofibrate, his lipids levels have returned to normal.

found a direct relationship between the time from onset of symptoms to diagnosis, the stage at presentation and the survival [3]. It is to be hoped that public campaigns to increase public awareness of the disease (including self-examination) will result in earlier diagnosis.

Diagnosis is confirmed by radical inguinal orchidectomy. Scrotal procedures, including trans-scrotal biopsy, are contra-indicated because of the risk of local recurrence or inguinal dissemination by altering the lymphatic drainage. The pathology report should include: (1) a description of all histological subtypes found (germ cell derivatives or not) (2) data concerning malignant involvement of the spermatic cord (free border) and testicular structures, and (3) assessment of the presence or absence of tumoral invasion in blood or lymphatic vessels. These are of special importance in planning treatment in early stages. In some instances, such as undifferentiated tumours with negative serum markers, immunohistochemistry and cytogenetics studies are valuable tools. The WHO histological classification of testicular GCT is given in Table 1 [4].

The essential investigations in staging the tumour are assays of AFP and B-HCG and radiological examinations. The latter should include a CT scan of chest, abdomen and pelvis. Other investigations depend on the previous findings and the planned therapy. A CT brain scan should be performed if there are very high levels of B-HCG or multiple lung metastasis. If chemotherapy is to be given, baseline measurement of creatinine clearance and lung function tests are necessary. Bipedal lymphography, which is unpleasant for the patient and sometimes technically difficult to perform, tends now to be abandoned in favour of CT scanning. Although in some circumstances lymphography can detect architectural abnormalities suggestive of metastases in normal size nodes, it does not appear to be more accurate than high-resolution CT imaging [5].

Several staging classification systems have been proposed for GCT but none is universally accepted. Most of them define three categories of disease: (1) confined to the testis, (2) retroperitoneal lymph node dissemination, and (3) supradiaphragmatic and/or visceral involvement. We employ the Royal Marsden Hospital staging criteria (Table 2) which affords simplicity and

Table 1. The WHO histological classification of testicular GCT [4].

Tumours of one histologic type
Seminoma
Spermatocytic seminoma
Teratoma: mature, immature or with malignant transformation
Embryonal carcinoma
Polyembrioma
Choriocarcinoma
Yolk sac tumours

Tumours of more than histologic type
Embryonal carcinoma and teratoma
Choriocarcinoma with or without embryonal carcinoma and/or teratoma (specify)
Other combinations (specify)

Table 2. The Royal Marsden Hospital staging system [6].

Stage I	No metastases evident outside testis
Stage IM	No clinical evidence of metastases but persistent elevation of serum markers (AFP, B-HCG) after orchidectomy
Stage II	Abdominal lymphadenopathy
A	<2 cm
B	2–5 cm
C	>5 cm
Stage III	Supradiaphragmatic lymphadenopathy
O	No abdominal disease
ABC	Abdominal node disease as in stage II
Stage IV	Extranodal metastases
L1	≤3 lung metastases
L2	>3 lung metastases all <2 cm diameter
L3	>3 lung metastases 1 or more >2 cm
H+	Liver involvement

incorporates a grading of abdominal and visceral metastases [6].

II. Management of stage I NSGCT

A widely advocated policy for clinical stage I NSGCT consists of retroperitoneal lymphadenectomy (RPLDN), with the aim of pathological staging and treatment. Patients with no tumour at operation (70%–75% of all cases) have a minimum risk of subsequent relapse (<10%) without further therapy. Those cases demonstrated to be truly stage II can be managed with 2 courses of adjuvant chemotherapy (relapse rate <2%) or observation (relapse rate 30%–40%). Both alternatives offer the same likelihood of survival (>95%) [7]. The refinements in surgical techniques have resulted in a substantial decrease in ejaculatory dysfunction, which is the most important complication of retroperitoneal lymph node dissection. Absence of anterograde ejaculation appeared in more than 90% of patients after bilateral radical procedures, while the current incidence is less than 5% in skilful hands using the nerve sparing technique and unilateral modified templates [8].

Some institutions, especially in Europe, have advocated a policy of observation without further therapy in patients without clinically apparent disease. The rationale for this approach is the high proportion of patients exposed to the morbidity of the lymphadenectomy without benefitting from it because they have already been cured with orchidectomy. Additionally, the 20%–30% of patients who relapse have an excellent prognosis with cisplatin based programs, when the diagnosis is established early [9]. The disadvantages of this policy are the need for frequent follow-up visits and some emotional distress to the patient who may feel at constant risk of relapse. Consequently, before deciding on a 'wait-and-see' policy the oncologist should ensure that the patient understands the position and that facilities are available for a rigorous follow-up schedule.

Several factors have been reported in surgical and observation series to predispose to the presence of undetectable retroperitoneal disease. A recent study of the MRC found four predictors of likelihood of relapse in this setting:(a) the presence of embryonal carcinoma, (b) the absence of yolk sac elements, (c) the presence of vascular invasion or (d) lymphatic invasion in the primary tumour [9]. In a subsequent study 101 patients with 3 or 4 risk factors (expected relapse rate on observation: 53%) were given two cycles of BEP, and after a median follow-up of 2 years only one has relapsed [10]. Therefore, short-course adjuvant chemotherapy in patients with high-risk pathological features is a safe and logical third possibility for management. Furthermore, the associated toxicity appears to be minimal [10]. The likelihood of post-orchidectomy relapse of a patient with two risk criteria, as in our case, is 20%, following the MRC model. With this basis no elective therapy is a reasonable alternative. The real significance of mature teratoma present in the primary remain uncertain in this context. Some authors would recommend staging RPLDN for these patients, as they predict a higher incidence of differentiated GCT also in the retroperitoneum. Other studies have, by contrast suggested that these patients have a lower risk of retroperitoneal disease.

At present, the chosen alternative for an individual stage I patient may vary, and it should be based on local urologist expertise with RPLDN, resources available for follow-up programs, tumour risk assignment and patient characteristics and preferences.

III. Chemotherapy for metastatic disease

There is no doubt that the availability of effective chemotherapeutic agents for metastatic NSGCT has dramatically changed the course of this disease. The most effective regimens are combinations of cisplatin – the most active single drug – with other agents such as vinblastine, etoposide, bleomycin, ifosfamide and actinomycin-D. Their use, with appropriate post-chemotherapy surgery, have yielded cure rates of over 85% in patients with advanced-stage disease during the last decade [11].

Was the chemotherapy program given to our patient optimal? The substitution of etoposide for vinblastine in the PVB regimen (cisplatin, vinblastine and bleomycin) has been shown in a randomized trial to decrease toxicity (mainly neuromuscular side effects) and to be associated with a possible survival gain in poor prognosis patients [12]. BEP is currently, therefore, a widely used regimen. We prefer to give the bleomycin as continuous infusion for 5 consecutive days (maximum cumulative dose: 450 U) instead of in weekly injections, in the hope of ameliorating the pulmonary toxicity.

Recently, it has been possible to recognize two prognostic subgroups of patients with metastatic testicular tumours in relation to the probability of complete remission and survival following cisplatin-containing chemotherapy (for review see 2). Sixty to 80% of the patients are included in the low-risk group. They usually present with low-burden metastatic disease and are highly curable (>90%). The remaining patients frequently have bulky disease and visceral involvement, and have a much worse prognosis (cure rate about 50%–60%). Current investigation is based on these findings. In low-risk patients, efforts are being made to decrease toxicity while maintaining the efficacy. Poor-risk patients are candidates for more intensive approaches in attempts to improve their outcome. In the good-risk setting, a randomized trial has shown that reduction of the number of cycles of BEP from 4 to 3 does not affect the outcome, although it reduces toxicity [13]. However, it is our policy, as well as that of other groups, to give two additional courses of chemotherapy after achievement of complete remission, instead of a predetermined number. Other approaches to reducing toxicity include omitting bleomycin and substituting cisplatin for carboplatin in the BEP regimen. With short follow-up, carboplatin has been associated with decreased disease-free survival in two randomized trials, and its use is discouraged [14]. Although four cycles of EP (cisplatin and etoposide) are as effective as four courses of VAB-6 using the MSKCC low-risk criteria, another three studies have not recommended the omission of bleomycin from the BEP combination [15].

In poor-risk patients, attempts to increase the efficacy of chemotherapy have been quite disappointing so far. An increase of the cisplatin dose to 200 m²/3 weeks, the use of alternating schedules, the introduction of ifosfamide in first-line schemes and the use of high-dose chemotherapy with bone marrow support have all been accompanied by greater toxicity but have not been shown to improve pronosis [16]. The results of further studies are awaited.

IV. Residual mass management

After completion of chemotherapy for GCT it is common to find persistent radiological abnormalities despite complete remission as judged by tumour markers. The almost universally accepted strategy in these circumstances is a surgical attempt to remove all residual masses with both therapeutical and prognostic aims. Pathological study of resected specimens shows fibrosis and/or necrosis in 30%–40% of the cases, mature teratoma in 30%–40% and viable tumour in the remaining 20%–30%. Their prognostic implications are clear [6]. Patients with fibrotic or teratoma containing masses rarely relapse provided that resection was complete. Thus, no additional therapy is needed for these patients. On the other hand, when viable malignant disease persists, two adjuvant courses of chemotherapy are usually given. With this approach, 60% of patients will remain disease-free, a figure which compares favourably with 9% without post-surgery chemotherapy [17].

Why is residual mass surgery indicated? First, viable chemo-refractory tumour can be removed and the patient benefit from further cytotoxic treatment. The latter, in our opinion, should be different from the regimen employed during the induction. Removal of differentiated teratoma which is unresponsive to chemotherapy is a second reason for surgery, since, when left in situ, the teratoma may grow, invade and compress surrounding tissues. Also, it may dedifferentiate to malignancy (of germ cell or non-germ cell histology) or result in a late recurrence [18]. Conversely, there is no clear advantage for resection of necrotic or fibrotic tissues. For this reason several investigators have tried to identify prognostic predictors of postsurgery histology. Most of the series have found an association between teratoma in the testicle and its presence in the residual mass. The finding of no benign or malignant tumour is more frequent when residual masses are of small size (e.g., <2 cm), those with high shrinkage of the original metastases (e.g., >90%), presurgery negative markers and, as mentioned, an absence of teratoma in the primary. Unfortunately, even when all these variables coincide in a patient, the chance of viable tumour or teratoma is 15%–20% [19]. Therefore, surgery to removal residual masses should be offered of any patient after chemotherapy, once markers are normalized.

V. Late post-treatment events

Are our patient's tinnitus, sexual dysfunction and hypercholesterolemia therapy related? The success of cisplatin combinations has resulted in an increasing number of long-term survivors among patients with advanced GCT. Concomitantly, several sequelae have been described and others presumably will be in the future.

Both cisplatin and vinblastine are known to produce peripheral neuropathy, predominantly sensory. Paresthesia is a common complaint during therapy but in most cases resolves in the succeeding months. Although only 10%–30% of patients remain symptomatic over the long term, the incidence of subclinical abnormalities is much higher, with 75% having abnormalities in conduction velocities and sensory action potentials [20]. A specific problem of cisplatin is ototoxicity, probably due to hair cell damage in the organ of Corti. Clinically, tinnitus is the predominant symptom (10%–30% of patients). High frequency hearing loss is easily demonstrable by audiometry although it seldom represents a problem for the patient. The degree of reduction in auditory function, as is the case for nephrotoxicity, seems to be related to the dose of cisplatin given and the mode of administration. The main renal consequence is a deterioration in glomerular function, measured as an average fall in GFR of 10%–30%. Among tubular disturbances hypomagnesemia is the most commonly reported [21].

It has recently been recognized that there may be an increased incidence of raised blood cholesterol levels in survivors treated with chemotherapy [22]. Raynaud's phenomenon and, less frequently, arterial hypertension and major vascular events, may also occur. Chronic pulmonary fibrosis is associated with bleomycin, especially when the cumulative dose exceeds 450 U.

Three factors may contribute to the decreased fertility which can affect GCT patients [23]. The first is ejaculatory dysfunction following retroperitoneal surgery. In specialized centres using current nerve sparing techniques, the incidence of permanent failure of ejaculation is less than 10%. Not uncommonly, a transient disturbance may occur, and some patients benefit from medical treatment (ephedrine, tricyclic antidepressants, etc.) or selective neural stimulation. Second, azo-oligospermia may occur and is frequently present at diagnosis. However, sperm count recovery is less frequent in patients treated with chemotherapy than in those with stage I disease who are followed without additional treatment. Third, some degree of Leydig cell dysfunction is present, as shown by normal serum testosterone levels with increased LH and FSH, as in our case. Our recommendation is to offer sperm banking to suitable patients before commencing cytotoxic treatment. Psychological morbidity, apart from anxiety and depression in 10% of the patients, also affects sexual activity. These disturbances, reported in 10%–40% of the cases, include impotence, premature ejaculation and loss of libido and sexual satisfaction [22].

Finally, an increased number of second malignancies arises in individuals treated for GCT (relative risk: 1.3–2). These include contralateral testicular tumours, solid tumours and haematological malignancies. Contralateral GCT appear in 3%–5% of survivors, usually within the 10 years following the first diagnosis. However, the risk, if any, is minimal in patients treated with chemotherapy, probably due to a protective effect against the pre-invasive lesion, in situ carcinoma [24]. Also a higher incidence of solid neoplasms has been reported (skin cancers, gastrointestinal tumours, lung tumours, urothelial carcinomas, etc.), particularly if radiotherapy is used. The actual incidence of leukaemia is unknown, but most cases involve patients treated with radiotherapy or etoposide [25]. A peculiar syndrome of non-therapy-induced haematological malignancies has been described in patients with primary mediastinal tumours. Both haematological and germ cell diseases seem to arise from a common progenitor [26].

Conclusion

The present case emphasizes the advantages of early diagnosis at presentation and relapse which correlates

104

with lower-burden disease in both circumstances. Careful follow-up is needed if RPLDN and chemotherapy are omitted in stage I. Once metastatic disease is present, the outcome is excellent if appropriate cisplatin chemotherapy is instituted and resection of residual masses undertaken when appropriate. Continuous follow-up should be offered to long-term survivors in order to detect and institute early management of late sequelae of treatment and other delayed complications.

The appropriate management of this highly curable disease requires the collaboration of several well-trained and experienced specialists. Given the rarity of GCT, both physicians and health service organizations should try to ensure that these tumours are treated in specialized centres [27].

Acknowledgement

Dr. Luis Paz-Ares is supported by a fellowship from the European Society of Medical Oncology (ESMO).

References

1. Einhorn LH. Treatment of testicular cancer: A new and improved model. J Clin Oncol 1990; 8: 1877–81.
2. Droz JP, Kramar A, Rey A. Prognostic factors in metastatic disease. Sem Oncol 1992; 19: 181–9.
3. Medical Research Council Working Party on testicular tumours. Prognostic factors in advanced non-seminomatous germ-cell testicular tumours: Results of a multicenter study. Lancet 1985; I: 8–11.
4. Mostofi FK, Sibin LH. Histological typing of testis tumors. International classification of tumors, No. 16. Geneva, World Health Organization, 1977.
5. Husband J. Advances in tumour imaging. In Horwich A (ed): Testicular cancer: Investigation and management. Chapman and Hall Medical: New York 1991; 2: 15–31.
6. Tait D, Peckham MJ, Hendry WF et al. Postchemotherapy surgery in advanced non-seminomatous germ cell tumours: The significance of histology with particular reference to differentiated (mature) teratoma. Br J Cancer 1984; 50: 601–9.
7. Williams SD, Stablein DM, Einhorn LH et al. Immediate adjuvant chemotherapy versus observation with treatment at relapse in pathological stage II testicular cancer. N Engl J Med 1987; 317: 1433–8.
8. Donahue JP, Thornhill JA, Foster RS et al. Retroperitoneal lymphadenectomy for clinical stage A testis cancer (1965–1989): Modifications of technique and impact on ejaculation. J Urol 1993; 149: 137–43.
9. Read G, Stenning SP, Cullen MH et al. Medical Research Council prospective study of surveillance for stage I testicular teratoma. J Clin Oncol 1992; 10: 1762–8.
10. Cullen MH on behalf of the Medical Research Council (MRC) Testicular Tumour Working Party. Short course adjuvant chemotherapy in high risk stage I non seminomatous germ cell tumours of the testis (NSGCTT): An MRC study report. Proc III Germ Cell Tumour Conference 1993; 3: 47 (Abstract).
11. Mead GM, Stenning SP, Parkinson MC et al. The Second Medical Research council study of prognostic factors in non-seminomatous germ cell tumors. J Clin Oncol 1992; 10: 85–94.
12. Williams SD, Birch B, Einhorn LH et al. Treatment of disseminated germ cell tumors with cisplatin, bleomycin and either vinblastine or etoposide. N Engl J Med 1987; 316: 1435–40.
13. Einhorn LH, Williams SD, Loehrer PJ et al. Evaluation of optimal duration of chemotherapy in favourable-prognosis disseminated germ cell tumors: A Southeastern Cancer Study Group protocol. J Clin Oncol 1989; 7: 387–91.
14. Bejorin DF, Sarosdy MF, Pfister DG et al. Randomized trial of etoposide and cisplatin versus etoposide and carboplatin in patients with good-risk germ cell tumors: A multiinstitutional study. J Clin Oncol 1993; 11: 598–606.
15. Levi JA, Raghavan D, Harvey V et al. The importance of bleomycin in combination chemotherapy for good-prognosis germ cell carcinoma. J Clin Oncol 1993; 11: 1300–5.
16. Paz-Ares L, Kaye SB. Intensive treatment schedules. Proc III Germ Cell Conference 1993; 3: 56.
17. Einhorn LH, Williams SD, Mandelbaum I et al. Surgical resection in disseminated testicular cancer following chemotherapeutic cytoreduction. Cancer 1981; 48: 904–10.
18. Paz-Ares L, Lianes P, Diaz-Puente M et al. Late relapses (LR) in malignant germ cell tumors (MCGT) treated with cisplatin-based chemotherapy. Proc Am Ass Cancer Res 1992; 34: 222 (Abstract).
19. Toner CG, Panicek DM, Heelan RT et al. Adjunctive surgery after chemotherapy for nonseminomatous germ cell tumors: Recommendations for patient selection. J Clin Oncol 1990; 8: 1683–94.
20. Hansen SW, Helweg-Larsen S, Trojaborg W. Long-term neurotoxicity in patients treated with cisplatin, vinblastine and bleomycin for metastatic germ cell cancer. J Clin Oncol 1989; 7: 1457–61.
21. Hansen SW, Groth S, Daugaard G et al. Long term side-effects on renal function and blood pressure of treatment with cisplatin, vinblastine and bleomycin in patients with germ cell cancer. J Clin Oncol 1988; 6: 1728–31.
22. Boyer M, Raghavan D. Toxicity of treatment of germ cell tumors. Sem Oncol 1992; 19: 128–42.
23. Fossa SD, Kreuser ED, Roth GJ et al. Long-term side effects after treatment of testicular cancer. Prog Clin Biol Res 1988; 357: 321–30.
24. von der Maase H, Rorth M, Walbom-Jorgesen S et al. Carcinoma in situ of contralateral testis in patients with testicular germ cell cancer. A study 27 cases in 500 patients. Br Med J 1986; 293: 1398–401.
25. Pedersen-Bjergaard J, Daugaard G, Hansen ST et al. Increased risk of myelodisplasia and leukaemia after etoposide, cisplatin, and bleomycin for germ cell tumours. Lancet 1991: 338: 359–63.
26. Rodriguez E, Mathew S, Reuter VE et al. Cytogenetic analysis of 124 prospectively ascertained male germ cell tumors. Cancer Res 1992; 52: 2285–91.
27. Harding MJ, Paul J, Gillis CR et al. Management of malignant teratoma: Does referral to a specialist unit matter? Lancet 1993; 341: 999–1002.

R. L. Souhami (ed.) The Teaching Cases from Annals of Oncology, 105–109, 1997.

A complicated case of metastatic teratoma
Growing teratoma syndrome and cerebral metastasis

P. D. Simmonds, G. M. Mead & J. M. A. Whitehouse

CRC Wessex Medical Oncology Unit, Royal South Hants Hospital, Southampton, U.K.

Key words: metastatic teratoma, growing teratoma syndrome, cerebral metastases

Introduction

Germ cell tumours of the testis are rare accounting for only 1% of all male malignancies, but have a special importance as they are by far the most common tumours in young men, their incidence is rapidly rising throughout the Western world and the majority are curable. Malignant teratomas (non seminomatous germ cell tumours) comprise about 50% of germ cell tumours, occurring at a median age of 27 years. Around half of these patients present with metastatic disease. Therapeutic advances over the past 20 years have seen cure rates for this disease rise to over 80%, but the management of patients with metastatic teratoma can be complex and commonly requires not only chemotherapy, but carefully timed surgical intervention as well. This case illustrates some of the unusual problems that may arise in patients receiving treatment for metastatic teratoma.

Case history

A 47-year-old man presented with a 3 month history of swelling of the right testis and lower backache. He had noted the more recent onset of a non-productive cough, not associated with dyspnoea. On examination there was a 3 cm left scalene mass and an enlarged, painful right testis. The chest was clear on auscultation. Testicular ultrasound examination showed a tumour occupying most of the right testis. The serum tumour markers alphafetoprotein (AFP) 708 kU/l (NR <10), human chorionic gonadotropin (HCG) 62 IU/l (NR <4) and lactate dehydrogenase (LDH) 1041 IU/l (N 200–400) were all elevated. Full blood count, serum electrolytes and creatinine and liver function tests were normal.

A right inguinal orchidectomy was performed and histological examination of the testis revealed a malignant teratoma intermediate (MTI/teratocarcinoma) with extensive areas of necrosis and obvious lymphatic and vascular invasion. A chest X-ray performed post operatively showed multiple (>20) pulmonary metastases bilaterally (Fig. 1) and computerized tomography (CT) of the abdomen revealed a 6 cm diameter left sided para-aortic mass. A CT scan of the brain was normal.

The patient was treated with BOP/VIP combination chemotherapy [1] comprising 3 cycles of bleomycin, vincristine and cisplatin at 10 day intervals followed by 3 cycles of etoposide, ifosfamide and cisplatin at 3 week intervals. Following chemotherapy the serum tumour marker levels had returned to normal and the left supraclavicular mass had resolved, as had all but one of the pulmonary nodules seen on chest X-ray prior to treatment (Fig. 2) – the latter lesion was noted to be enlarging. Chest and abdominal CT scans showed 3 pulmonary lesions in the right lower lobe, the largest measuring 2 cm in diameter and a residual 2 cm left para-aortic nodal mass with resolution of all other abnormalities. A repeat CT scan of the brain again showed no abnormality.

The patient underwent a combined right thoracotomy and laparotomy 5 weeks after the completion of chemotherapy. A 2 cm mass and adjacent necrotic

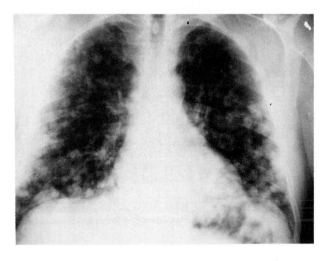

Fig. 1. Chest X-ray taken at presentation showing multiple pulmonary metastases.

tumour were completely resected from the right lower lobe of the lung and a mass of para-aortic nodes extending from the left renal vessels to the bifurcation of the aorta was also completely excised. Histological examination of the lung nodule showed differentiated teratoma containing malignant glandular and stromal elements with frank adenocarcinomatous foci within the nodule; there was, however, no invasion of the surrounding lung parenchyma by this process. The retroperitoneal nodes contained necrotic tumour together with several areas of differentiated teratoma without malignant change, but with cytological atypia.

On routine follow-up 4 months later the patient was found to have rising serum markers (AFP 15, HCG 17) and clinically had developed a left homonymous hemianopia. A CT scan of the brain revealed a 3.5 cm diameter right occipital lobe metastasis (Fig. 3).

CT scans of the chest and abdomen were also performed which showed no evidence of recurrent disease

at these sites. A craniotomy and excision of the occipital metastasis was performed and there was subsequent near-complete resolution of the left hemianopia and the serum marker levels fell to normal. Histological examination of the resected tissue revealed metastatic germ cell tumour composed of malignant teratoma undifferentiated (MTU/embryonal carcinoma) and yolk sac tumour. Post operatively cranial irradiation was given to a dose of 54 Gray. The patient remains alive with no evidence of disease 11 months after the completion of cranial irradiation.

Discussion

Malignant teratomas are histologically diverse and often include benign as well as several malignant components. The benign elements (teratoma differentiated) comprise mature tissues and commonly include glandular structures and cartilage. The neoplastic elements may include recognisable areas of seminoma, trophoblastic tissue (the source of HCG) and yolk sac tumour (the source of AFP) as well as undifferentiated elements. Any of these neoplastic elements may be present in pure form and all are capable of metastasising. Two histological classifications of malignant teratomas are currently in use (Table 1).

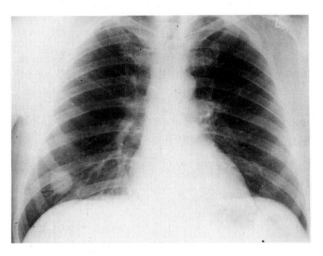

Fig. 2. Chest X-ray at the completion of chemotherapy showing a solitary residual lesion which was subsequently noted to enlarge.

Table 1. Pathological classification of teratomas/non-seminomatous germ cell tumours.

British Testicular Tumour Panel Classification	WHO Classification
Teratoma differentiated (TD)	Mature teratoma
Malignant teratoma undifferentiated (MTU)	Embryonal carcinoma
Malignant teratoma intermediate (MTI)	Teratocarcinoma
Malignant teratoma trophoblastic (MTT)	Choriocarcinoma
Yolk sac tumour	Yolk sac tumour

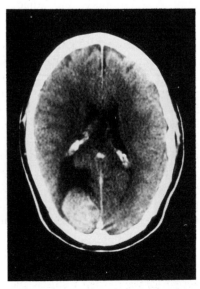

Fig. 3. Cerebral CT scan showing a solitary metastasis in the right occipital lobe at the time of relapse.

Teratomas metastasize in a predictable fashion, initially spreading either via the testicular lymphatics to the paraaortic nodes [2] and subsequently to nodes in the mediastinum and neck or by vascular invasion with subsequent haematogenous spread, mainly to the lungs and less often to liver, bone or brain. The degree of dissemination is an important indicator of prognosis and should be established prior to commencing treatment. The staging investigations that should be performed include (i) a thorough physical examination, paying particular attention to the supraclavicular fossa, abdomen and chest, (ii) serum tumour markers (AFP, HCG, LDH) – one or both of the serum tumour markers AFP or HCG will be elevated in 80%–90% of patients with teratoma; these markers are sensitive indicators of active disease and can reliably be used to assess patients response to treatment, (iii) chest X-ray and (iv) CT scan of the chest and abdomen. A cerebral CT scan need only be performed in those patients with evidence of CNS dysfunction or those who are at increased risk of cerebral metastases (multiple pulmonary metastases, very high HCG level, choriocarcinoma).

The basis of treatment for metastatic teratoma is cisplatin combination chemotherapy followed by surgical excision of residual disease. A variety of different prognostic models have been developed to try to predict the outcome of patients with metastatic teratoma. The absence of an agreed international system for defining prognostic groups had made it difficult to compare data derived from different trials. Those factors which are generally accepted to adversely affect prognosis include (i) extensive disease (particularly involvement of the liver, CNS and bone), (ii) markedly elevated pretreatment levels of AFP, HCG, or LDH and (iii) extragonadal primary tumour [3]. Using such prognostic factor models, patients can be divided into 2 or 3 risk groups. Those in the good prognosis group (approximately two thirds of cases) will have a failure free survival of approximately 90% whilst those in the poor prognosis group have an approximately 60% failure free survival with currently available treatment [4].

The standard chemotherapy regimen for metastatic teratoma is BEP (bleomycin, etoposide and cisplatin) which has been given according to a variety of different schedules [5, 6]. Patients with good prognosis disease should receive 3 or 4 courses of BEP [6, 7]. Attempts to reduce the toxicity of this treatment by substituting carboplatin for cisplatin [8] or deleting bleomycin [9] has led to an increase in subsequent relapse rates and cannot be recommended.

The management of patients with poor prognosis disease remains controversial. A number of phase II studies have suggested that these patients may benefit from more intensive chemotherapy [1, 10, 11] and a randomised National Cancer Institute (NCI) trial [12] comparing PVB (cisplatin 100 mg/m^2, vinblastine, bleomycin) with PVeBV (cisplatin 200 mg/m^2, etoposide, bleomycin, vinblastine) showed a survival advantage for the later treatment arm. It is likely, however, that this result was due to the introduction of etoposide rather than the increased dose of cisplatin as a subsequent randomised trial of 157 patients with advanced disease defined by Indiana criteria comparing 4 cycles of standard BEP with 4 cycles of BEP using double dose cisplatin (200 mg/m^2) showed no difference in efficacy [13]. Preliminary results of a randomised trial comparing BEP with VIP has shown no clear difference in outcome between patients in the 2 treatment arms [14] and similarly, a randomised trial comparing 4 cycles of PVeBV with 2 cycles of the same treatment followed by high dose chemotherapy with autologous bone marrow rescue showed no improvement in survival for the patients who received the more intensive treatment [15]. As more intensive initial therapy has not yet been shown to increase survival, the standard treatment for poor prognosis teratoma remains 4–6 cycles of BEP [5, 6]. The present MRC/EORTC trial for poor

prognosis teratoma is comparing BEP with BOP-VIP. The BOP-VIP regimen was designed to increase the dose intensity for cisplatin by an initial induction phase with a short interval (10 days) between treatments and also to introduce in a sequential fashion further highly effective drugs (etoposide and ifosfamide) [1]. The outcome of this trial is awaited with interest.

At the completion of chemotherapy, all initial sites of disease should be reassessed. Residual masses are commonly present, particularly in patients with bulky disease at presentation. CT scanning can accurately define the site and size of these masses but not their composition [16]. Such residual masses are most commonly found in the retroperitoneum, but may also occur in the mediastinum, lungs and elsewhere. It is not uncommon for residual masses to persist at more than one site. Patients who have residual masses present at the completion of chemotherapy can be divided into 2 groups: (i) those patients with persistently elevated or rising serum markers who have residual malignant disease and in general should be treated with salvage chemotherapy and (ii) the majority of patients in whom the serum marker levels have returned to normal who have residual mass(es) which may be composed of necrotic debris/fibrosis, teratoma differentiated, viable carcinoma or any combination of these – such masses should be surgically resected. If the primary tumour is still in situ, orchidectomy is also recommended post chemotherapy [17].

Excision of residual masses serves to remove residual teratoma differentiated (TD, mature teratoma) and carcinoma and it identifies those patients with residual viable carcinoma who require further treatment. TD is thought to be relatively resistant to the effects of chemotherapy and so survives whilst the adjacent malignant tumour is destroyed. TD may grow locally and obstruct or invade adjacent structures and become unresectable; less commonly it may dedifferentiate giving rise to germinal or non-germinal malignancies [18]. The prognosis after resection of residual masses has been shown to relate to the histology of the resected mass and the completeness of the resection [19]. Those patients with only necrotic tumour/fibrosis or completely excised TD are almost always cured, whereas patients with residual malignant teratoma which has been completely excised have a high probability of disease progression and should empirically receive a further 2 cycles of cisplatin based chemotherapy following which over 50% will remain disease free [20]. Patients who are found to have nongerminal malignant elements (sarcoma/carcinoma) within masses composed predominantly of TD also have a high risk of developing recurrent disease subsequently [21]. Where the surgical resection is incomplete the majority of patients will relapse.

No criteria have yet been determined which can accurately predict those patients who will have only necrotic debris/fibrosis in their residual mass. Thus, all patients with residual retroperitoneal masses identified by CT scan (>1.0 cm) should undergo exploration of the retroperitoneum and excision of the residual mass; a full retroperitoneal lymph node dissection is probably not necessary in this situation [22]. Similarly, all residual mediastinal masses identified at the completion of chemotherapy should be resected. A small proportion of patients with retroperitoneal metastases at presentation, but no abnormality seen in the retroperitoneum on a post chemotherapy CT scan will have microscopic disease (TD or carcinoma) in the retroperitoneal nodes [23], however, it is generally agreed that operating on all these patients would subject too many to unnecessary surgery. Non-resolving pulmonary lesions visible on chest X-ray should also be resected. It is important that all residual lung nodules are removed as different pathological findings may be seen in separate nodules [24].

The 'growing teratoma syndrome' [25] describes the situation where masses composed entirely of TD are seen to enlarge in patients with normal or falling serum markers who are undergoing or have completed chemotherapy. Thus growing teratoma may become apparent during chemotherapy (where an initial reduction in the size of the lesion may be seen followed by enlargement later in the course of treatment) or after a 'disease free' interval. Growing teratoma lesions usually occur at metastatic sites involved at presentation, most frequently in the retroperitoneum and chest. Complete surgical excision is necessary for long term survival. Patients with growing teratoma usually have coexistent malignant teratoma and should therefore receive at least 4 cycles of cisplatin containing chemotherapy prior to surgical resection which should be performed as soon as possible after completion of chemotherapy. Excision of growing teratoma masses is often difficult, particularly in the retroperitoneum and early exploration optimises the chances of complete resection. Rarely it may be necessary to excise a rapidly enlarging mass prior to the completion of chemotherapy.

Cerebral metastases from teratoma occur uncommonly. Less than 5% of patients with disseminated teratoma will have cerebral metastases at presentation [26, 27]. With previously treated disease which is refractory to chemotherapy, CNS metastases are more frequent and 10%–15% of patients with disseminated teratoma have been shown to develop cerebral metastases during the course of their disease despite chemotherapy [26, 28]. Isolated CNS relapse after effective chemotherapy is rare, but may occur because the CNS can act as a sanctuary sites for germ cell tumours as cytotoxic drugs penetrate this area less well than systemic sites due to the presence of the blood brain barrier. However, the overall incidence of CNS disease in patients with germ cell tumours is too low to warrant routine prophylactic treatment. When serum markers rise after returning to normal with chemotherapy, patients who do not have evidence of recurrent disease in the abdomen or chest should always have a cerebral CT scan performed, even if they are asymptomatic, to exclude CNS disease. If the CT scan is normal, a CSF HCG level should also be performed. If the ratio of CSF:serum HCG level is >1:60 this is suggestive of CNS disease [27].

The presence of cerebral metastases in patients with teratoma does not preclude cure. Those patients with cerebral metastases at presentation and those with isolated relapse in the CNS should be treated with curative intent. For patients who present with cerebral metastases, cure rates of greater than 50% have been reported using standard BEP/PVB chemotherapy combined with whole brain irradiation [29], or POMB-ACE chemotherapy combined with intrathecal methotrexate [30]. Those patients who have received successful systemic chemotherapy and subsequently relapse with a solitary cerebral metastasis should have this surgically excised where feasible and then receive whole brain irradiation [29]. Where the location of the metastasis precludes excision or there are multiple metastases, whole brain irradiation alone should be given. It has also been recommended that concomitant cisplatin based chemotherapy be given to these patients as CNS relapse may herald systemic relapse [29]. Patients who develop CNS disease in the setting of progressive disease elsewhere are probably not curable and should be treated with palliative radiotherapy with or without further chemotherapy.

Summary

All patients presenting with metastatic teratoma should be regarded as potentially curable and this case demonstrates the multiple treatment modalities which are often needed in the management of such patients. Increasing experience with cisplatin based combination chemotherapy has led to the development of prognostic factors which are used to determine the intensity of treatment given to individual patients. Surgical intervention plays a very important role in the management of residual disease at the completion of chemotherapy. Recognition of the growing teratoma syndrome and the importance of early surgical excision is illustrated by this case. Isolated CNS relapse may occur because the CNS may act as a sanctuary site in patients receiving systemic chemotherapy, but does not preclude long term disease free survival.

References

1. Lewis CR, Fossa SD, Mead G et al. BOP/VIP – a new platinum intensive chemotherapy regimen for poor prognosis germ cell tumours. Ann Oncol 1991; 2: 203–21.
2. Donohue JP, Zachary JM, Maynard BR. Distribution of nodal metastases in nonseminomatous testis cancer. J Urol 1982; 128: 315–20.
3. Mead GM, Stenning SP. Prognostic factors for metastatic germ cell cancers treated with platinum based chemotherapy: The international germ cell cancer collaborative group (IGCCCG)

project to standardise risk criteria. Proc ASCO 1994; 13: 251 (Abstr).

4. Mead GM, Stenning SP, Parkingson MC et al. The second Medical Research Council study of prognostic factors in non-seminomatous germ cell tumours. J Clin Oncol 1992; 10: 85–94.

5. Williams SD, Birch R, Einhorn LH et al. Treatment of disseminated germ cell tumours with cisplatin, bleomycin and either vinblastine or etoposide. N Engl J Med 1987; 316: 1435–40.

6. Dearnley DP, Horwich A, A'Hern R et al. Combination chemotherapy with bleomycin etoposide and cisplatin (BEP) for metastatic testicular teratoma: Long term follow-up. Eur J Cancer 1991; 27: 684–91.

7. Einhorn LH, Williams SD, Loehrer PH et al. Evaluation of optimal duration chemotherapy in favorable prognosis disseminated germ cell tumours: A Southeastern Cancer Study Group protocol. J Clin Oncol 1989; 7: 387–91.

8. Bajorin DF, Sarosdy MF, Pfister DG et al. Randomized trial of etoposide and cisplatin versus etoposide and carboplatin in patients with good risk germ cell tumours: A multi-institutional study. J Clin Oncol 1993; 11: 598–606.

9. Loehrer PJ, Elson P, Johnson DH et al. A randomized trial of cisplatin plus etoposide with or without bleomycin in favourable prognosis disseminated germ cell tumours: An ECOG study. Proc ASOC 1991; 10: 169 (Abstr).

10. Cullen MH, Harper PG, Woodroffe CM et al. Chemotherapy for poor risk germ cell tumours. An independent evaluation of the POMB/ACE regimen. Br J Urol 1988; 62: 454–60.

11. Horwich A, Brada M, Nicholls J et al. Intensive induction chemotherapy for poor risk non-seminomatous germ cell tumours. Eur J Cancer Clin Oncol 1989; 25: 177–84.

12. Ozols RF, Ihde DC, Linehan WM et al. A randomized trial of standard chemotherapy v. a high-dose chemotherapy regimen in the treatment of poor prognosis non-seminomatous germ cell tumours. J Clin Oncol 1988; 6: 1031–40.

13. Nichols CR, Williams SD, Loehrer PJ et al. Randomized study of cisplatin dose intensity in poor risk germ cell tumours: A Southeastern Cancer Study Group and Southwest Oncology Group protocol. J Clin Oncol 1991; 9: 1163–72.

14. Loehrer PJ, Einhorn LH, Elson P et al. Phase III study of cisplatin plus etoposide with either bleomycin or ifosfamide in advanced stage germ cell tumours: An Intergroup trial. Proc ASCO 1993; 12: 261 (Abstr).

15. Chevreau C, Droz JP, Pico JL et al. Early intensified chemotherapy with autologous bone marrow transplantation in first line treatment of poor risk non-seminomatous germ cell tumours. Eur Urol 1993; 23: 213–8.

16. Stomper PC, Jochelson MS, Garnick MB et al. Residual abdominal masses after chemotherapy for non-seminomatous testicular cancer: Correlation of CT and histology. AJR 1985; 145: 743–6.

17. Greist A, Einhorn LH, Williams SD et al. Pathological findings at orchiectomy following chemotherapy for disseminated testicular cancer. J Clin Oncol 1984; 9: 1025–7.

18. Ulbright TM, Loehrer PJ, Roth LM et al. The development of non germ cell malignancies within germ cell tumours. A clinicopathologic study of 11 cases. Cancer 1984; 54: 1824–33.

19. Jansen RLH, sylvester R, Sleyfer DT et al. Long term follow up of non seminomatous testicular cancer patients with mature teratoma or carcinoma at post chemotherapy surgery. Eur J Cancer 1991; 6: 695–8.

20. Fox EP, Weathers TD, Williams SD et al. Outcome analysis for patients with persistent non-teratomatous germ cell tumour in pot chemotherapy retroperitoneal lymph node dissections. J Clin Oncol 1993; 11: 1294–9.

21. Davey DD, Ulbright TM, Loehrer PJ et al. The significance of atypia within teratomatous metastases after chemotherapy for malignant germ cell tumours. Cancer 1987; 59: 533–9.

22. Hendry WF, A'Hern RP, Hetherington JW et al. para-aortic lymphadenectomy after chemotherapy for metastatic non-seminomatous germ cell tumours: Prognostic value and therapeutic benefit. Br J Urol 1993; 71: 208–13.

23. Fossa SD, Ous S, Lien HH, Stenwig AE. Post chemotherapy lymph node histology in radiologically normal patients with metastatic non-seminomatous testicular cancer. J Urol 1989; 141: 557–9.

24. Toner GC, Panicek DM, Heelan RT et al. Adjunctive surgery after chemotherapy for nonseminomatous germ cell tumours: Recommendations for patient selection. J Clin Oncol 1990; 8: 1683–94.

25. Jeffery GM, Theaker JM, Lee AHS et al. The growing teratoma syndrome. Br J Urol 1991; 67: 195–202.

26. Williams SD, Einhorn LH. Brain metastases in disseminated germinal neoplasms: Incidence and clinical course. Cancer 1979; 44: 1514–6.

27. Kaye SB, Bagshawe KD, McELwain TJ et al. Brain metastases in malignant teratoma: A review of four years experience and an assessment of the role of tumour markers. Br J Cancer 1979; 39: 217–23.

28. Logothetis CJ, Samuels ML, Trindade A. The management of brain metastases in germ cell tumours. Cancer 1982; 49: 12–8.

29. Spears WT, Morphis JG, Lester SG et al. Brain metastases and testicular tumours: Long term survival. Int J Radiat Oncol Biol Phys 1991; 22: 17–22.

30. Rustin GJS, Newlands ES, Bagshawe KD et al. Successful management of metastatic and primary germ cell tumours in the brain. Cancer 1986; 57: 2108–13.

R. L. Souhami (ed.) The Teaching Cases from Annals of Oncology, 111–116, 1997.

Gestational choriocarcinoma

M. Bower, C. Brock, R. A. Fisher, E. S. Newlands & G. J. S. Rustin

Trophoblastic Tumour Screening and Treatment Centre, Department of Medical Oncology, Charing Cross Hospital, London, U.K.

Key words: choriocarcinoma, gestational trophoblastic disease, hCG, hydatidiform mole

Case history

In December 1992 a 27-year-old primagravida woman had a baby girl by normal vaginal delivery. The third trimester of pregnancy was complicated by mild pre-eclamsia which settled after delivery. Five weeks later the patient experienced vaginal bleeding which persisted intermittently until she attended hospital 3 months post partum when a urinary hCG pregnancy test was negative and a pelvic ultra-sound scan showed a thickened uterine wall. The bleeding continued but she did not represent until she had a heavy vaginal bleed 8 months post partum. She felt pregnant, with malaise and nausea, and her urinary pregnancy test was positive. A uterine dilatation and curettage was undertaken and the histology revealed choriocarcinoma.

She was referred to Charing Cross Hospital. She remained fatigued and nauseous and had left sided pleuritic chest pain without a cough or haemoptysis or bleeding. Examination on admission was unremarkable. A chest X-ray demonstrated a solitary metastasis in the right midzone. Pelvic ultrasonography with Doppler study showed a bulky retroverted uterus with a 4.0 × 3.5 cm mass in the fundus which had abnormal blood flow, and reduced uterine artery perfusion indices (0.9–1.0: normal range >2.0).

According to the WHO trophoblastic disease prognostic scoring index [1] (Table 1) she fell into the high risk treatment group and therefore started treatment with EMA/CO chemotherapy [2] (Table 2) together with intrathecal methotrexate 12.5 mg alternate weeks as CNS prophylaxis. The CSF hCG measurement was 248 iu/l compared with a simultaneous serum level of 156,455 iu/l. The serum: CSF hCG ratio was therefore greater than 60:1. Ratios <60:1 indicate the presence of intracerebral metastases [3].

After 2 cycles of EMA/CO her pv bleeding & chest pain had resolved and serum hCG had fallen to 724 iu/l with a CSF hCG of 3 iu/l. She experienced the expected side effects of nausea & vomiting, which were controlled by ondansetron and dexamethasone; mucositis and sore eyes which responded to increased folinic acid rescue and hypromellose eye-drops; alopecia and myelosuppression. Following the third cycle the right lung metastasis had decreased in size; however, the serum hCG plateaued around 1,000 iu/l indicating serological evidence of drug resistance. Therefore the chemotherapy was changed to EP/EMA alternating weekly (Table 2). Radioimmunolocalisation scanning with ^{131}I tagged monoclonal antibodies directed against hCG have been used to identify sites of active disease in women with elevated serum levels but normal radiology [4] (Fig. 1) but her scan was negative. Since the single pulmonary metastasis was the only known site of disease a right thoracotomy was performed and the metastasis resected but there was not viable tumour at histology. Following a rapid post-operative recovery, the serum hCG began to rise. Re-staging imaging scans were performed; a cerebral MRI was normal, and pelvic ultrasonography demonstrated a normal sized uterus with residual abnormal blood flow. However, a body CT indicated that a left apical lung metastasis had

Table 1. Prognostic scoring scheme for GTD.

	Score			
	0	1	2	6
Age	<39 years	>39 years		
Pregnancy	Hydatidiform mole	Abortion/ unknown	Term	
Interval (months)	<4	4–7	7–12	>12
Serum hCG	10^3–10^4 iu/l	<10^3 iu/l	10^4–10^5 iu/l	>10^5 iu/l
ABO (F × M) blood group		A×O	B×A or O	
		A×A	AB×A or O	
		O×A or unknown		
Number of metastases	0	1–4	5–8	>8
Site of metastases	Lung Vagina	Spleen Kidney	GIT Liver	Brain
Largest mass (uterine volume)	<3 cm <100 ml	3–5 cm 100–250 ml	>5 cm >250 ml	
Number of prior chemotherapy treatments	0		1	2+

Low risk: 0–5
High risk: 9+

Table 2. GTD chemotherapy regimens used in this case.

GTD high risk regimen

EMA
Day 1
Actinomycin D	0.5 mg i.v. bolus
Etoposide	100 mg/m² i.v.
Methotrexate	300 mg/m² i.v.

Day 2
Actinomycin D	0.5 mg i.v.
Etoposide	100 mg/m² i.v.
Folinic acid	15 mg PO/IM bd for 2 days starting 24 h after MTX

CO
| Vincristine | 0.8 mg/m² i.v. bolus (max 2 mg) |
| Cyclophosphamide | 600 mg/m² i.v. |

Repeat EMA/CO alternating weekly to marker CR plus a further 6–8 weeks therapy

EP/EMA for drug resistant choriocarcinoma

| Etoposide | 100 mg/m² i.v. |
| Cisplatin | 75 mg/m² i.v. |

EP alternates with standard EMA schedule weekly

Conditioning chemotherapy pre-transplant

Day 8	Etoposide	600 mg/m² i.v.
	Carboplatin	10 (EDTA clearance + 25) mg i.v.
Day 6	Etoposide	600 mg/m² i.v.
	Carboplatin	10 (EDTA clearance + 25) mg i.v.
	Cyclophosphamide	60 mg/kg i.v.
	Mesna	60 mg/kg i.v.
Day 4	Etoposide	600 mg/m² i.v.
	Carboplatin	10 (EDTA clearance + 25) mg i.v.
	Cyclophosphamide	60 mg/kg i.v.
	Mesna	60 mg/kg i.v.
Day 0	Reinfuse bone marrow	

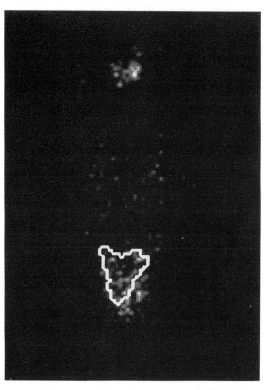

Fig. 1. Posterior planar views of an anti-hCG antibody localization scan from a different patient. The green outline represents the bladder derived from a simultaneously imaged ⁹⁹ᵐTc-DTPA scan. Antibody localised in tumour can be seen below the bladder to the right. Non-specific uptake of iodine in the thyroid can also been seen. By courtesy of Professor R. H. J. Begent.

developed. This was again the only site of disease but in view of the difficulty in controlling the disease the possible role of chemotherapy dose intensification with autologous progenitor cell rescue was raised. Prior to her second thoracotomy, she received 3 g/m² cyclophosphamide followed by G-CSF and peripheral stem cell harvesting.

The left sided apical metastasis was resected and active tumour was demonstrated histologically in one nodule. The serum hCG fell from 1219 iu/l pre-operatively to 479 iu/l post-operatively. She received a further cycle of EP chemotherapy but the hCG continued to rise suggesting resistance to platinum. The uterus was bulky with abnormal vascularity on ultrasound and in view of the drug resistance and absence of other sites of demonstrable disease, a hysterectomy was performed. There was no histologically viable choriocarcinoma. The hysterectomy failed to reduce the serum hCG. In the absence of radiological evidence for a site of active disease further surgery was impossible and the disease had been found to be resistant to all conven-

tional chemotherapy schedules for trophoblastic disease. A trial of biological therapy with α-interferon 3 MU s/c od and oral 13-cis retinoic acid 1 mg/kg/day was commenced in an attempt to encourage the tumour to differentiate. This treatment was badly tolerated and was ceased. Subsequently she noted paraesthesia and mild weakness in both legs and developed urinary retention. The neurology progressed rapidly with bilateral leg weakness with loss of sensation upto both knees, over the sacral area and the right anterior abdominal wall at T10/T11 dermatome. Her legs were areflexic, but there was no spinal tenderness. An MRI scan confirmed T11 vertebral body involvement which extended to the middle of both adjacent vertebral bodies, there was also an extra-dural tumour causing secondary compression. The serum hCG was 2003 iu/l. Dexamethasone was commenced and an anterior decompression performed, involving a T11 vertebrectomy via a left thoracotomy, with insertion of a Moss cage with rib bone-graft and Webb-Mosely fusion. Histologically the extra-dural tumour was metastatic choriocarcinoma and the vertebral body comprised necrotic metastatic choriocarcinoma. The serum hCG had fallen to 762 iu/l post-operatively; however, some of the decline was due to dilution by peri-operative blood transfusions.

The serum hCG rose post-operatively and a repeat chest X-ray demonstrated new pulmonary metastases.

Further chemotherapy was commenced with 5-fluorouracil, an agent not previously employed for this patient and which has anecdotal efficacy in drug resistant trophoblastic tumours. The regime used was 5-FU (3500 mg/m^2 over 48 h) as a continuous two-day infusion given weekly. Three courses of 5-FU were administered which produced an initial fall in the serum hCG. Four weeks following the neurosurgery she developed haemoptysis with no associated chest pain nor evidence of venous thrombosis. The CXR showed progression of the metastases.

Conditioning chemotherapy was commenced with a regime used for relapsed germ cell tumours which includes high doses of etoposide, carboplatin and cyclophosphamide (Table 2). One day after PBSC infusion she had a fresh haemoptysis followed by sudden dyspnoea without chest pain. It was felt that this episode was due to bleeding into her pulmonary metastases as she had been on prophylactic heparin and was thrombocytopaenic. Her condition continued to deteriorate and she required elective intubation and ventilation before transfer to ITU. She developed multiorgan failure. She had episodes of paroxysmal atrial flutter which stabilised with intravenous amiodarone, but by day 6 post PBSC infusion she required boluses of adrenaline to help maintain her BP, and finally required full inotropic support with adrenaline and noradrenaline by day 10. Her liver enlarged progressively, eventually reaching her umbilicus and she developed a 4-cm palpable spleen. The hepatic function deteriorated and she became anuric. Ultrasonography showed several metastases in the right and caudate lobes of the liver plus a small amount of ascites, both kidneys showed evidence of diffuse renal disease. Haemofiltra-

tion was commenced which improved her uraemia but her urine output never recovered. The effect of haemofiltration upon the clearance of hCG is unknown and changes in the serum half-life of hCG could alter the kinetics significantly. Therefore hCG levels were assayed in both the serum and dialysate. In fact on the three days that she was dialysed, the dialysate from 10–15 iu/l giving a haemofiltration clearance for hCG of 10–35 mcl/min compared with a normal urinary clearance of hCG of approximately 100 ml/min. Serum hCG assays and the treatment schedules for this patient are shown in Fig. 2.

By day 11 her gas exchange had deteriorated and despite maximal inotropic support she deteriorated and died. At post mortem there were numerous metastases in both lungs, which were haemorrhagic and congested. There were also metastases in the liver and on the surface of the kidneys. There was a large retroperitoneal metastasis beneath the diaphragm to the right of the vertebral column and the brain was oedematous with numerous metastases, the largest in the right frontal lobe.

Discussion

Introduction

Gestational choriocarcinoma arises from trophoblastic epithelium and in contrast to hydatidiform moles, neither embryonic elements nor villi are present. The lack of villous structures distinguishes choriocarcinoma from invasive hydatidiform mole morphologically; however, the reliance upon persistently elevated hCG

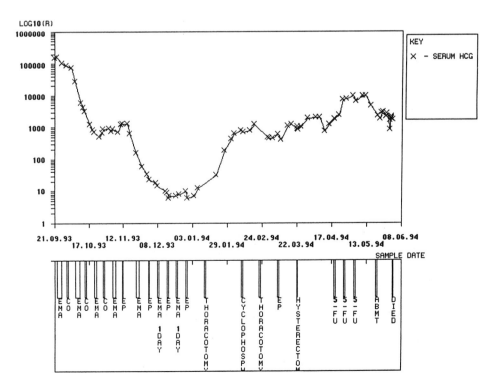

Fig. 2. Graph of serum hCG for this patient. Graph demonstrating the serum hCG level and treatments for the patient described in this case report.

levels and the frequent absence of tissue for histology often makes it impossible to differentiate between invasive mole and choriocarcinoma, so the term 'gestational trophoblastic disease' (GTD) is used to cover both diagnoses. The clinical presentation of invasive mole and choriocarcinoma may be indistinguishable.

Epidemiology/aetiology

The incidence of choriocarcinoma in population based studies varies from 0.05 to 0.23/1000 live births [5]. Although racial origin has been found to influence the risk of hydatidiform moles this relationship is less clear for choriocarcinoma where the most important risk factor is a history of hydatidiform mole. Around 40%–60% of patients with choriocarcinoma have a history of a molar pregnancy, although a substantial proportion either follow a normal full-term pregnancy or a spontaneous abortion [6]. Increased maternal age at diagnosis is the only other well established risk factor [5].

Molecular biology

Gestational trophoblastic tumours are unique in cancer biology as they include paternally derived genetic material that is absent from the patient's genotype, a fact which may be exploited for diagnosis. Gestational choriocarcinoma may arise following a monospermic or dispermic complete hydatidiform mole (CHM) [7], a triploid partial hydatidiform mole (PHM) [8], or a normal biparental pregnancy [9–11]. Comparison of genetic polymorphisms in the patient and her partner with those of the tumour can be used to distinguish gestational from non-gestational tumours by demonstrating the presence of paternal genes in the tumour [12], and to determine the causative pregnancy in cases of gestational tumours [10, 11, 13, 14].

Establishing a diagnosis of choriocarcinoma in women with metastatic malignancy and a raised hCG is of great importance as the differential diagnosis includes carcinomas with trophoblastic differentiation (most commonly lung, bladder and gastric cancers), although non-trophoblastic tumours are rarely associated with hCG levels above 1000 iu/l. These carcinomas are incurable in the presence of widespread metastases and should be treated palliatively, whilst metastatic gestational choriocarcinoma remains curable despite dissemination. In patients with GTD it is useful to establish the responsible pregnancy, since both the nature of the causative pregnancy and the time interval between that pregnancy and diagnosis of the tumour are factors in determining the prognosis of the patient and hence the chemotherapy administered. Molecular genetic studies have shown that the immediately antecedent pregnancy may not be the causative pregnancy in some cases of choriocarcinoma, particularly where there is a history of molar pregnancy [12–14].

Genetic diagnosis was carried out on DNA prepared from blood samples from the patient and her husband and from pathological blocks of tissue from the first thoracotomy and removed at post mortem. Comparison of informative DNA polymorphisms in the tumour with those in parental DNA showed that both tissue from the lung metastases and from the post mortem tissue contained alleles which were paternally derived (Fig. 3), confirming that the tumour was gestational. In DNA from the lung metastases two further alleles were present which corresponded to the maternal alleles. The presence of both maternal alleles in DNA prepared from a gestational tumour generally results from contamination of the tumour tissue by normal host cells, which are difficult to exclude when tumours are small and heavily infiltrated by patient's cells. Comparison of the relative proportion of the two maternal alleles in the tumour with those in the maternal sample makes it possible to determine whether either maternal allele is present in excess indicating that the allele constitutes DNA both from the tumour and from contaminating patient cells. For five informative polymorphisms one maternal allele was present in excess suggesting that a maternal contribution was present in the tumour and thereby demonstrating that the tumour had arisen in a pregnancy resulting from a normal conception.

The DNA prepared from the post mortem sample was refractory to amplification by PCR for some of the pairs of primers used. However, three polymorphisms were informative. In each case only a single allele com-

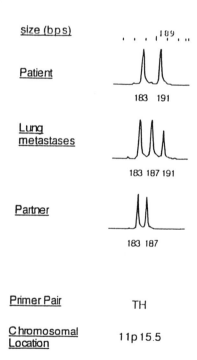

Fig. 3. DNA polymorphisms identified in the patient, tumour and her partner. This figure shows an electrophoretogram of DNA samples from the patient, her partner and metastatic lung tissue amplified with primers for a short tandem repeat sequence on chromosome 11p15. It demonstrates the presence of a paternal allele (187bp) in the tumour sample. The less abundant maternal allele (191bp) is contributed by contaminating non-malignant host cells.

patible with a maternal allele, was found showing that the DNA prepared from the tumour was free of contaminating host cells. For one set of primers two alleles were present, one maternally and the other paternally derived showing that the tumour had arisen in a biparental conception. For a second primer pair the tumour was homozygous for an allele present in both parents; for the third primers only a single maternal allele was present indicating loss of the paternal allele. Genetic analysis of choriocarcinoma has shown that they are generally aneuploid [9, 10, 15] and show duplication loss and rearrangement of chromosomes. Thus, unequal representation or loss of parental alleles would be expected, particularly in metastatic tumour samples. However, it was possible to clearly demonstrate that the tumour was gestational and had arisen in a biparental conception.

Tumour marker role in choriocarcinoma

Clinically active choriocarcinoma is excluded as a diagnosis by a normal serum hCG (<2 iu/l) although very elevated levels may be missed by conventional one-step radioimmunoassays [16]. In trophoblastic disease the hCG molecules in the urine and the serum include not only the intact molecule and α and β subunits, but also nicked and degraded core fragments which may not be detected by some assays. The normal serum half-life of hCG is 36 h and the molecule is excreted in the urine. For patients requiring renal support the clearance of hCG in the dialysate must be measured in order to follow the progress of treatment by the kinetics of the fall in tumour marker levels.

Grossly elevated hCG levels may be responsible for the development of clinically overt thyrotoxicosis due to ligand-receptor cross-reactivity between hCG and TSH. This effect has been demonstrated for testicular germ cell tumours with serum hCG levels in excess of 200,000 iu/l [17] although specific anti-thyroid treatment is rarely necessary.

Serum hCG levels are essential for following treatment and monitoring remission as well as for diagnosis. A normal hCG level is compatable with a tumour burden of up to 10^5 trophoblastic cells [18] and thus chemotherapy is continued for a number of cycles after a normal range value has been achieved. This marker should be measured regularly following the completion of treatment as rising markers may herald relapse before signs or symptoms develop. Late recurrences occasionally occur in trophoblastic tumours and so tumour marker follow-up is for life.

Treatment (including role of surgery and second line & experimental therapies)

The treatment of GTD is determined by a number of prognostic factors that stratify patients into low, medium and high risk groups. This is based upon a prognostic scoring system originally introduced by Bag-

shawe [6] and subsequently adopted by the World Health Organisation (WHO) [1] (Table 1). Initial treatment for high risk GTD at Charing Cross hospital is with a weekly combination chemotherapy schedule EMA/CO achieving an 80% complete clinical response rate and 82% survival with minimal toxicity in 76 high-risk patients who had received no prior therapy [2]. In patients who fail to achieve normal hCG levels with EMA/CO, tumours are generally only relatively drug resistant and a switch to platinum containing treatments will allow complete remission in approximately 40% of these patients. At Charing Cross the EP/EMA regimen is used in these circumstances. There is unpublished anecdotal evidence supporting the use of 5-fluorouracil in drug-resistant choriocarcinoma, and similarly a very small number of patients have received high dose chemotherapy with autologous progenitor cell rescue although no cases have reached publication. Choriocarcinoma cell growth in vitro is influenced by numerous cytokines [19] and this is the rationale behind the use of interferon and retinoids in this patient. An alternative approach for drug resistant tumour is to initiate a search for sites of residual disease with a view to surgical resection.

The role of surgery in the treatment of choriocarcinoma is generally restricted to resection of isolated foci of drug-resistant tumour and the prevention of haemorrhagic complications. Thoracotomy with pulmonary wedge resection or partial lobectomy is frequently undertaken for drug resistant lung metastases in GTD. However, the radiographic appearance lag behind the serological evidence of response. Resection of pulmonary metastases may induce remission in a few women with drug-resistant disease and in these cases it is important to exclude other sites of disease. Post operative serological remission and normal hCG levels a fortnight following surgery of an isolated pulmonary nodule predict a good outcome.

Disease within the CNS occurs in 8%–15% of patients with metastatic GTD, and is associated with a worse prognosis [6]. These metastases are highly vascular with a tendancy to haemorrhage accounting for a significant proportion of the early deaths. Early resection of brain metastases followed by combination chemotherapy is successful in the management of most patients with CNS involvement [20]. However, the surgical approach is rarely of benefit for drug-resistant lesions except for the emergency management of compressive or haemorrhagic complications.

Since the publication of this clinical case, the use of high dose chemotherapy followed by autologous bone marrow transplantation has been reported for five women with metastatic platinum-resistant gestational trophoblastic tumours. Two (40%) achieved complete remission of whom one relapsed after 2 months and one remains disease free after >5 years [21].

Rare presentations

The diagnosis of CNS metastases of GTD should be included in the differential diagnosis of any woman of reproductive age with a cerebral haemorrhage or CNS metastases with an unknown primary and a serum hCG should be measured in these patients. In addition hCG should be measured in women with unexplained pulmonary hypertension or multiple pulmonary emboli. Rarely choriocarcinoma may grow in the pulmonary arterial bed causing pulmonary artery obstruction resulting in multisegmental or unilateral loss of vascular markings and right ventricular enlargement and hypertrophy.

Long term side effects

Even in the presence of metastases, GTD is generally curable with chemotherapy [2], however great psychological pressures are felt by patients and their partners. These stresses include the loss of a pregnancy, a potentially life-threatening diagnosis, treatment with chemotherapy and/or surgery, and the delay of future pregnancy. It is not surprising that mood disturbances, sexual dysfunction and concerns over fertility occur in many patients and their partners [22]. In an analysis of 445 women treated at the Charing Cross Hospital 97% of those who wished to become pregnant succeeded and 86% of these had at least one live birth [23].

The incidence of second malignancies in 1,394 patients treated with chemotherapy for GTT was 37 compared to an expected rate of 24. The greatest increase in second tumours was myeloid leukaemia (relative risk 16.6) and all 5 patients who developed leukaemia had received etoposide as part of their treatment [24]. The overall results are reasonably reassuring although caution should be exercised in the use of etoposide unless it forms an essential part of patient management.

Further analysis of the risk of second tumours following chemotherapy for PTD has revealed that the increased risk was confined to women receiving combination chemotherapy and included significantly increased risks of colon cancer, breast cancer and melanoma (relative risks = 4.6, 5.8 & 3.4, respectively) as well as AML.

References

1. World Health Organisation Scientific Group. Gestational trophoblastic diseases. In Technical Report Series No. 692. Geneva: WHO 1983.
2. Newlands ES, Bagshawe KD, Begent RHJ et al. Results with the EMA/CO (etoposide, methotrexate, actinomycin D, cyclophosphamide, vincristine) regime in high risk gestational trophoblastic tumours, 1979 to 1989. Br J Obstet Gynaecol 1991; 98: 550–7.
3. Bagshawe KD, Harland S. Immunodiagnosis and monitoring of gonadotrophin-producing metastases in the central nervous system. Cancer 1976; 38: 112–8.
4. Begent R. Radioimmunolocalization of germ cell tumours. In Jones WG, Milford Ward A, Anderson CK (eds): Germ Cell Tumours II. Oxford: Pergamon Press 1986; 159–62.
5. Baltazar JC. Epidemiological features of choriocarcinoma. Bull WHO 1976; 54: 523.
6. Bagshawe KD. Risk and prognostic factors in trophoblastic neoplasia. Cancer 1976; 38: 1373–85.
7. Fisher RA, Lawler SD, Povey S et al. Genetically homozygous choriocarcinoma following pregnancy with hydatidiform mole. Br J Cancer 1988; 58: 788–92.
8. Bagshawe KD, Lawler SD, Paradinas FJ et al. Gestational trophoblastic tumours following initial diagnosis of partial hydatidiform mole. Lancet 1990; 335: 1074–6.
9. Wake N, Tanaka K-I, Chapman V et al. Chromosomes and cellular origin of choriocarcinoma. Cancer Res 1981; 41: 3137–43.
10. Chaganti RSK, Kodura PRK, Chakraborty R et al. Genetic origin of a trophoblastic choriocarcinoma. Cancer Res 1990; 50: 6330–33.
11. Osada H, Kawata M, Yamada M et al. Genetic identification of pregnancies responsible for choriocarcinomas after multiple pregnancies by restriction fragment length polymorphism analysis. Am J Obstet Gynecol 1991; 165: 682–8.
12. Fisher RA, Newlands ES, Jeffreys AJ et al. Gestational and non-gestational trophoblastic tumours distinguished by DNA analysis. Cancer 1992; 69: 839–45.
13. Suzuki T, Goto S, Nawa A et al. Identification of the pregnancy responsible for gestational trophoblastic disease by DNA analysis. Obstet Gynecol 1993; 82: 629–34.
14. Fisher RA, Soteriou B, Meredith L et al. Previous hydatidiform mole identified as the causative pregnancy of choriocarcinoma following birth of normal twins. Int J Gynecol Cancer 1995; 5: 64–70.
15. Sheppard DM, Fisher RA, Lawler SD. Karyotypic analysis and chromosome polymorphisms in four choriocarcinoma cell lines. Cancer Genet Cytogenet 1985; 16: 251–9.
16. O'Reilly SM, Rustin GJS. Mismanagement of choriocarcinoma due to a false low HCG measurement. Int J Gynecol Cancer 1993; 3: 186–8.
17. Giralt SA, Dexeus F, Amato R et al. Hyperthyroidism in men with germ cell tumors and high levels of beta-human chorionic gonadotrophin. Cancer 1992; 69: 1286–90.
18. Searle F, Boden J, Lewis JCM et al. A human choriocarcinoma xenograft in nude mice; a model for the study of antibody localization. Br J Cancer 1981; 44: 137–44.
19. Steller MA, Mok SC-H, Yeh et al. Effects of cytokines on epidermal growth factor receptor expression by malignant trophoblast cells in vitro. J Reprod Med 1994; 39: 209–16.
20. Rustin GJS, Newlands ES, Begent RHJ et al. Weekly alternating etoposide, methotrexate and actinomycin/vincristine and cyclophosphamide for the treatment of CNS metastases of choriocarcinoma. J Clin Oncol 1989; 7: 900–3.
21. Lotz J-P, André T, Donsimoni R et al. High dose chemotherapy with ifosfamide, carboplatin and etoposide combined with autologous bone marrow transplantation for the treatment of poor-prognosis germ cell tumors and metastatic trophoblastic disease in adults. Cancer 1995; 75: 874–85.
22. Wenzel LB, Berkowitz RS, Robinson S et al. Psychological, social and sexual effects of gestational trophoblastic disease on patients and their partners. J Reprod Med 1994; 39: 163–7.
23. Rustin GJS, Booth M, Dent J et al. Pregnancy after cytotoxic chemotherapy gestational trophoblastic tumours. Br Med J 1984; 288: 103–6.
24. Newlands ES, Rustin GJS, Holden L et al. Incidence of second tumours in patients treated with cytotoxic chemotherapy for gestational trophoblastic tumours (GTT) at Charing Cross Hospital 1958–1990. Proc VII World Congress on Gestational Trophoblastic Diseases, Hong Kong 1994.

R. L. Souhami (ed.) The Teaching Cases from Annals of Oncology, 117–119, 1997.

Male breast cancer

I. Besznyák & S. Eckhardt

Department of Surgery and Clinical Oncology, National Institute of Oncology, Budapest, Hungary

Key words: breast cancer, male breast cancer

Case history

A 71-year-old male patient had been aware for 3 years of a slowly-growing nodule in his left breast that began to produce a discharge in the 3 months prior to his presentation. The discharge became progressively blood-stained. Nevertheless, he consulted a doctor only one week before admission. Physical examination revealed an ulcerated mass retracting the nipple (Fig. 1) and involving the entire glandular substance. Axillary lymph nodes were clinically enlarged. Mastectomy with axillary block dissection was performed. The tumour proved to be a ductal invasive carcinoma (Fig. 2) positive for oestrogen and progesterone receptor by radio-immunoassay determination. Twelve of eighteen lymph nodes examined contained tumour metastasis. The patient was given postoperative radiotherapy /50 Gy/ to the chest wall and regional lymph node areas and received adjuvant tamoxifen in the dosage of 20 mg daily for a period of 18 months. He died three years after postoperative radiotherapy. The cause of death was not related to tumour. No autopsy was done.

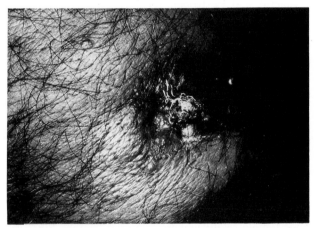

Fig. 1. Macroscopic image of the exulcerated breast cancer.

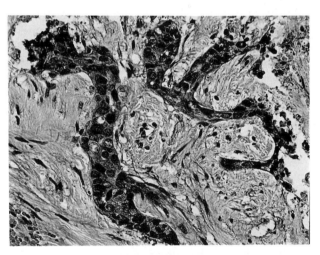

Fig. 2. Microphotogram of the tumour. Irregular nests of solid tumour cells in abundant connective tissue stroma. Size and staining character of cell nuclei are different. Nuclear grade 2. Hematoxylin-eosin stain. Original magnification ×300.

Discussion points

1. Epidemiology, etiopathology in male breast cancer

Recognition for the first report of male breast carcinoma should be given to the 14th century British physician John of Erderne. He discovered an enlarging mass beneath the right nipple of a priest in Colostone. A local barber-surgeon promised cure but John 'would let no cutting come there nigh' [11].

Male breast cancer is a rare disease, accounting for 1% of all breast cancers and 0.25% to 0.8% of male malignancies. In contrast to breast cancer in women, the incidence in men is not increasing. According to a WHO database [13] reviewing 25 European countries (not including the Soviet Union and a few small countries such as Andorra, Iceland and Liechtenstein) in the late 1980s, about 550–600 death per year from male breast cancer were certified in these countries. The variation was relatively limited, most age-standardized rates being within the range of 1.5 to 3.0 per million. These European data show the relatively highest incidence in France, Hungary, Austria, Scotland and Portugal while the lowest incidence is encountered in Italy, Finland, Sweden and Greece.

Most male breast cancers occur at around 60 years of age – about a decade later than in women. In men, the oestrogen content of the plasma originates partly from testicular secretions, and partly from transformation of the androgen precursors. In its development the importance of elevated plasma oestrogen levels, genetic factors [20], diffuse hepatic disease, Klinefelter syndrome, long-lasting or high-dose oestrogen therapy/ prostatic carcinoma, has been suggested [18]. A role for them has not yet been proved, for instance, a higher plasma oestrogen level is not always associated with male breast cancer [19]. Cohen et al. [5] suggested that the use of artificial light might change melatonin rhythms in a population, suppressing the usual nighttime high levels, and eventually leading to increases in prolactin and oestrogen receptor/ER-positive breast cancer rates. Evidence from the laboratory [10] indicates that the presence of melatonin can suppress the growth of ER-positive tumours. Male breast cancers are predominantly ER-positive and might be susceptible to these changes in melatonin. According to Matanoski et al. [16] the excess of male breast cancer which has been observed in workers potentially exposed to electro-magnetic fields (EMF) may support the theory that EMF exposure can change melatonin diurnal rhythms and thus lead to changes in the incidence of specific cancers. Familial occurrence of the disease is very rare among males. Nevertheless, approximately 60% of men affected by this malignancy have female relatives with mammary cancer. Since the discovery of BRCA-2 this observation might be explained by the potential presence of this gene in both sexes [21]. Suppressor gene alterations, especially those of p53 might also be detected [3].

2. Diagnosis and differential diagnosis in male breast cancer

The diagnosis – provided it is made – does not cause a problem in most cases. In spite of this a considerable number of patients consult a physician only in an advanced stage. The clinical and pathological TNM classification and staging of male breast cancer are the same as those used in female breast cancer. Due to the smaller size of the male breast the carcinoma often infiltrates the covering skin and the pectoral fascia as in the case described here. Most frequently, the tumour is localized on the subareolar region, sometimes deforming and ulcerating the nipple and causing discharge. Axillary lymph node metastases appear earlier than with female breast cancer. In the majority of tumours larger than 2 cm, axillary metastasis is already present. Thirty-eight of our 59 patients had axillary lymph node metastasis already at the time of surgery, in 3 cases distant metastasis was also present.

In addition to biochemical profile, investigation should include full blood count, chest x-ray and a Technetium 99 bone scan. The oestrogen and progesterone receptor content of the tumour tissue may be assessed.

Most male breast cancers are receptor-positive [19]. Twenty-five of 27 of our patients were oestradiol receptor-positive while progesterone receptor-positivity was present in 9 of 16 tumours. In a report of Ribeiro et al. [19] serum oestradiol, testosterone, follicle-stimulating hormone and luteinizing hormone estimates in ten patients with male breast cancer showed no significant difference from estimates made in 31 matched controls. No additional knowledge was gained in the analysis of the hormone profile of the patients. The profile was normal in all patients except for one with Klinefelter's syndrome.

The differential diagnosis includes primary cancer of the skin covering the breast, gynecomastia, and the inflammatory breast lesions. Histologic examination reveals ductal invasive carcinoma in 90% of the cases but other types also occur, as in the female breast.

3. Management of male breast cancer

Therapy of the disease is primarily surgical. While this used to mean Halsted's radical mastectomy, nowadays simple mastectomy with axillary block disection is the treatment of choice. We regard this latter as indispensable for determining the precise extent of the disease and the further therapeutic management. In cases where the pectoral fascia or the pectoral musculature are infiltrated these tissues must be excised. Due to the small size of the male breast, less radical surgery, which has become widely used in the treatment of female breast cancer, cannot be considered.

There is no consensus with regard to postoperative management. In view of the rarity of the disease, prospective, randomized studies have not been conducted. The earlier exclusive use of postoperative radiotherapy is now being complemented with, or often replaced by, adjuvant chemo- and hormone therapy, primarily based on the favourable therapeutic effect achieved in female breast cancer.

Adjuvant chemotherapy has usually consisted of CMF. According to Gateley and Mansel [8] the adjuvant chemotherapy with twelve cycles of cyclophosphamide, methotrexate and 5-fluorouracil in 24 men with axillary node metastases produced an estimated 5-year survival of over 80%. Twenty of 24 patients had no evidence of recurrent disease after a median follow-up time of 46 months. A review of the literature suggests that alkylating agents and doxorubicin are the most effective agents in the treatment of male breast cancer, although only a few drugs have been adequately tested [4]. We agree with Patel et al. [17] that the low incidence of this disease clearly necessitates multi-institutional or large cooperative studies to clearly define the role of adjuvant therapies in male breast cancer patients.

Kinne and Hakes [12] have summarized the literature of hormonal manipulation in male breast cancer.

The rate of overall response to hormonal treatment is 51% and rises to 71% in instances of oestrogen receptor-positivity. They warn, however, that the literature in this area is sparse and most reports on ablative procedures are from an earlier era when response criteria were ill-defined.

Ribero and Swindell [19] in 1976 initiated adjuvant tamoxifen treatment in stage II and operable stage III male breast cancer. The treatment duration was initially one and then two years. There were no serious side effects. The actuarial survival of the tamoxifen-treated patients is 61% at 5 years compared to 44% for historical controls.

Inoperable breast cancer used to be treated primarily by radiotherapy with surgical endocrine ablation by orchiectomy or adrenalectomy. Nowadays, in view of its lack of side effects, tamoxifen should be used as first-line treatment in advanced disease, and surgical endocrine ablation should be reserved for those patients who do not respond to tamoxifen or other methods of hormone manipulation. Growing experience underscores the effect of sexual hormone status on tumour response.

Responses to antioestrogens, antiandrogens, aminogluthetimide have been seen, and buserelin [6, 14, 15, 17] remains the major agent of palliation in disseminated male breast cancer.

4. Prognosis and survival

The prognosis of male breast cancer seems slightly poorer than that of female breast cancer. This may be due to the fact that the disease is already in an advanced stage at first detection. However, the prognosis of male breast cancer is possibly worse than that of female breast cancer of the same stage. Adami et al. [1] found that male breast cancer occurring in the elderly has a worse prognosis.

Borgen et al. [4] found the actuarial 5-year relapse-free survival to be 68% and the actuarial 5-year overall survival 85%. The relapse-free survival at 5 years for axillary node-negative patients was 87% and for node-positive patients 30%. In the study of Guinee et al. [9] the survival rate at 10 years was 84% for patients with histologically-negative nodes, 44% for those with one to three positive nodes, and 14% for the group with four or more histologically-positive nodes [9].

In our population (59 patients) the mean survival was 80.3 months and only 39 months in node-positive patients. Two-thirds of these patients died within 5 years compared with only 5% of the axillary node-negative patients. Only node-negative patients survived for ten years.

References

1. Adami HO, Hakulinen T, Ewertz M et al. The survival pattern in male breast cancer. An analysis of 1492 patients from the Nordic countries. Cancer 1989; 64: 1177–82.
2. Anderson DE, Badzioch MD. Breast cancer risk in relatives of male breast cancer patients. J Natl Cancer Inst 1992; 84: 1114–7.
3. Anelli A, Tania FMA, Youngson B et al. Mutations of the p53 gene in male breast cancer. Cancer 1995; 75: 2233–8.
4. Borgen PI, Wong GY, Vlamis V et al. Current management of male breast cancer. Ann Surg 1992; 215: 451–9.
5. Cohen M, Lippman M, Chapner B. Role of pineal gland in aetiology and treatment of breast cancer. Lancet 1978; 2: 814–6.
6. Crichlow RW, Galt SW. Male breast cancer. Surg Clin North Amer 1990; 70: 1165–77.
7. Demeter JG, Waterman NG, Verdi GD. Familial male breast carcinoma. Cancer 1990; 65: 2342–3.
8. Gateley CA, Mansel RE. Male breast cancer. Surgery /internat. edit./ 1991; 13: 2186–7.
9. Guinee VF, Olsson H, Moller T et al. The prognosis of breast cancer in males. Cancer 1993; 71: 154–61.
10. Hill SM, Blask DE. Effects of the pineal hormone melatonin on the proliferation and morphological characteristics of human breast cancer cells (MCF-7) in culture. Cancer Res 1988; 48: 6121–6.
11. Holleb Al, Freeman HP, Farrow JH. Cancer of male breast. NY State Med J 1968; 68: 544–53.
12. Kinne D, Hakes T. Male breast cancer. In Harris JR, Hellman JS, Henderson C et al. (eds): Breast diseases, Vol. 2. Lippincott JP: Philadelphia 1991; 782–90.
13. La Vecchia C, Levi F, Lucchini F. Descriptive epidemiology of male breast cancer in Europe. Int J Cancer 1992; 51: 62–6.
14. Lopez M, Di Lauro L, Papaldo P et al. Chemotherapy in metastatic male breast cancer. Oncology 1985; 42: 205–9.
15. Lopez M, Di Lauro L, Lazzaro B et al. Hormonal treatment of disseminated male breast cancer. Oncology 1985; 42: 345–9.
16. Matanoski GM, Breysse PN, Elliott EA. Electromagnetic field exposure and male breast cancer. Lancet 1991; 337: 737–7.
17. Patel HZ, Buzdar AU, Hortobágyi GN. Role of adjuvant chemotherapy in male breast cancer. Cancer 1989; 64: 1583–5.
18. Pejovic LMH, Cabanne MN, Bouchardy C et al. Risk factors for male breast cancer; a Franco-Swiss case-control study. Int J Cancer 1990; 45: 661–5.
19. Ribeiro R, Swindell R. Adjuvant tamoxifen for male breast cancer (MBC). Br J Cancer 1992; 65: 252–4.
20. Stephens RL, Schimke RN. Case report; breast cancer in males – A genetic consideration. Am J Med Sci 1992; 304: 91–2.
21. Wooster R, Neuhausen SL, Mangion Y et al. Localization of a breast cancer susceptibility gene, BRCA 2, to chromosome 13g 12–13 BRCAZ chr 13q 12–13. Science 1994; 266: 120–2.

R. L. Souhami (ed.) The Teaching Cases from Annals of Oncology, 121–131, 1997.
© 1997 *Kluwer Academic Publishers. Printed in the Netherlands.*

First-line systemic therapy for metastatic breast cancer and management of pleural effusion

F. Perrone, C. Carlomagno, S. De Placido, R. Lauria, A. Morabito & A. R. Bianco
*Division of Medical Oncology, Department of Molecular and Clinical Endocrinology and Oncology, School of Medicine, University
'Federico II', Naples, Italy*

Key words: metastatic breast cancer, chemotherapy, endocrine therapy, pleural effusion

Case report

S.A. was a 35-year-old woman when, in October 1988, she discovered a nodule in her right breast and was referred to a surgeon. She had a family history of breast cancer and was nulliparous. Physical examination revealed a stony hard nodule of 2.5 cm in diameter in the upper medial quadrant of her right breast. Mammography confirmed a breast mass and cytological examination was positive for malignant cells. Chest X-ray, bone scan, liver ultrasonography and complete blood chemistry all yielded normal results. The patient then underwent a modified radical mastectomy. Histological examination showed infiltrating ductal carcinoma without axillary nodal involvement (pT2G2N0, stage I). A hormone receptor assay was not performed and no adjuvant therapy was given after surgery. She had no recurrence during the next 52 months. In February 1993, the now-40-year-old patient was referred to our institution for the first time with a persistent non-productive cough and dyspnea. Physical examination revealed right-sided dullness to percussion, decreased vocal fremitus and breath sounds. There was expansion of the right hemithorax with an absence of diaphragmatic movement. Chest X-ray (Fig. 1a, b) revealed a middle-basal opacification in the right hemithorax with mediastinal shift to the left and a solid mass in the middle zone of the right lung. Thoracentesis was performed, and cytological examination of the effusion demonstrated malignant cells in pleural fluid. Chest computed tomography (CT) showed a solid mass in the right lung and enlargement of mediastinal lymph nodes (Fig. 2a, b). Bone scan showed increased radionuclide uptake in the sternum but sternal X-ray revealed no osteolytic or osteoblastic lesions. Results of a liver scan and mammography of the left breast were negative.

The patient was eligible for a phase I trial of high-dose chemotherapy for advanced breast cancer. She received 4 courses of chemotherapy with epirubicin (82.5 mg/m^2) and cyclophosphamide (2.250 mg/m^2)

plus G-CSF support at three-week intervals. In June 1993, the restaging procedures showed a partial remission of disease. The chest X-ray revealed persistence of blunting of the costophrenic angle; thoracic CT scan showed a disappearance of lung and nodal metastases; bone scan showed a reduction of sternal uptake; liver scan and mammography results remained negative.

The patient continued on chemotherapy for six courses of standard EC (epirubicin 60 mg/m^2, cyclophosphamide 600 mg/m^2). She developed amenorrhea with the first cycle of chemotherapy. At the end of chemotherapy (October 1993) she was put on endocrine treatment with tamoxifen (30 mg/day). At the present time (2 years later) her disease has not progressed and she is continuing on tamoxifen therapy.

Systemic therapeutic approach to metastatic breast cancer

General issues

Despite innumerable studies, there are no definite guidelines as to the best therapeutic strategy for metastatic breast cancer. As a general rule, the therapeutic approach should be based on systemic treatment because this is a systemic disease. In certain situations local therapy may be essential (e.g., bone metastasis which is painful or likely to cause a fracture, spinal cord compression, life-threatening pleural or pericardial effusions and brain metastasis). In these clinical situations, local therapies (surgery or radiotherapy) may be used before, during, or after systemic treatment.

Metastatic breast cancer may be considered moderately responsive to both chemo- and endocrine therapy. At first-line treatment, the response rate is 40%–60% with chemotherapy and 30% to 70% after endocrine therapy in unselected and estrogen receptor-positive patients, respectively.

The two end-points, both tumor-related, most

122

widely used to estimate the activity or efficacy of therapies are response rate (an approximate measure of the tumor shrinkage after the treatment) and time to progression. Treatment for metastatic breast cancer is rarely evaluated by using patient-oriented end-points such as survival and quality of life. The relationships between tumor- and patient-oriented end-points have not been completely clarified. Analyses of quality-of-life scores have demonstrated a direct correlation between quality of life and response, i.e., higher the response rate the better the quality of life, regardless of the toxic effects of treatment [1, 2] or of its duration [3]. The rate of symptom relief (so-called 'subjective response'), which is a component of quality-of-life analysis, usually exceeds the response rate [4]. The relationships between response rate and survival are more controversial and subject to bias. The longer survival reported for patients who experience objective responses does not necessarily demonstrate that response prolongs survival. This is because the prognostic characteristics of longer-surviving patients (good performance status, absence of co-morbidity, less aggressive disease) are such that they are more likely to obtain a response than are those with shorter survivals. Thus, analysis of patient survival by tumor response can be biased and misleading rather than helpful [5]. However, a meta-analysis of randomised trials has suggested a significant direct relationship between response rate and survival (the higher the response rate the longer the median survival) and that 37% of the

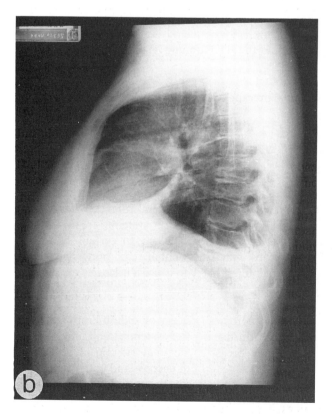

Fig. 1. Pre-treatment postero-anterior (a) and lateral (b) chest X-ray showing right pleural effusion, and a solitary nodule in the mid-zone of the right lung.

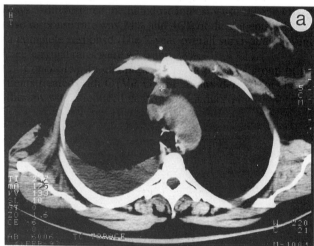

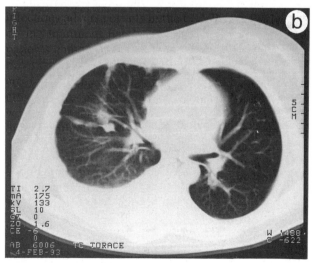

Fig. 2. Pre-treatment chest CT scan without (a) and with (b) e.v. enhancement showing right pleural effusion, mediastinal metastatic lymph nodes and a solid mass with infiltrating margins.

variation seen in survival can be explained by variation in the response rate [6] as an independent variable.

Which therapy should be used first, endocrine or cytotoxic?

In general, the therapeutic decision-making process for metastatic breast cancer is an exclusion-based strategy. It is easier to determine which treatment is likely to be useless than which may be effective. Because cure is unlikely and palliation is the major goal, one should aim at obtaining the best result with minimum toxicity. Thus, a general rule could be that the first-line approach should be endocrine treatment unless it is contra-indicated. In case of factors contra-indicating endocrine treatment the alternative should be chemotherapy. What are these factors?

Firstly, a life-threatening disease with aggressive visceral dissemination and multi-organ involvement. There is some evidence that patients with involvement of soft tissues and bone are more likely to respond to endocrine therapy than those with visceral (lung and liver) involvement.

Secondly, the presence on tumor cells of receptors for steroid hormones is a strong predictor of responsiveness to endocrine therapy in metastatic breast cancer [7–9]. Thus, for receptor-negative patients endocrine treatment could be supplanted by chemotherapy as the first treatment, although the absence of steroid receptors does not totally preclude any activity of endocrine treatment [10, 11].

Thirdly, young premenopausal patients have rapidly disseminating disease, with multi-organ involvement, more frequently than do older postmenopausal patients. However, they usually have a better performance status, with no or minor comorbidity and a better tolerance for haematologic and cardiac toxic effects of chemotherapy than older patients. Consequently, endocrine treatment is usually not the first choice for young premenopausal patients, although young age and premenopausal status are not absolute contra-indications for endocrine therapy as first-line treatment. Estrogen production by the ovaries may be easily stopped either surgically with ovarian ablation, or pharmacologically with LHRH antagonist analogues that ultimately inhibit hypophyseal gonadotropin release. After the cessation of ovarian activity, patients are fully postmenopausal, regardless of age.

Finally, more patients are now relapsing during or shortly after adjuvant tamoxifen, because of the trend towards prolonging tamoxifen therapy for 5 years or more after surgery and extending it to node-negative patients [12, 13]. After 2 years of adjuvant tamoxifen, a decreased activity (14% response rate) of first-line endocrine treatment (tamoxifen ± fluoxymesterone) as compared with that in relapsed patients who had received no adjuvant tamoxifen (54% response rate) was reported by Fornander et al. [14]. Similar results were obtained in the Guy's-Manchester study [15].

The choice of first-line treatment can also be dictated by factors that contra-indicate chemotherapy as opposed to endocrine therapy.

The first of these factors is age. Although chronological age might not correspond to biological age, clinical trials and guidelines on chemotherapy often use the age of 70 as a threshold for eligibility; this threshold is lower in trials of high-dose chemotherapy. A patient above 70 years of age with metastatic breast cancer may have cardiac co-morbidity that is incompatible with anthracycline therapy. Her bone marrow tolerance may be lower so that longer intervals between chemotherapy cycles or dose reductions are required, with a decreased dose-intensity and chemotherapy activity. There may be ambulatory problems due to chronic diseases, which can hamper chemotherapy delivery or frequent staging and restaging procedures. However, these are relative, and not absolute, contra-indications.

Chemotherapy is sometimes contra-indicated for patients who have relapsed during adjuvant chemotherapy or shortly after its completion. This principle is less stringent than for endocrine treatment, because chemotherapy regimens with some degree of non-cross resistance can be used, and also because breast cancer which relapses during adjuvant chemotherapy is usually a very aggressive disease and thus not amenable to endocrine therapy. Independently of the disease-free interval, there is conflicting data on the effect of previous adjuvant chemotherapy on first-line chemotherapy for metastatic disease. Some studies have found that previous adjuvant chemotherapy does not affect the rate of response to either endocrine or cytotoxic first line treatment [16–18] and, by contrast, that previous adjuvant CMF lowers the response rate to first-line treatment with both endocrine and cytotoxic therapy [19].

Finally, patients may not agree to undergo chemotherapy because of side effects, especially hair loss. Although doctors should do their best to give each patient the optimal treatment, the choice of first-line treatment may depend on the patient's wish rather than on the expected response rate or time to progression.

When cytotoxic therapy is indicated, which regimen is the best?

The options for first-line chemotherapy are much more numerous than for endocrine therapy, which makes the choice more difficult. When possible it is desirable to enter patients into clinical trials (Fig. 3). Randomised phase III studies are essential to determine which treatment regimens and dose levels are most active. Phase I and phase II studies are of two types. Those aimed at determining the maximum tolerable dose and testing the toxicity and activity of new compounds should be limited to a second- or third-line approach to metastatic breast cancer, because the chance of response is less than 5% [20]. Those aimed at defining maximum tolerable dose and testing the toxicity and activity of known

124

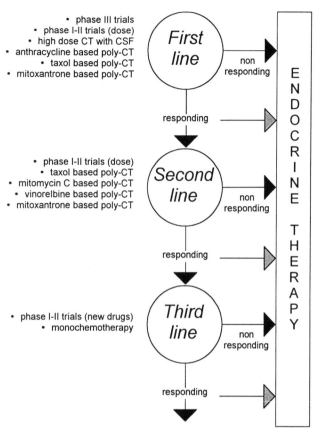

Fig. 3. Flow chart of cytotoxic therapy options for metastatic breast cancer (CT = chemotherapy; CSF = colony-stimulating factors).

active drugs (or combinations of drugs) given with supportive strategies (CSF, PBSC, chemoprotectants) which overcome the standard-dose limiting toxic effects [21] can reasonably be proposed as first-line treatment because there is little risk of offering inadequate treatment.

Studies on tumor-bearing animals treated with alkylating agents [22] pointed to a direct relationship between dose intensity (i.e., the amount of drug per time unit) and the percentage of tumor shrinkage (tumor response), and between total dose and duration of responses (time to progression) and survival. If this is true in human cancer, a high response rate might be expected with the high dose-intensity strategy, and prolonged survival with the high total dose approach.

The former expectation has been suggested in breast cancer by a number of studies which, unfortunately, are mostly non-randomised phase II trials. Verification of efficacy from randomised trials is still required. The use of high-dose chemotherapy (HD-CT) with autologous bone marrow transplantation (ABMT) rapidly increased between 1989 and 1992 in North America [23]. In 1992, in a review of published non-randomised studies [24], both the objective response rate (70% vs. 39%) and the complete response rate (36% vs. 8%) were increased after high-dose treatment with bone marrow support, as compared indirectly with standard-dose chemotherapy. In the same year, it was concluded that the HD-CT + ABMT strategy provides substantial

benefit but with untenable costs [25]. A survival advantage has been reported [26] for metastatic breast cancer patients responding to standard-dose induction chemotherapy who underwent HD-CT consolidation with ABMT, but only as compared with historical data of the SWOG database. Median survival was 21–24 months versus 10 months, and the 2-year disease-free survival rate was 17%–26% versus 5%. Historical comparisons have often been misleading in cancer therapy. Autotransplant with peripheral hematologic progenitor cells has made dose intensification easier because of its lower toxicity and higher activity [27].

However, chemotherapy of increased intensity may be administered without stem cell rescue. This can be done by shortening the interval between cycles of standard-dose chemotherapy or by increasing single doses, plus CSF support. With the first strategy (accelerated chemotherapy) the dose intensity may increase by about only 1.5 times. Nevertheless, in a randomised trial on 62 metastatic breast cancer patients, there was an increased response rate (68.9% vs. 41.6%, p = 0.09) with 'accelerated CEF' (cyclophosphamide, epirubicin, fluorouracil) recycling every 2 weeks plus GM-CSF support versus 'standard CEF' recycling every 3 weeks without CSF [28]. The patient described here was part of a recently completed study [29] in which, by modifying the schedule and the amount of single doses of epirubicin and cyclophosphamide with CSF support, the dose intensity was more than 3 times the standard dose intensity; the response rate was very high, with 33 objective responses among 39 treated patients (84.6%; 95% confidence limits: 73.3%–95.9%). These observations indicate that response rate is increased by increased dose intensity. The impact on survival is not clear.

The relationship between total dose and time to progression or survival is still debated. Randomised studies on this topic have yielded conflicting results. Coates et al. [3] randomised 305 patients to continuous chemotherapy (until progression or 18th month of treatment), or intermittent chemotherapy (i.e. stopping after 3 cycles and restarting the same treatment upon disease progression). Median time to progression (6.0 vs. 4.0 months, p < 0.001) and survival (10.7 vs. 9.4 months, p = 0.07) were longer for patients treated with continuous chemotherapy. The patients' quality of life, measured with seven linear analogue self-assessment scores, improved during the first three cycles, when all patients were treated. Thereafter, scores (for physical well-being, mood, appetite, patient-indicated and doctor-indicated quality of life indexes) worsened in association with intermittent chemotherapy; this finding may be partly explained by the lower response rate (32% vs. 49%, p = 0.02) obtained with the intermittent chemotherapy; furthermore, recent evidence suggests that retreatment of patients with the same induction therapy after progression of disease is not beneficial [30]. Harris et al. [31] compared the efficacy of short-term (4 cycles) with continuous (until progression) mitoxantrone in a randomised trial with 132 patients; no difference was observed in median time to progression (6 vs. 5 months) and median survival (12 vs. 11 months). However, both the low response rate (30%) and the short median survival (overall, less than 1 year) suggest that single-drug therapy with mitoxantrone was less active than standard 3-drug combinations and a kind of threshold effect may not be discounted since any benefit of prolonging treatment might be evident only with more active treatments. In contrast with Harris and in agreement with Coates, Ejlertsen et al. [32] in a trial with 318 patients randomised to 6 months vs. 18 months of FEC reported a significant advantage in median time to progression (10 vs. 14 months) and median survival (18 vs. 23 months) for patients receiving 18 months of chemotherapy. Both the survival outcome and response rate (52%) of that trial are comparable with other studies.

Excluding clinical trials, optimal first-line chemotherapy could be a combination of drugs including cyclophosphamide, methotrexate, 5-fluorouracil, doxo- or epi-doxorubicin. In general, combination regimens containing anthracyclines have been shown to induce an overall higher response rate than those without anthracyclines (Table 1). Also, prolongation of time to progression has been reported with FEC as compared to CMF [33, 34]. The advantage in survival for anthracycline-treated patients is probably small, if any, so that randomised trials do not show statistically significant differences [34]. On the other hand, myelosuppression, vomiting, alopecia and cardiotoxicity are more frequent with anthracycline-containing regimens. Thus, the choice of initial chemotherapy for metastatic breast cancer should be based on a balance between planned activity and toxicity. Many physicians prefer including adriamycin (A) or its analogue epirubicin (E) in the first-line polychemotherapy scheme, the most common association being with cyclophosphamide and fluorouracil (FAC, FEC), unless previous adjuvant treatment with an anthracycline had been administered. In the latter case regimens without anthracyclines are preferable.

Recently, the doxorubicin-taxol combination was found to be active [35]. In view of its high activity as a

single drug [36], taxol holds promise also for patients not eligible for anthracycline-based chemotherapy. Many trials are ongoing to define taxol-based regimens that do not include anthracyclines; promising results have been obtained with the taxol-cyclophosphamide and taxol-cisplatin combinations [37]. Mitoxantrone is also an active drug for metastatic breast cancer; the combination of mitoxantrone with cyclophosphamide and fluorouracil (CNF) has recently been compared in a randomised trial with the FAC scheme [38]: the response rate was the same (68%) and median survival was similar (19 vs. 18 months), while the median time to progression was not reported. Furthermore, mitoxantrone has some activity also in patients pre-treated with an adjuvant anthracycline [39]. Vinorelbine is also active in metastatic breast cancer [40] and a 74% response rate has been reported in a series of 89 stage IV breast cancer patients treated with a vinorelbine-plus-adriamycin combination [41].

In summary, a wide variety of chemotherapy regimens have activity in advanced breast cancer. The use of more dose-intensive regimens is still under investigation. The choice of first regimen depends on many factors including activity and toxicity profile and whether the patient has received adjuvant treatment.

When endocrine treatment is indicated, which drug should be used first?

A flow chart for endocrine treatment of metastatic breast cancer is illustrated in Fig. 4. In premenopausal women either tamoxifen or oophorectomy will be the initial approach of choice [42]. Although the two treatment modalities are equally effective, ovarian ablation by surgery, radiation or LH-RH analogues remains the classical treatment. In postmenopausal women, tamoxifen is usually given as first-line treatment because of its activity and low incidence of side effects. Progestins are also active and in some cases are preferable to tamoxifen. The two progestins now available are medroxyprogesterone acetate (MPA) and megestrol acetate (MA). Randomised trials of these drugs have shown that high-dose administration induces higher response rates than low- or standard-dose [43, 44] and that high-dose MA prolongs time to progression and survival when compared with standard dose [44].

Randomised clinical trials have compared tamoxifen with either MPA or MA (Table 2). In the study of van Veelen et al. [45] 129 postmenopausal patients received either tamoxifen 40 mg/daily or MPA 900 mg/daily, both orally. The overall response rate was somewhat higher in the MPA arm (35% with tamoxifen and 44% with MPA) and, in the subgroup of patients with bone metastasis, the difference was statistically significant (23% vs. 44%). Data on time to progression were not reported, but there was no significant difference in median survival. The Swiss Group for Clinical Cancer Research [10] published a similar phase III study involving 119 postmenopausal patients receiving first-

Table 1. Randomised trials of polychemotherapy without or with anthracyclines in metastatic breast cancer.

Author [ref.]	Treatment arms		No. of pts	Response rate (%)		
	Without	With		Without		With
Smalley [33]	CMFVP	vs. FAC	113	37	vs.	64
Bull [87]	CMF	vs. FAC	78	62	vs.	82
Muss [88]	CMFVP	vs. CAFVP	148	57	vs.	58
Tormey [89]	CMF±P	vs. AV	331	60	vs.	56
Tormey [90]	CMFVP	vs. CAFVP	216	50	vs.	71
Cummings [91]	CMFP	vs. FAC	155	53	vs.	53
Aisner [92]	CMF	vs. CAF±VP	260	37	vs.	56
Madsen [93]	CMF	vs. CAF	344	37	vs.	56

line endocrine treatment. Tamoxifen 20 mg/day orally was compared with the high-dose MPA schedule (1 g/day i.m. 5 days/week for 4 weeks and then 500 mg twice a week) previously reported to be active [43]. MPA induced a higher response rate than tamoxifen (50% vs. 30%) with a non-significantly longer time to progression (8.8 vs. 5.4 months) and survival (28 vs. 20 months). On the other hand, MPA was associated with more toxic effects, namely hypertension, weight gain and tremor.

Gill et al. [11] reported a phase III study with 184 postmenopausal patients randomised to tamoxifen 40 mg/daily or standard-dose MA (160 mg daily) or a combination of the two. There were no significant dif-

ferences in response rate, median time to progression or survival. Recently, Muss et al. [9] reported a study comparing tamoxifen 20 mg/day with high-dose oral MPA (1 g/day) in 182 randomised patients. The response rate was significantly lower with tamoxifen than with MPA (17% vs. 34%), the differences being due mainly to the response of bone metastases; no significant difference was evident in median time to progression (5.5 and 6.3 months) or median survival. One-third of the patients treated with first-line MPA suffered significant weight gain.

In summary, high-dose MPA may be associated with a higher response rate than tamoxifen, especially in bone metastasis, but there is little difference in time to progression or survival.

Pharmacologic and clinical activity of aromatase inhibitors have recently been reviewed [46]. Among first-generation compounds, aminogluthetimide is the most widely used in metastatic breast cancer as second- or third-line treatment; usually it is associated with corticosteroid replacement therapy to overcome inhibition of the physiologic surrenalic enzymatic pathway. Recently, second-generation compounds have been produced that are more selective than aminogluthetimide and do not require the coadministration of corticosteroids. Of these new agents, formestane [47, 48], fadrazole [49] and Arimidex [50] have shown activity against metastatic breast cancer. Although early phase III trials comparing these new drugs with either tamoxifen or progestins have recently been presented [50, 51], further larger randomised trials are still needed to confirm the efficacy of these compounds and to elucidate their possible role as alternatives to tamoxifen and progestins.

The treatment of metastatic pleural effusion in breast cancer

Pleural effusion is a frequent occurrence in breast cancer; indeed about 50% of patients with metastatic disease will develop a malignant pleural effusion at some time during their illness [52–54]. In malignant disease, pleural effusion is an exudate (protein content > 3 g/dl) and is due to pleural metastasis that disrupts the capil-

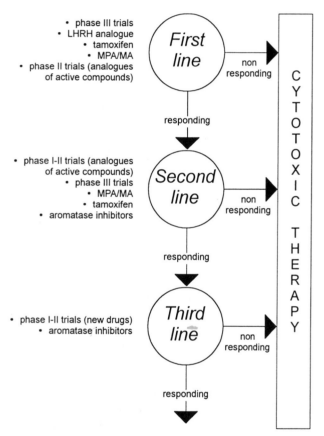

Fig. 4. Flow chart of endocrine therapy options for metastatic breast cancer (LHRH = luteinising hormone releasing hormone; MPA = medroxy-progesterone acetate; MA = megestrol acetate).

Table 2. Randomised trials comparing tamoxifen with progestins in first-line therapy of metastatic breast cancer.

Author [ref.]	Arms	No. pts	Response rate	Median TTP (months)	Median survival (months)
van Veelen [45]	TM vs. hd-MPA	68 vs. 61 postmenopausal	35% vs. 44%	23 vs. 17	26 vs. 20
Castiglione-Gertsch [10]	TM vs. hd-MPA	64 vs. 55 postmenopausal	30% vs. 50% (p = 0.023)	5.4 vs. 8.8 (p = 0.051)	20 vs. 28 (n.s.)
Gill [11]	TM vs. MA	58 vs. 60 postmenopausal	26% vs. 37%	7.7 vs. 3.8	n.r. (n.s.)
Muss [9]	TM vs. hd-MPA	91 vs. 91	17% vs. 34% (p = 0.01)	5.5 vs. 6.3 (n.s.)	24 vs. 33 (p = 0.09)

lary endothelium, impairs resorption and causes inflammatory changes, thus contributing to the accumulation of the fluid in the pleural space. In most cases (60%–70%) the pleural effusion is ipsilateral to the mastectomy, leading to the postulation that is the result of loco-regional spreading through lymphatic vessels rather than a hematogenous metastasis [55, 56]. However, data from a recent study that evaluated by thoracoscopy the intrathoracic involvement at first presentation of pleural effusion, suggest that malignant pleural effusion is due to systemic spread to the visceral pleura [57]. About 75% of patients with pleural effusion are symptomatic, the most common symptoms being dyspnea, cough and chest pain. The severity of symptoms depends on the rapidity with which the fluid has accumulated rather than its total amount.

Assessment of the response to therapy is difficult [58] without an agreed-upon definition. Variability in response assessment makes it difficult to compare the results of published studies. The most accepted and widely used criteria for response assessment are those published by Paladine [59]: a complete response is no further reaccumulation of fluid for longer than 30 days; a partial response is minimal fluid recurrence as noted by X-ray, but not symptomatic and not requiring further thoracentesis within 30 days; failure is reaccumulation of fluid within 30 days requiring thoracentesis.

The primary aims in management are early diagnosis and rapid relief of symptoms. In most solid tumours, the majority of patients with pleural effusion will die within six months [60]. In contrast, the reported median survival time of patients with pleural effusion due to breast cancer ranges from 6 to 16 months [53, 61]. Consequently, the therapeutic approach, beyond the rapid relief of symptoms, should aim at long-lasting remission.

The choice of the optimal strategy for the treatment of the pleural effusion in breast cancer patients is influenced by the following factors: a) the presence and degree of the symptoms; b) the overall condition of the patient (sites of metastasis, performance status, whether the patient is likely to benefit from chemo- or endocrine therapy); c) life expectancy; d) the possible side effects of each treatment considered.

In patients with asymptomatic limited pleural effusion, as determined by X-ray or CT scan, the best systemic therapy chosen on the basis of the state of their disease, is the preferred one. For symptomatic pleural effusion, some form of local treatment is required in addition to systemic therapy.

Overall responses to systemic therapy as first treatment for pleural effusion range between 18% and 50% [62–64]. Nevertheless, systemic therapy as the initial treatment for breast cancer patients with pleural effusion can be considered only in patients with a moderate amount of fluid who have a good chance of response. When patients show no response, or if they are initially unlikely to have a response to systemic therapy, local treatment should be started.

The most useful local treatments are: 1. *Thoracentesis*. Fine needle evacuation of fluid accumulated in the pleural space alone is ineffective in controlling malignant pleural effusions [52, 65]. It should be used only for diagnostic purposes and when rapid relief of symptoms is required. Multiple thoracenteses increase the risk of complications such as pneumothorax and empyema [54], and of inducing loculations and adhesions which could cause the failure of further sclerosing treatment due to the inability of the lung to expand [66].

2. *Thoracostomy tube drainage.* The complete evacuation of pleural fluid by placement into the pleural space of a chest tube connected to an underwater-seal drainage system has yielded contradictory results ranging from no control [52] to 50% control of pleural effusion [65]. However, this technique alone is no longer used because it is not as effective as pleurodesis.

3. *Pleurodesis*. Thoracostomy tube drainage plus the instillation of a sclerosing agent into the pleural space is the most widely used local treatment for malignant pleural effusion [53, 54, 59, 66]. Over the past 30 years, many substances have been used to obtain pleurodesis. Although quinacrine, nitrogen mustard and radioactive isotopes have been able to control pleural effusion in more than 50% of cases [52, 53, 65, 67, 68], all of these are now of merely historical interest, having been replaced by more effective and less toxic agents. Tetracycline, talc and bleomycin are the most widely used sclerosing agents. The best agent is still a matter of debate as they differ slightly in technique of administration, cost and toxic effects. In addition, their mechanism of action is still unclear. In many institutions tetracycline intrapleural administration is the treatment of choice because of its efficacy, low cost, minimal toxicity and ease of manipulation [54, 62, 69–71]. The optimal dose of tetracycline is not clear; the most widely used dose is 500 mg dissolved in 50–100 ml of saline solution, but there is some evidence that ≥ 1 gr may be more effective [70].

Bleomycin is an alternative to tetracycline. In uncontrolled trials it controls more than 60% of malignant pleural effusions, with very limited side effects [59, 72]. For bleomycin there is not a dose-response correlation, so the dose of 60 mg, which is effective and relatively non-toxic, can be recommended for routine use [72]. Whereas tetracycline acts by provoking fibrosis in the pleural space consequent to the inflammatory reaction, bleomycin does not induce a very strong inflammatory reaction and about 45% of it is adsorbed systemically, suggesting that its action in controlling pleural effusion could be due, at least partially, to an antineoplastic effect [73, 74]. In addition to its good performance in the uncontrolled trials, bleomycin induced a better response than tetracycline in a randomised trial [75]. In conclusion, bleomycin seems to be very effective in controlling malignant pleural effusions, even though its use is restricted by a higher cost and somewhat greater systemic toxicity than those associated with tetracycline.

The instillation of sterile talc powder through the thoracostomy tube is a very effective method for obtaining pleurodesis, and over 80% of subjects obtained objective response with this procedure in both uncontrolled [67, 76, 77] and randomised trials [67, 78]. However, the high degree of discomfort for patients, due to chest pain and general anesthesia, limit its widespread application.

Another category of substances used to control pleural effusion because of their action as simple irritants and as modifiers of the immune response, are the biologic agents. One of the first agents tested was the *Corynebacterium parvum* that controls malignant pleural effusion in about 50% of cases [79, 80]; however, it frequently causes chest pain and fever.

More recently, beta-interferon (β-INF) and interleukin-2 (IL-2) have been used to obtain pleurodesis. After evacuation of pleural effusion by simple needle thoracentesis, β-INF is introduced through the thoracentesis needle into the pleural space. The starting dose is generally 5 million units. The treatment can be repeated twice in instances of recurrence at intervals of one week, with the dosage increased up to 15 million. The response is generally assessed within one month of the last thoracentesis. Thus far, this strategy does not seem to be as effective as other sclerosing agents and the results obtained are not consistent [81, 82].

The use of IL-2 alone [83] or in combination with LAK cells [84] seems to have better results, but further studies are required to confirm early reports.

The success of the pleurodesis technique depends on: i) complete drainage of the effusion before instillation of the sclerosant; ii) efficacy of the sclerosing agent; and iii) completeness of lung reexpansion.

4. Pleural-peritoneal shunt. In patients in whom the lung cannot completely reexpand after fluid evacuation ('trapped lung') due to loculated effusion, adhesions or fibrotic cortex, pleurodesis is usually unsuccessful. In this setting, a pleural-peritoneal shunt can be an effective alternative. This technique, which requires the insertion of a shunt to permit the discharge of the pleural effusion into the peritoneal cavity [85], was first described in the mid-80s. The early reports show this treatment to be an effective and safe strategy of palliation for patients who fail or are not likely to respond to pleurodesis [66].

5. Pleurectomy. The stripping of the parietal pleura has been reported to control the pleural effusion in more than 80% of cases [52, 86]. However, it is infrequently used because of its high morbidity (about 29% postoperative complication) and mortality (about 9%), and of the availability of alternative techniques which are as effective but less toxic.

needle thoracentesis that allowed both cytological diagnosis and partial relief of symptoms. She was young and premenopausal; the ER status of her primary tumor was unknown. Staging revealed multiple-site disease with visceral involvement in the lung and mediastinum and a pleural effusion. Bone scan positivity, unconfirmed by X-ray, was considered suggestive of bone metastasis. No further evaluation of the sternum was made because the results would not have affected the therapeutic strategy. The patient had never received chemotherapy and she was eligible for a clinical trial on high-dose chemotherapy with G-CSF support. Local treatment of pleural effusion was not considered because of a good chance of her response to systemic therapy. The dose-intensive treatment rapidly induced the complete disappearance of symptoms, which had already been reduced by thoracentesis. After restaging, a partial response was recorded. This assessment is difficult because residual fibrosis after the disappearence of an effusion produces a radiologic pattern (blunting of the costophrenic angle) similar to the persistence of a small amount of fluid. Based on the good response achieved with the experimental high-dose approach, the patient continued on standard-dose chemotherapy to reach a high total dose of chemotherapy, with the aim of prolonging the duration of response. After the end of first-line chemotherapy, she was considered to be in stable remission.

Figure 3 outlines the possibilities for treating patients with endocrine therapy after response to chemotherapy. Whether this strategy improves survival is not known, and clinical trials are required to address this question. We are of the opinion that first-line endocrine treatment should always be considered for patients who completed their first-line chemotherapy and are still responding. It may happen, as in the case reported above, that reassessement of the disease leads to a re-evaluation of initiating endocrine treatment. In our case, visceral metastases disappeared, a menopausal status was induced and, although the receptor status was unknown, this did not contra-indicate endocrine treatment. Furthermore, a complete or partial response to chemotherapy is a sign of a significant reduction of tumor burden but not cure. Consequently, continuing therapy is reasonable. Any surviving tumor cells are probably resistant to chemotherapy but they might still be responsive to endocrine treatment. Based on these considerations, endocrine therapy may prolong the disease-free interval without adding significant toxicity. In the case reported, tamoxifen was selected instead of progestins because the patient was overweight and the side effects of progestins would not have been acceptable at that moment.

Discussion of the clinical case

When the patient was originally referred to our institution, the diagnostic procedure was initiated with a fine-

References

1. Tannock IF, Boyd NF, De Boer G et al. A randomized trial of two dose levels of cyclophosphamide, methotrexate, and

fluorouracil chemotherapy for patients with metastatic breast cancer. J Clin Oncol 1988; 1377-87.

2. Baum M, Priestman T, West RR et al. A comparison of subjective responses in a trial comparing endocrine with cytotoxic treatment in advanced carcinoma of the breast. In Mouridsen HT, Palshof T (eds): Breast Cancer – Experimental and Clinical Aspects. Oxford: Pergamon Press 1980; 223-6.

3. Coates A, Gebski V, Bishop JF et al. Improving the quality of life during chemotherapy for advanced breast cancer. N Engl J Med 1987; 317: 1490-5.

4. Brunner KW, Sonntag RW, Martz G et al. A controlled study in the use of combined drug therapy for metastatic breast cancer. Cancer 1975; 36: 1208-19.

5. Andersen JR, Cain KC, Gelber RD. Analysis of survival by tumor response. J Clin Oncol 1983; 11: 710-9.

6. A'Hern RP, Ebbs SR, Baum MB. Does chemotherapy improve survival in advanced breast cancer? Br J Cancer 1988; 57: 615-8.

7. Byar DP, Sears ME, McGuire WL. Relationships between estrogen receptor values and clinical data in predicting the response to endocrine therapy for patients with advanced breast cancer. Eur J Cancer 1979; 15: 299-310.

8. Brooks SC, Saunders DE, Singhakowinta A et al. Relation of tumor content of estrogen and progesterone receptors with response of patients to endocrine therapy. Cancer 1980; 46: 2775-8.

9. Muss HB, Case LD, Atkins JN et al. Tamoxifen versus high-dose oral medroxyprogesterone acetate as initial endocrine therapy for patients with metastatic breast cancer: A Piedmont Oncology Association study. J Clin Oncol 1994; 12: 1630-8.

10. Castiglione-Gertsch M, Pampallona S, Varini M et al. Primary endocrine therapy for advanced breast cancer: To start with tamoxifen or with medroxyprogesterone acetate? Ann Oncol 1993; 4: 735-40.

11. Gill PG, Gebski V, Snyder R et al. Randomized comparison of the effects of tamoxifen, megestrol acetate or tamoxifen plus megestrol acetate on treatment response and survival in patients with metastatic breast cancer. Ann Oncol 1993; 4: 741-4.

12. Early Breast Cancer Trialists' Collaborative Group. Systemic treatment of early breast cancer by hormonal, cytotoxic, or immune therapy. Lancet 1992; 339: 1-15, 71-85.

13. Fisher B, Costantino J, Redmond C et al. A randomized clinical trial evaluating tamoxifen in the treatment of patients with node-negative breast cancer who have estrogen receptor-positive tumors. N Engl J Med 1989; 320: 479-84.

14. Fornander T, Rutqvist LE, Glas U. Response to tamoxifen and fluoxymesterone in a group of breast cancer patients with disease recurrence after cessation of adjuvant tamoxifen. Cancer Treat Rep 1987; 71: 685-8.

15. Rubens RD. Effects of adjuvant systemic therapy on response to treatment after relapse. Cancer Treat Rev 1993; 19: 3-10.

16. Buzdar AU, Legha SS, Hortobagy GN et al. Management of breast cancer patients failing adjuvant chemotherapy with adriamycin-containing regimens. Cancer 1981; 47: 2798-802.

17. Valagussa P, Tancini G, Bonadonna G. Salvage treatment of patients suffering relapse after adjuvant CMF chemotherapy. Cancer 1986; 58: 1411-7.

18. Buckner JC, Ingle JN, Everson LK et al. Results of salvage hormonal therapy and salvage chemotherapy in women failing adjuvant chemotherapy after mastectomy for breast cancer. Breast Cancer Res Treat 1989; 13: 135-42.

19. Houston SI, Richiards MA, Bentley AE et al. The influence of adjuvant chemotherapy on outcome after relapse of patients with metastatic breast cancer. Eur J Cancer 1993; 29A: 1513-8.

20. Decoster G, Stein G, Holdener EE. Responses and toxic deaths in phase I clinical trials. Ann Oncol 1990; 1: 175-81.

21. Merrouche Y, Gatimel G, Clavel M. Hematopoietic growth factors and chemoprotectants: Should we move toward a two-step

process for phase II clinical trials in oncology? Ann Oncol 1993; 4: 471-4.

22. Skipper HE. Dose intensity versus total dose of chemotherapy: An experimental basis. In De Vita VT, Hellman S, Rosenberg SA (eds): Advances in Oncology. Philadelphia: JP Lippincott 1990; 43-64.

23. Antman KS, Armitage JO, Horowitz MM et al. Autotransplants for breast cancer in North America. Proc Am Soc Clin Oncol 1994; 13: #69.

24. Eddy DM. High-dose chemotherapy with autologous bone marrow transplantation for the treatment of metastatic breast cancer. J Clin Oncol 1992; 10: 657-70.

25. Hillner BE, Smith TJ, Desch CE. Efficacy and cost-effectiveness of autologous bone marrow transplantation in metastatic breast cancer. JAMA 1992; 267: 2055-61.

26. Livingstone RB. High-dose consolidation for stage IV breast cancer. In American Society of Clinical Oncology Educational Book. Dallas 1994; 74-9.

27. Bregni M, Siena S, Bonadonna G, Gianni AM. Clinical utilisation of human haematopoietic progenitors elicited in peripheral blood by recombinant human granulocyte colony-stimulating factor. Eur J Cancer 1994; 30A: 235-8.

28. Ardizzoni A, Venturini M, Sertoli MR et al. Granulocyte-macrophage colony-stimulating factor (GM-CSF) allows acceleration and dose intensity increase of CEF chemotherapy: A randomised study in patients with advanced breast cancer. Br J Cancer 1994; 69: 385-91.

29. Perrone F, Lauria R, Carlomagno C et al. High-dose chemotherapy with epirubicin and cyclophosphamide plus hemopoietic colony-stimulating factors in locally advanced or metastatic breast cancer. A phase I-II trial. Eur J Cancer 1993; 29A(6): #S57.

30. Falkson G, Gelman R, Glick J et al. Reinduction with the same cytostatic treatment in patients with metastatic breast cancer: An Eastern Cooperative Oncology Group study. J Clin Oncol 1994; 12: 45-9.

31. Harris AL, Cantwell BMJ, Carmichael J et al. Comparison of short-term and continuous chemotherapy (mitozantrone) for advanced breast cancer. Lancet 1990; 335: 186-90.

32. Ejlertsen B, Pfeiffer P, Pedersen D et al. Decreased efficacy of cyclophosphamide, epirubicin and 5-fluorouracil in metastatic breast cancer when reducing treatment duration from 18 to 6 months. Eur J Cancer 1993; 29A: 527-31.

33. Smalley RV, Carpenter J, Bartolucci A et al. A comparison of cyclophosphamide, adriamycin, 5-fluorouracil (CAF) and cyclophosphamide, methotrexate, 5-fluorouracil, vincristine, prednisone (CMFVP) in patients with metastatic breast cancer. Cancer 1977; 40: 625-32.

34. Colajori E, Ackland S, Anton A et al. I.v. FEC with epirubicin 50 mg/m^2 d 1,8 prolongs time to progression with respect to i.v. CMF d 1,8 given at equimyelosuppressive doses as front-line chemotherapy of metastatic breast cancer: A randomized multinational multicentric phase III trial. Proc Am Soc Clin Oncol 1995; 14: 114, #156.

35. Holmes FA. Combination chemotherapy with taxol (paclitaxel) in metastatic breast cancer. Ann Oncol 1994; 5(Suppl 6): S23-7.

36. Holmes FA, Walters RS, Theriault RL et al. Phase II trial of taxol, an active drug in the treatment of metastatic breast cancer. J Natl Cancer Inst 1991; 83: 1797-805.

37. O'Shaughnessy JA, Cowan KH. Current status of paclitaxel in the treatment of breast cancer. Breast Cancer Res Treat 1994; 33: 27-37.

38. Alonso MC, Tabernero JM, Ojeda B et al. A phase III randomized trial of cyclophosphamide, mitoxantrone, and 5-fluorouracil (CNF) versus cyclophosphamide, adriamycin, and 5-fluorouracil (CAF) in patients with metastatic breast cancer. Breast Cancer Res Treat 1995; 34: 15-24.

39. Perrone F, De Placido S, Carlomagno C et al. Mitomycin C and mitoxantrone in anthracycline-pretreated advanced breast can-

cer patients. A phase II study. Am J Clin Oncol (CCT) 1994; 17: 218–22.

40. O'Reilly S, Kennedy MJ, Rowinsky EK et al. Vinorelbine and topoisomerase 1 inhibitors: Current and potential roles in breast cancer chemotherapy. Breast Cancer Res Treat 1994; 33: 1–17.

41. Spielman M, Dorval T, Turpin F et al. Phase II trial of vinorelbine/doxorubicin as first line therapy of advanced breast cancer. J Clin Oncol 1994; 12: 1764–70.

42. Jonat W, Kaufmann M, Blamey RW et al. A randomized study to compare the effect of the luteinising hormone-releasing hormone (LHRH) analogue goserelin with or without tamoxifen in pre- and perimenopausal patients with advanced breast cancer. Eur J Cancer 1995; 31A (2): 137–42.

43. Cavalli F, Goldhirsch A, Jungi F et al. Randomized trial of low- versus high-dose medroxyprogesterone acetate in the induction treatment of postmenopausal patients with advanced breast cancer. J Clin Oncol 1984; 2: 414–9.

44. Muss HB, Case LD, Capizzi RL et al. High- versus standard-dose megestrol acetate in women with advanced breast cancer: A phase III trial of the Piedmont Oncology Association. J Clin Oncol 1990; 8: 1797–805.

45. van Veelen H, Willemse PHB, Tjabbes T et al. Oral high-dose medroxyprogesterone acetate versus tamoxifen. Cancer 1986; 58: 7–13.

46. Goss PE, Gwyn KMEH. Current perspectives on aromatase inhibitors in breast cancer. J Clin Oncol 1994; 12: 2460–70.

47. Coombes RC, Hughes SWM, Dowsett M. 4-hydroxy-androstenedione: A new treatment for postmenopausal patients with breast cancer. Eur J Cancer 1992; 28A: 1941–5.

48. Bajetta E, Zilembo N, Buzzoni R et al. Endocrinological and clinical evaluation of two doses of formestane in advanced breast cancer. Br J Cancer 1994; 70: 145–50.

49. Raats J, Falkson G, Falkson HC. A study of fadrazole, a new aromatase inhibitor in postmenopausal women with advanced metastatic breast cancer. J Clin Oncol 1992; 10: 111–6.

50. Jonat M, Howell A, Blomqvist CP et al. A randomized trial of the new specific aromatase inhibitor Arimidex versus megestrol acetate in the treatment of postmenopausal women with advanced breast cancer. Proc Am Soc Clin Oncol 1995; 14: 108, #130.

51. Thurliman B, Beretta K, Bacchi M et al. First-line fadrozole versus tamoxifen in advanced breast cancer: Prospective randomized study SAKK 20/88. Proc Am Soc Clin Oncol 1995; 14: 98, #90.

52. Anderson CB, Philpott GW, Ferguson TB. The treatment of malignant pleural effusions. Cancer 1974; 33: 916–22.

53. Raju R, Kardinal C. Pleural effusion in breast carcinoma: Analysis of 122 cases. Cancer 1981; 48: 2524–7.

54. Evans TRJ, Stein R, Pepper J et al. A randomised prospective trial of surgical against medical tetracycline pleurodesis in the management of malignant pleural effusions secondary to breast cancer. Eur J Cancer 1993; 29A (3): 316–9.

55. Weichselbaum R, Marck A, Hellman S. Pathogenesis of pleural effusion in carcinoma of the breast. Int J Radiat Oncol Biol Phys 1977; 2: 963–8.

56. Thomas JM, Redding WH, Sloane JP. The spread of breast cancer. Importance of the intrathoracic lymphatic route and its relevance to treatment. Br J Cancer 1979; 40: 540–4.

57. Fentiman JS, Rubens RD, Hayward JL. The pattern of metastatic disease in patients with pleural effusion secondary to breast cancer. Br J Surg 1982; 69: 193–8.

58. Miller AB, Hoogstraten B, Staquet M et al. Reporting results of cancer treatment. Cancer 1981; 47: 207–14.

59. Paladine W, Cunningham T, Sponzo R et al. Intracavitary bleomycin in the management of malignant effusions. Cancer 1976; 38: 1903–8.

60. Chernow B, Sahn SA. Carcinomatous involvement of the pleura. Am J Med 1977; 63: 695–702.

61. Fentiman IS, Millis R, Sexton S et al. Pleural effusion in breast cancer. A review of 105 cases. Cancer 1981; 47: 2087–92.

62. Contegiacomo A, Fiorillo L, De Placido S et al. The treatment of metastatic pleural effusion in breast cancer: Report of 25 cases. Tumori 1987; 73: 611–6.

63. Rosato FE, Wallach MW, Rosato EF. The management of malignant effusion from breast cancer. J Surg Oncol 1974; 6: 411–6.

64. Di Lorenzo D, Zaniboni A, Simoncini E et al. Estrogen and progesterone receptors in neoplastic cells of metastatic pleural effusion of breast carcinoma of before and after tamoxifen therapy. Correlation with the clinical response. Chemioterapia 1986; 5: 232–6.

65. Izbicki R, Weyhing BT, Baker L et al. Pleural effusion in cancer patients. A prospective randomized study of pleural drainage with the addition of radioactive phosphorous to the pleural space vs. pleural drainage alone. Cancer 1975; 36: 1511–8.

66. Petrou M, Kaplan D, Goldstraw P. Management of recurrent malignant pleural effusions. Cancer 1995; 75: 801–5.

67. Fentiman IS, Rubens RD, Hayward JL. Control of pleural effusion in patients with breast cancer. Cancer 1983; 52: 737–9.

68. Bayly TC, Kisner DL, Sysert A et al. Tetracycline and quinacrine in the control of malignant pleural effusions: A randomized trial. Cancer 1978; 41: 1188–92.

69. Dryzer SR, Allen ML, Strange C et al. A comparison of rotation and nonrotation in tetracycline pleurodesis. Chest 1993; 104: 1763–6.

70. Gravelyn TR, Michelson MK, Gross BH et al. Tetracycline pleurodesis for malignant pleural effusions. A 10-year retrospective study. Cancer 1987; 59: 1973–7.

71. Zaloznik AJ, Oswald SG, Langin M. Intrapleural tetracycline in malignant pleural effusions. A randomized study. Cancer 1983; 51: 752–5.

72. Ostrowski MJ. An assessment of the long-term results of controlling the reaccumulation of malignant effusions using intracavitary bleomycin. Cancer 1986; 57: 721–7.

73. Alberts DS, Chen HSG, Mayersohnm et al. Bleomycin pharmacokinetics in man: Intracavitary administration. Cancer Chemother Pharmacol 1979; 2: 127–32.

74. Vargas FS, Wang NS, Lee HM et al. Effectiveness of bleomycin in comparison to tetracycline as pleural sclerosing agent in rabbits. Chest 1993; 104: 1582–4.

75. Ruckedeschel JC, Moores D, Lee JY et al. Intrapleural therapy for malignant pleural effusion: A randomized comparison of bleomycin and tetracycline. Chest 1991; 100: 1528–35.

76. Sanchez-Armer A, Rodriguez-Panadero F. Survival and talc pleurodesis in metastatic pleural carcinoma, revisited. Report of 125 cases. Chest 1993; 104: 1482–5.

77. Sorensen PG, Svendsen TL, Enk B. Treatment of malignant pleural effusion with drainage, with and without instillation of talc. Eur J Respir Dis 1984; 65: 131–5.

78. Fentiman IS, Rubens RD, Hayward JL. A comparison of intracavitary talc and tetracycline for the control of pleural effusions secondary to breast cancer. Eur J Cancer 1986; 22: 1079–82.

79. Ostrowski MJ, Priestman TJ, Houston RF et al. A randomized trial of intracavitary bleomycin and corinebacterium parvum in the control of malignant pleural effusions. Radiother Oncol 1989; 14: 19–26.

80. Hillerdal G, Kiviloog J, Nou E et al. Corynebacterium parvum in malignant pleural effusion. A randomized prospective study. Eur J Resp Dis 1986; 69: 752–7.

81. Cascinu S, Isidori PP, Fedeli A et al. Experience with intrapleural natural beta interferon in the treatment of malignant pleural effusions. Tumori 1991; 77: 237–8.

82. Rosso R, Rimoldi R, Salvati F et al. Intrapleural natural beta interferon in the treatment of malignant pleural effusions. Oncology 1988; 45: 253–6.

83. Lissoni P, Barni S, Ardizzoia A et al. Intracavitary administration of interleukin-2 as palliative therapy for neoplastic effusions. Tumori 1992; 78: 118–20.

84. Yasumoto K, Miyazaki K, Nagasima A et al. Induction of lymphokine-activated killer cells by intrapleural instillations of

recombinant interleukin-2 in patients with malignant pleurisy due to lung cancer. Cancer Res 1987; 47: 2184–7.

85. Cimochowski GE, Joyner LR, Fardin R et al. Pleuroperitoneal shunting for recalcitrant pleural effusions. J Thorac Cardiovasc Surg 1986; 92: 866–70.

86. Martini N, Bains M, Beattle EJ. Indication for pleurectomy in malignant effusion. Cancer 1975; 35: 734–8.

87. Bull JM, Tormey DC, Li SH et al. A randomized comparative trial of adriamycin versus methotrexate in combination drug therapy. Cancer 1978; 41: 1649–57.

88. Muss HB, White DR, Richards F et al. Adriamycin versus methotrexate in five-drug combination chemotherapy for advanced breast cancer. Cancer 1978; 42: 2141–8.

89. Tormey DC, Gelman R, Band PR et al. Comparison of induction chemotherapies for metastatic breast cancer. Cancer 1982; 50: 1235–44.

90. Tormey DC, Weinberg WE, Leone LA et al. A comparison of intermittent versus continuous and of adriamycin versus methotrexate five drug chemotherapy for advanced breast cancer. A cancer and leukemia group B study. Am J Clin Oncol (CCT) 1984; 7: 231–9.

91. Cummings FJ, Gelmans R, Horton J. CAF versus CMFVP in metastatic breast cancer. Analysis of prognostic factors. J Clin Oncol 1985; 3: 932–40.

92. Aisner J, Weinberg V, Perloff M et al. Chemotherapy versus chemoimmunotherapy (CAF vs. VAFVP vs. CMF each +/− MER) for metastatic carcinoma of the breast: A CALGB study. J Clin Oncol 1987; 5: 1523–33.

93. Madsen EL, Andersson M, Mouridsen HT et al. A randomised study of CAF + tamoxifen versus CMF + tamoxifen in disseminated breast cancer. Proceedings of the 5th breast Cancer Working Conference, Leuven, 1991.

R. L. Souhami (ed.) The Teaching Cases from Annals of Oncology, 133–136, 1997.

Brain metastases in small-cell lung cancer

U. Lassen, P. E.G. Kristjansen & H. H. Hansen

Department of Oncology, Rigshospitalet, Finsen Center, Copenhagen, Denmark

Key words: small-cell lung cancer, brain metastases

Introduction

Approximately 10% of the patients with small-cell lung cancer (SCLC) present with brain metastases at the time of diagnosis [1] and another 40% develop symptomatic CNS involvement during or after treatment [2]. At autopsy approximately 50% will have brain metastases [3], and the cumulative risk of developing brain metastases at two years' survival is 50%–80% [2, 4]. The prognosis after a cerebral relapse is poor, with a median survival below three months [1, 5], whereas the isolated prognostic impact of CNS involvement at initial diagnosis is minimal [6]. A small fraction of patients will benefit from radiotherapy or chemotherapy and become long-term survivors despite their CNS involvement [7].

Case history

A 61-year-old female, formerly a heavy smoker, presented with a one-month history of worsening dyspnea, back pain, anorexia and an unintended weight loss of four kilograms. Chest X-ray revealed a mass at the left hilar region and a widening of the upper mediastinum. At ultrasonography of the abdomen liver metastases were suspected, and a liver biopsy showed SCLC; both broncoscopy and bilateral bone marrow examination confirmed this diagnosis. Her performance status was 2 according to the Zubrod score, and she received protocolled combination chemotherapy containing cisplatin, carboplatin, vincristine and teniposide alternating with cyclophosphamide and epirubicin in a four-week schedule. Immediately after the first cycle the patient had an episode of a generalized seizure and unconsciousness. A clinical neurological examination revealed no focal neurologic signs and a cranial CT scan did not indicate brain metastasis. Chemotherapy was continued and at her three-month reevaluation when the initial staging procedures were repeated the patient was in complete remission (CR). Treatment was discontinued after six months of therapy, and her final evaluation still showed CR. At this time her perfor-

mance status was 0, and she was asymptomatic. The patient was thereafter followed once a month. After four months she presented with back pain, dyspnea and coughing. Lactate dehydrogenase (LDH) and the transaminases were increasing, and both ultrasonography of the liver and chest X-ray showed pathological lesions. Second-line chemotherapy with oral etoposide was initiated and her pain and pulmonary symptoms were alleviated. LDH and the transaminases were normalized, and a chest X-ray after four weeks again showed complete response with no signs of tumor. After six months of therapy, still with complete local tumor control, the patient presented with nausea, vertigo, emesis and ataxia. Brain metastases were suspected and a CT scan showed multiple bilateral lesions in the cerebrum and cerebellum. The patient received high-dose corticosteroids and cranial irradiation, 20 Grays in four fractions of five Grays. Again, the patient responded rapidly as the neurological symptoms completely disappeared. Chest X-ray was still normal and the patient had no pulmonary symptoms. Treatment with oral etoposide was continued and the steroid dose was decreased. However, after five further months the patient deteriorated, with signs of increased intracranial pressure. The steroid dose was increased without effect, and the patient died. No signs of thoracic or abdominal progression were found and the chest X-ray finding was still normal. Autopsy was not performed.

Clinical findings

The clinical pattern of brain metastasis is very broad. Symptoms of increased intracranial pressure such as headache, nausea, emesis and vertigo are frequent. Other possible manifestations include focal neurological symptoms such as hearing loss or visual disturbance, double vision, hemiparesis or numbness. Patients may also present with seizures, ataxia, behavioral disturbances or in rare cases diabetes insipidus [3, 8, 9]. In some cases the symptoms are very discrete and difficult to distinguish from psychological reactions to the cancer diagnosis or difficulties in coping with hospitalization, or from side effects of the treatment, e.g. neurotoxicity due to vinca alkaloids, cisplatin or prophylactic cranial irradiation (PCI) [10]. Paraneoplastic neurologic syndromes such as the Lambert-Eaton syndrome occur in 1%–5% of patients with SCLC [11], and symptoms such as muscle weakness and pain, cranial nerve paresis and autonomic disorders may often lead to a suspicion of brain metastasis. Spinal cord compression, and leptomeningeal carcinomatosis (LMC) can both produce symptoms such as paresis, numbness or ataxia, and difficulties in the differential diagnosis versus intracranial lesions may occur. A clinical neurological examination will often help in distinguishing between these entities. However, the symptoms of leptomeningeal carcinomatosis can be very diffuse and discrete, and in most cases leptomeningeal metastases are concomitant with cerebral or cerebellar metastatic lesions.

Diagnosis

In patients with SCLC, neurologic disorders are caused by brain metastases in 75%, and there is more than one cause in an additional 8% [8]. When a patient with SCLC shows neurological symptoms or signs a careful clinical neurological examination should be performed. However, the diagnosis of brain metastases cannot be based on clinical examination alone and must be supplemented with imaging procedures of the brain. Contrast CT scan has a predictive value of 71%–84% [4, 8], whereas the clinical evaluation alone has a predictive value of 65%–93% [3, 4]. Gadolinium-DTPA enhanced magnetic resonance imaging (MRI) has been shown to be superior to CT in assessment of brain metastases [12], and this is of special interest if the palliative intervention includes surgery. Brain metastases of SCLC are most often multiple and frequently located in the posterior fossa [3]. In neither instance is neurosurgery recommended.

If brain imaging procedures fail to detect metastases, other possible causes of the neurological symptoms must be excluded. The detection of leptomeningeal carcinomatosis is difficult because the symptoms can be very vague and diffuse. Most often patients suffer from neurological symptoms such as pareses or numbness related to more than one level of the neuraxis [4]. This is in contrast to spinal cord compression whereby most often one dominant level is found. Cytologic analysis of cerebrospinal fluid (CSF) after a lumbar puncture is the prime analysis although pathologic structures along the spinal cord may be observed with MRI. The diagnosis of LMC relies on the presence of tumor cells in CSF. The positive and negative predictive values of the neurological examination are 57% and 95%, respectively [4], while the predictive value of CSF cytology is only approximately 50%, even though the predictability increases with an increasing number of lumbar punctures. Elevated CSF protein and low CSF glucose levels tend to occur in metastatic neurologic disease [4] and substantiates the suspicion of LMC when other findings are negative.

As both scans and CSF cytology may be negative despite unequivocal signs and symptoms of metastatic neurologic disease the neurologic examination plays a central role in assessment of CNS metastases. The diagnostic methods are complementary and if brain metastases are strongly suspected despite negative test results, other non-invasive imaging modalities are now available. Positron emission tomography (PET) is a functional imaging modality in which uptake of radiotracers is used to quantitate and visualize metabolic events based on computer tomography. PET has turned out to be a useful diagnostic tool in the assessment of primary brain tumors [13]. The method has been extrapolated to metastatic brain tumors, but further studies are needed [14].

Treatment

With the present therapeutic potential, the goal of the treatment of brain metastases in SCLC is palliation even though a few patients do become long-term survivors. Brain relapse implies a poor prognosis with a medium survival of only a few months in untreated patients [1, 5]. Patients with brain metastases as the sole site of metastasis at the time of diagnosis were also previously considered to have a poor prognosis, but as diagnostic methods have become more sensitive, the negative prognostic impact of initial brain metastasis has disappeared [15]. The performance characteristics of the newest CT and MRI scanners provide a spatial resolution of 0.5–1.0 mm which allows detection of asymptomatic metastases. Small brain metastases may have little or no influence on morbidity, and as the response of initial brain metastases is similar to that of extracranial metastases to chemotherapy [16], the initial treatment strategy of combination chemotherapy should not be altered. Patients with initial symptomatic brain metastases usually receive corticosteroids, which effectively alleviate the patients but which might influence the drug delivery to the brain parenchyma. Steroids decrease the brain-to-tumor capillary permeability and animal studies suggest that steroids decrease brain uptake of methotrexate [17]. A widely accepted hypothesis of failure in the systemic treatment of brain metastases has been that due to the blood brain barrier (BBB) the brain is a pharmacologic sanctuary [18]. However, BBB is often disrupted in the tumor and the widely used cytotoxic agents such as epipodophyllotoxin derivates, platinum compounds, bleomycin and nitrosoureas reach brain tumors in adequate concentrations [19]. This might explain the more favorable prognosis of initial brain metastases [16, 20]. However, drug concentrations in peritumoral areas with intact BBB is lower, resulting in treatment failure of infiltrating tumor cells [19]. Several attempts have been made to overcome this problem [18]. Intra-arterial chemotherapy or osmotic disruption of BBB have produced improved treatment responses, and high-dose administration of etoposide has yielded increased response rates at the expense of substantial toxic effects in the treatment of brain relapses from SCLC [16, 21].

Whole-brain radiotherapy (WBRT) is the treatment of choice for brain relapse in SCLC. The fractionation schedules have varied in different studies, but have usually been 20–40 Gy in fractions of 2–3 Gy [22]. Treatment with doses of 40 Gy given in small fractions tend to improve median survival only slightly, and because the treatment period increases in proportion to the number of fractions the clinical benefit of the survival improval is questionable. The response of WBRT varies as the evaluation parameters of retrospective studies are variable, but complete symptomatic remissions seem to range from 25%–70% [22]. Concurrent treatment with corticosteroids improves the symptomatic remission, which often occurs within a few hours after administration [12, 17]. Anticonvulsants should be administered prophylactically if patients have had seizures [12].

Second-line chemotherapy in patients with brain relapse produces response rates comparable to those of the therapy for extracranial relapse [16]. The duration of response is a few months and the toxicity can be substantial, especially if the patient has received combination chemotherapy prior to the relapse. Significant palliation and improval of quality of life with minimal toxicity is best obtained with high-dose corticosteroids immediately after the diagnosis of the brain relapse and rapid onset of WBRT at a dose of 20–30 Gy in 1–2 weeks. In order to minimize side effects steroid tapering should commence following discontinuation of WBRT.

Prophylactic cranial irradiation

Prophylactic cranial irradiation (PCI) is a frequent component of different treatment programs in SCLC patients after a CR is obtained. But even in this subgroup of patients the exact role of PCI remains disputable. No statistically significant impact on survival has been demonstrated, although it is clear that the likelihood of brain metastasis is reduced. It appears that delayed radiotherapy at early detection of CNS relapse is as effective as early PCI for all patients [22–24]. In the latter case only a minority received cranial irradiation.

Conclusion

This case appears to represent the relatively rare event of an isolated brain relapse leading to the death of the patient. Proponents of PCI would argue that this patient would have benefited from that approach, and perhaps also that a prolonged WBRT with 'curative'

intent might have yielded a longer survival in this patient. From another point of view, this case reflects clinical reality in SCLC. It is a systemic disease, in which CRs are frequently obtained, but cure, unfortunately, in only a minority. Another important benchmark of SCLC is biological and clinical heterogeneity leading to variable and asyncronous responses at different anatomical disease sites. Effective circumvention of resistance mechanisms and, foremost, the development of new more powerful therapeutic agents are needed before the cure rate can exceed 10%.

References

1. Nugent JL, Bunn PA, Matthews MJ et al. CNS metastases in small-cell bronchogenic carcinoma. Increasing frequency and changing pattern with lengthening survival. Cancer 1979; 44: 1885–93.
2. Bunn PA, Nugent JL, Matthews MJ. Central nervous system metastases in small-cell bronchogenic carcinoma. Semin Oncol 1978; 5: 314–22.
3. Hirsch FR, Paulson OB, Hansen HH, Vraa-Jensen J. Intracranial metastases in small-cell carcinoma of the lung. Correlation of clinical and autopsy findings. Cancer 1982; 50: 2433–7.
4. Pedersen AG. Diagnostic procedures in the detection of CNS metastases from small-cell lung cancer. In Hansen HH (ed): Lung Cancer: Basic and Clinical Aspects. Boston: Martinus Nijhoff 1986; 153–82.
5. Carmichael J, Crane JM, Bunn PA et al. Results of therapeutic cranial irradiation in small-cell lung cancer. Int J Radiat Oncol Biol Phys 1988; 14: 455–9.
6. Østerlind K. Prognostic factors in small-cell lung cancer: An analysis of 874 consecutive patients. In Hansen H (ed): Lung Cancer: Basic and Clinical Aspects. Boston: Martinus Nijhoff 1986; 129–52.
7. Giannone L, Johnson DH, Hande KR, Greco FA. Favorable prognosis of brain metastases in small-cell lung cancer. Ann Intern Med 1987; 106: 386–9.
8. Sculier JP, Feld R, Evans WK et al. Neurologic disorders in patients with small-cell lung cancer. Cancer 1987; 60: 2275–83.
9. Lucas CF, Robinson B, Hoskin PJ et al. Morbidity of cranial relapse in small-cell lung cancer and the impact of radiation therapy. Cancer Treat Rep 1986; 70: 565–70.
10. Johnson BE, Becker B, Goff WB et al. Neurologic, neuropsychologic, and computed cranial tomography scan abnormalities in 2- to 10-year survivors of small-cell lung cancer. J Clin Oncol 1985; 3: 1659–67.
11. Bauer J, Kuntzer T, Leyvraz S. Paraneoplastic neurologic syndromes. Ann Oncol 1995; 6: 291–6.
12. DeAngelis LM. Management of brain metastases. Cancer Invest 1994; 12: 156–65.
13. Di Chiro G. Positron emission tomography using {18-F}Fluorodeoxyglucose in brain tumors. A powerful diagnostic and prognostic tool. Invest Radiol 1986; 22: 360–71.
14. Grifeth LK, Rich KM, Dehdashti F et al. Brain metastases from non-central-nervous system tumors: Evaluation with PET. Radiology 1993; 186: 37–44.
15. Dearing MP, Steinberg SM, Phelps R et al. Outcome of patients with small-cell lung cancer: Effect of changes in staging procedures and imaging technology on prognostic factors over 14 years. J Clin Oncol 1990; 8: 1042–9.
16. Kristensen CA, Kristjansen PEG, Hansen HH. Systemic chemotherapy of brain metastases from small-cell lung cancer: A review. J Clin Oncol 1992; 10: 1498–502.
17. Jarden JO, Dhawan V, Poltorak A et al. Positron emission tomographic measurement of blood-to-brain and blood-to-

tumor transport of {81}-Rb: The effect of dexamethasone and whole-brain radiation therapy. Ann Neurol 1985; 18: 636–46.

18. Greig NH. Chemotherapy of brain metastases: Current status. Cancer Treat Rev 1984; 11: 157–86.

19. Donelli MG, Zucchetti M, D'Incalci M. Do anticancer agents reach the tumor target in the human brain? Cancer Chemother Pharmacol 1992; 30: 251–60.

20. van Hazel GA, Scott M, Eagan RT. The effect of CNS metastases of the survival of patients with small-cell cancer of the lung. Cancer 1983; 51: 933–7.

21. Black PM. Brain tumors (first of two parts). N Engl J Med 1991; 324: 1471–6.

22. Kristjansen PEG. Prophylactic cranial irradiation. In Johnson BE, Johnson DH (eds): Lung Cancer. New York: Wiley-Liss, Inc. 1995; 303–18.

23. Arriagada R, Le Chevalier T, Borie F et al. Prophylactic cranial irradiation for patients with small-cell lung cancer in complete remission. J Natl Cancer Inst 1995; 87: 183–90.

24. Bunn PA, Kelly K. Prophylactic cranial irradiation for patients with small-cell lung cancer (Editorial). J Natl Cancer Inst 1995; 87: 161–2.

R. L. Souhami (ed.) The Teaching Cases from Annals of Oncology, 137–143, 1997.

The role of surgery in small-cell lung cancer: A case history

C. D. Colder & P. E. Postmus

Department of Pulmonology, Free University Hospital, Amsterdam, The Netherlands

Key words: small-cell lung cancer, chemoradiotherapy, solitary pulmonary nodule, staging, primary surgery, adjuvant surgery

Introduction

Lung cancer is a still-growing health care problem throughout the world. Despite major efforts in the last three decades there has been only a very small improvement in prognosis with a current overall five-year survival of 15%.

About 20%–25% of the patients with lung cancer present with small-cell lung cancer (SCLC) and their prognosis is even worse than that of those with non-small-cell lung cancer (NSCLC). The cornerstone of treatment of patients with SCLC is chemotherapy. Local treatment with either surgery or radiotherapy has yielded only poor results. Later, for those patients with a so-called limited disease, it was found in a meta-analysis that adding radiotherapy resulted in a small improvement of survival at three years [1]. This is in contrast to the situation in patients with NSCLC, for whom surgery in the early stages of the disease offers the only chance for cure.

With the described approach the prognosis today of patients with SCLC is a median survival of approximately one year and a five-year survival of about 5%. Even after five years these patients are still at risk of dying of SCLC or secundary NSCLC [2].

Given this very unfavourable prognosis, the role of surgery has been reassessed in the past decade. This has led to the view that there may be a role for surgery in SCLC in selected cases. The following case history will demonstrate one of the situations in which a patient with SCLC seems to benefit from surgery.

Case history

A 74-year-old man presented in November 1993 with a history of one year of increased cough with hemoptysis over the previous two or three months. There was no dyspnea. He had been coughing for years and suffered from one episode of bronchitis every year, which was usually treated with antibiotics. He was otherwise healthy and was not on any medication. He had stopped smoking several years previously, after 50 years of smoking heavily. He had worked as a printer.

On examination he was in good physical condition, and examination of the lungs and heart was normal. There was no lymphadenopathy.

Chest X-ray showed two small calcified lesions in the left lung (Figure 1). The rest of the lungfields, the heart, hila and mediastinum were normal.

Pulmonary function tests showed; FVC 2.64 L (predicted 4.13), FEV1 1.36 L (predicted 3.05), FEV1/FVC 0.52 and RV 3.36 L (predicted 2.62), indicating a moderate chronic obstructive pulmonary disease (COPD) with emphysema. Results of other investiga-

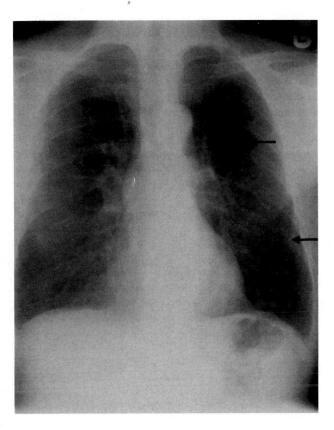

Fig. 1. Chest X-ray on first visit; no abnormalities except two calcified lesions (arrows).

tions, including full blood count, serum electrolytes and renal and liver function tests, were all within normal limits. Aspergillus serology was negative. Sputum cultures were sterile and M. Tuberculosis was not found. Flexible bronchoscopy revealed no endobronchial abnormalities. Cytology of sputum and washings was negative.

The conclusion was that the patient suffered from a moderate COPD and the hemoptysis was explained by forceful clearing of the throat. He was treated with inhalation therapy, consisting of inhalation corticosteroids and beta-agonists.

During follow-up the cough persisted and high resolution CT-scanning of the thorax was performed in search of bronchiectasis. This showed a small, smooth lesion in the left lower lobe, suggesting bronchiectasis with mucus impaction (Figure 2). Chest X-ray and CT were repeated after three months and showed slight expansion of the lesion (Figure 3). Bronchoscopy again showed no abnormalities. Cytology of washings and brushings and transbronchial biopsy were all negative.

Thoracotomy was performed in September 1994. Examination of the frozen tissue section showed SCLC and a lobectomy with mediastinal node sampling was performed. Postoperative recovery was uneventful. Postoperative pathologic staging classified the tumour as a T1N0 SCLC. Results of additional staging procedures such as abdominal ultrasound and bone scan were negative.

In the months following the thoracotomy our patient recieved five courses of chemotherapy consisting of cyclophosphamide (1000 mg/m²), doxorubicin (45 mg/m²) and etoposide (3 × 100 mg/m²). Because of a severe leukocytopenia with septicemia after the first course of chemotherapy the dose was reduced to 75% in the second to fifth courses. This was well tolerated and there were no further complications.

At this time the patient is in excellent health with no signs of recurrent disease.

Discussion of the case history

This case history presents the problem of a solitary pulmonary nodule (SPN) without cytologic or histologic diagnosis. In our patient it was an oval lesion with a diameter of ± 1 cm, which increased in size over a period of 3 months. This was an indication of malignancy and so a thoracotomy was performed. During the operation the diagnosis was made on the frozen tissue section and after verification by additional histologic investigation SCLC was concluded. Since SCLC is known to metastasize early systemic therapy was thought to be indicated and so chemotherapy was administered.

The diagnosis of SCLC is very uncommon in SPN, which accounts for less than 5% of cases. The typical presentation of SCLC is a centrally localized tumour with perihilair infiltration and quite often enlarged hilar and mediastinal lymph nodes. The typical bronchoscopic picture is that of a mucosa with a cobblestone feature, due to submucosal growth of the tumour.

The problem of the SPN

This problem is not uncommon in daily practice. A SPN is usually defined as a spherical or oval density with a diameter of up to 4 to 6 cm, mostly surrounded by normal lung. A SPN is detected in approximately in 1:500 consecutive chest X-rays [3].

Although the differential diagnosis of the SPN is extensive, the most clinically relevant question is whether the nodule is benign, and thus inconsequential, or (potentially) malignant, and requiring treatment.

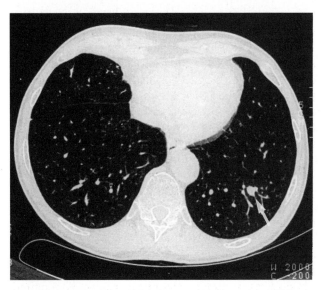

Fig. 2. First HR-CT-scan of the thorax, showing a smooth lesion in the left lower lobe (Ø 1 cm, arrow).

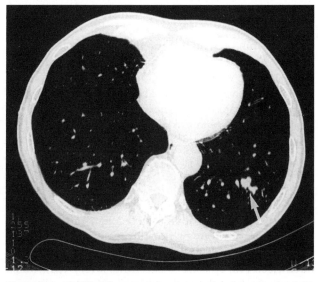

Fig. 3. Second HR-CT-scan of the thorax, showing growth of the lesion (arrow).

Comparison with earlier or consecutive chest X-rays or CT-scans might be of help in the distinction between benign and malignant. If the nodule was found two years earlier and has not grown since it is probably benign. If it shows growth in a period of three months or more (as in our patient), malignancy should be suspected.

Furthermore, the X-ray pattern may be of some help, although it is very difficult to conclude that a nodule is benign. If calcification is found with a benign pattern (see Figure 4) or fat is shown in the lesion, it is safe to conclude that it is a benign lesion. Other calcification patterns indicate malignancy until proven otherwise [3, 4]. The pulmonary window of high resolution CT is of help to define the edges of the nodule [5]. If they are lobulated or smooth benignity is indicated. If they are irregular or spiculated malignancy is indicated (see Figure 5).

Bronchoscopy rarely shows abnormalities in patients with a SPN. Because the diagnostic yield of cytology of brushes and biopsy is low (20%–40%, depending on size of the nodule), it is of little help in the distinction between benign and malignant. In case of doubt it is justified to perform a more invasive procedure such as percutaneous transthoracic needle aspiration biopsy (PTNAB) during fluoroscopy or under CT guidance. Although this can help in the distinction between benign and malignant, with a diagnostic yield of up to 85%, it is often not possible to make a classifying, histologically correct diagnosis with this procedure [6]. In selected cases a standard thoracotomy or a video-assisted thoracoscopy (VATS) is indicated.

Recently, with positron emission tomography scanning (PET) with radioactive fluoro-deoxyglucose (FDG), a nuclear technique has become available which shows promise in distinguishing the benign from the malignant SPN. Several studies from different PET centers throughout the world report a sensitivity, specificity and accuracy of, respectively, 85%–90%, 85%–95% and 85%–90% [7, 8].

It is advisable to use a systematic approach in the diagnostic work-up of the SPN as shown in Figure 6 in order to avoid needless, potentially harmful procedures. The exact position of PET-FDG in this approach has yet to be defined.

In the general population the incidence of malignancy in SPN is about 5%–20%, depending on the size of the nodule; in surgical series, from which many obviously benign lesions have been excluded, it is about 30% to 50%. In areas endemic for histoplasmosis, coccidioidomycosis or tuberculosis these percentages are considerably lower [3].

Smoking history, age, size of the nodule and prevalence of malignancy in the population from which the patient originates, are important factors in estimating the chance of malignancy in a SPN [9].

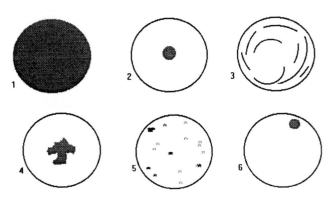

Fig. 4. Patterns of calcification: 1 = diffuse; 2 = central; 3 = laminar, concentric; 4 = popcorn; 5 = stippled; 6 = eccentric; 1–4 indicate benignity; 5 and 6 indicate malignancy. Redrawn from Webb [4].

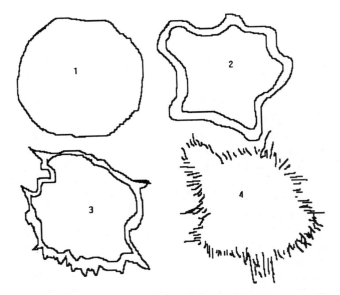

Fig. 5. Edges of the SPN: 1 = sharp and smooth; 2 = moderately smooth, lobulated; 3 = irregular undulations or slight spiculation; 4 = grossly irregular with spiculation; 1 and 2 indicate benignity; 3 and 4 indicate malignancy. Redrawn from Siegelman et al. [5].

The staging of SCLC

Since the early 1970s SCLC has been regarded as a systemic disease because of its propensity to early dissimination. This has resulted in a systemic approach in therapy. Along with this the staging procedures have been altered for SCLC, because the exact anatomical staging, as in the TNM-system, is needed only when decisions on therapy are altered by stage of disease. In most cases of SCLC, the staging system developed by the Veterans Administration Lung Cancer Study Group (VALCSG) is sufficient. It divides the disease into two stages; 'limited' and 'extensive' (Table 1). Diagnostic work-up is focused on excluding metastasis other than ipsilateral lymph nodes [6, 10–12]. More recently, because of the reevaluation of radiotherapy and surgery, the TNM-system was adjusted to replace the VALCSG-system in order to make comparison more accurate in case of additional local treatment, where a more exact anatomical staging is required (Table 1) [6, 10, 11].

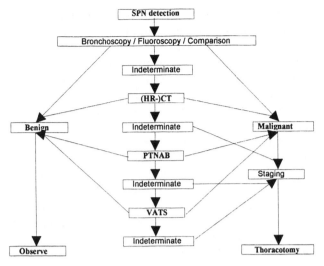

Fig. 6. Systematic approach of the SPN: HR-CT = high-resolution computed tomography; PTNAB = percutaneous transthoracic needle aspiration biopsy; VATS = video-assisted thoracoscopy.

Table 1. Staging of SCLC.

Limited	With or without ipsilateral or contralateral
= stage I, II, IIIA + B (TNM)	mediastinal or ipsilateral supraclavicular lymph node metastasis (can all be encompassed in one radiation field)
Extensive = stage IV (TNM)	Any disease at sites beyond the definition of limited disease

In normal daily practice the procedures listed in Table 2 are sufficient to distinguish between limited and extensive disease. If any abnormalities appear in these routine examinations, further steps can be taken to rule out distant tumour. If one of these procedures demonstrates metastases the patient is staged as having extensive disease.

If patients are selected for a (neo)adjuvant loco-regional treatment or a clinical trial a more thorough screening may be undertaken (Table 2). Some of the investigations may of course already have been done as part of diagnosis. Mediastinal lymph nodes, bone, bone marrow, liver, adrenals and the brain are known sites of early metastasis and are thus objects of investigation.

Using some or all of these procedures about 30% of patients with SCLC are staged as having limited disease. Most have mediastinal nodal involvement (N2 or N3 disease = stage IIIA or B) [6]. Less than 5% present with stage I.

When there is an operative diagnosis of SCLC (as in our patient), the staging procedures are completed postoperatively [10, 11]. After treatment of any kind the patient should be restaged according to pretreatment staging in order to evaluate the effect [6, 10, 11].

PET-FDG shows promising results in staging. With the whole-body scanning technique it is possible to assess the N and M stage at the same time with greater precision (accuracy: ± 90%) than with the conventional procedures [12].

Stage of disease is an important prognostic factor in

Table 2. Staging procedures in SCLC.

Procedure	Daily practice	Additional local therapy		Clinical trial
		Radiation	Surgery	
General				
Physical exam.	+	+	+	+
Full blood count	+	+	+	+
Biochemistry	+	+	+	+
Cytology/histology	+	+	+	+
Local tumour				
Chest X-ray	+	+	+	+
Chest CT	–	+	+	+
Bronchoscopy	–	–	+	+
Mediastinoscopy	–	–	+	–[a]
Pleural tap	–	+	+	+[a]
Supraclav. node cyto/ histology	–	–	+	+[a]
Distant tumour				
Bone marrow biopsy/ aspiration	–	+	+	+
Bone scan	+[b]	+	+	+
Abdominal CT or ultra- sound	+[b]	+	+	+
Brain CT	–	+	+	+

[a] Only if other findings are doubtfull and positive result affects treatment.
[b] Often performed routinely in daily practice but in fact not strictly necessary if no additional therapy is contemplated.

SCLC, together with performance score, number of sites involved, sex, weight loss and some laboratory abnormalities (elevated alkaline phosphatase or LDH, low albumin) [11, 13, 14].

The treatment of SCLC

Chemo-radiotherapy

During the period 1975–1990 chemotherapy became the cornerstone of therapy of SCLC. The use of a combination of several active drugs has become standard and several combinations are being used in daily practice nowadays (Table 3) [6, 10, 11, 15].

Although this therapy has improved prognosis from a median survival of six to twelve weeks to one year, it has not lead to a high cure rate. In patients with extensive disease median survival is around nine months with five years' survival ⩽2%. In most patients palliation is the goal of treatment [15]. In patients with limited disease median survival is around 15 months with a two-year survival rate of approximately 20% and a long-term disease free survival in 5%–10% of the patients. Despite a good initial rate of response to chemotherapy (80%–90%, 30%–50% of them complete), most patients relapse after therapy. Most relapses appear at the site of bulky disease before therapy [6, 10, 11, 15].

After the introduction of chemotherapy, thoracic

Table 3. Typical combination chemotherapy regimens in SCLC.

PE	
Cisplatin	75 mg/m^2 day 1
Etoposide	100 mg/m^2 day 1, 2, 3
CAV	
Cyclophosphamide	1000 mg/m^2 day 1
Doxorubicin	50 mg/m^2 day 1
Vincristine	1.4 mg/m^2 day 1, 8
CDE	
Cyclophosphamide	1000 mg/m^2
Doxorubicin	45 mg/m^2 day 1
Etoposide	100 mg/m^2 day 1, 3, 5

irradiation was abandoned as a monotherapy for SCLC because chemotherapy was clearly superior. However, the fact that a fair percentage (± 33%) of relapses occur at the site of the primary tumour, an improved local control might have an impact on the course of the disease. Since SCLC is proven to be very radiosensitive, thoracic irradiation has been added as adjuvant therapy during the past two decades. A meta-analysis based on up-dated individual patient data on all trials whether published or not has shown a better three-year survival for patients with limited disease treated with a combination of chemotherapy and thoracic irradiation [1]. Patients with extensive disease probably do not benefit from radiotherapy. It has been suggested that early irradiation combined with chemotherapy improves prognosis [16].

Nowadays patients with limited disease are therefore treated with a combination of chemotherapy and radiotherapy, and those with extensive disease receive chemotherapy for palliation.

Surgery

SCLC-SPN
Surgery was abandoned in the 1970s as a therapy for SCLC, after early the British Medical Research Council Trial [17] demonstrated no survival advantage for surgery over that of radiotherapy, and because of the success of chemotherapy. Since then several reports on surgery in SCLC have been published which give the impression that one group does seem to benefit from surgery. These are the patient in whom SCLC presents as a solitary pulmonary nodule (SCLC-SPN), as did the patient in our case report. Diagnosis is often only made peri- or post-operatively, which is the reason why surgeons continued to operate on these patients.

Pooled data from several studies demonstrate a five-year survival rate of 40% to 53% for these patients (pathologically staged T1–2N0M0) [18, 19]. The suggestion in the literature is that either the smaller tumour burden or a fundamental biological difference is responsible for the difference in survival [18–20]. The literature shows that about 2%–4% of SCLC present as a SCLC-SPN, which makes it a rather rare entity [18, 19].

Although their survival is much better than that of the general population with SCLC, it is not as good as the one for stage I NSCLC. This underscores the systemic nature of SCLC and suggests a need for chemotherapy. General advice with respect to these patients therefore is to give adjuvant chemotherapy, although there are no controlled trials supporting this advice.

Primary surgery
Given the still very poor prognosis with chemo-radiotherapy a number of studies have reassessed the role of surgery as a means of local control in resectable, limited, centrally localized, disease (so-called 'very limited' disease). Surgery has been followed by adjuvant combination-chemotherapy and if appropriate irradiation [21–29] (Table 4).

Survival rates for this so-called primary surgery show a considerable spread for stages I and II. The rates range from 22% to 67% and from 20% to 50%, respectively. For stage III the results were poor with low rates of five-year survival. However, most of these studies are retrospective and the number of patients included is small. In most studies the results were compared with the ones in patients treated with chemo-radiotherapy including clinically unresectable stages of disease (IIIA and IIIB). Furthermore, the fact that only the patients in the best condition and the earliest stages of disease are operated on must lead to misinterpretation. In the study of the Finsen Institute by Østerlind et al. [23], for instance, there was no difference in long-term survival in operable, resected patients compared to operable, non-resected patients.

Of note is the percentage of resected tumour with a histological diagnosis of SCLC mixed with NSCLC. In about 10%–15% of the operations in the cited studies a mixed tumour was resected. The percentage of mixed tumour in chemo-radiotherapy studies is unclear. Patients with mixed SCLC-NSCLC may more often be resectable than patients with pure SCLC. This could have a positive influence on survival, as the prognosis for NSCLC, when resected, is better than for SCLC.

Thus, although a benefit of primary surgery seems to be demonstrated in most studies for the lower stages of

Table 4. Results of primary surgery with adjuvant chemotherapy.

Author study	No. patients		Five-year survival (%)		
		Stage	I	II	III
Shields [21]	132		44	20	2.5
Merkle [22]	170		23	NR	0
Østerlind [23]	52		22	28	
Shepherd [24]	63		48	24	24
Karrer [25]	112		62[a]	50	41[a]
Hara [26]	36		67	36	0
Prasad [27]	97		35	23	0
Shepherd [28]	119		NR	28	19
Smit [29]	20		50		12

NR = not reached.
[a] Three-year survival.

disease, the above mentioned facts make comparison and interpretation hazardous.

Adjuvant surgery

Because of the possibility that chemotherapy may reduce some tumours to the point of operability, chemotherapy followed by so-called 'adjuvant surgery' is an appealing approach in limited, centrally localized SCLC. However, there are very few reports on trials with induction chemotherapy and adjuvant surgery. Initially a significantly longer survial for stages I and II was reported [30–32] (Table 5). In one study the operated patients ($n = 38$) had a significantly longer median survival than those who were eligible for surgery but did not undergo thoracotomy ($n = 19$) [32].

However, a recently published large prospective, randomized trial showed no significant difference in survival for the early stages of disease (I and II) [33]. The two-year survival for both arms in the study (chemotherapy *versus* chemotherapy followed by adjuvant surgery) was ± 20% (Table 5).

The long-term results of this trial have not yet been reported. This study also showed no prolonged survival for 'salvage' surgery [33]. This is surgery in patients with residual disease after chemotherapy (i.e., partial responders) or patients with a relapse only in the primary site after a complete response. Earlier reports suggested that stage I patients could benefit from this kind of operation [34].

In 4%–37% the histological diagnosis after resection is that of mixed SCLC-NSCLC or even of pure NSCLC (Table 5). This may again have an influence on the results of adjuvant surgery.

Table 5. Results of adjuvant surgery in limited SCLC.

Author	No. patients			NSCLC[a] % resected patients	Survival	
	Total	Resp. to chemotherapy (%)	Resected (%)		Median (months)	Two-year (%)
Baker [30]	37	19 (51)	19 (51)	37	NS[b]	65
Williams [31]	57	31 (54)	25 (44)	4	33	48
Shepherd [32]	72	57 (79)	38 (53)	16	22	50
Ladd [33]	328	217 (66)	146 (44) 70R[c]	11	16[d]	20[d]

[a] NSCLC in pathological examination after chemotherapy and resection.
[b] Not stated.
[c] 146 patients were resectable and randomized. 70 were resected and 76 were not resected (control group).
[d] Median survival and two-year survival were the same for both arms of the study.

Conclusion

The cornerstone in the treatment of patients with SCLC is chemotherapy alone in extensive-stage disease and chemotherapy combined, when possible, with early, thoracic irradiation in limited-stage disease.

It is difficult to assess the role of surgery in SCLC, mostly because so few patients present with resectable, limited disease. The patient with SCLC presenting as a SPN (peripherally localized stage I SCLC) clearly benefits from primary surgery. In these patients adjuvant chemotherapy may be helpful in view of the systemic nature of SCLC, but a prospective, randomized trial is not at hand to support this view.

The role of primary surgery, combined with adjuvant chemo-radiotherapy, in centrally localized stage I and II SCLC is not yet clear. When performed, it should preferably be done in the setting of prospective, randomized trials and only after complete and careful clinical staging.

No benefit of adjuvant surgery in stages I and II after chemo-radiotherapy has been shown in a randomized trial in spite of encouraging phase II data.

References

1. Pignon JP, Arriagada R, Ihde DC et al. A meta-analysis of thoracic radiotherapy for small-cell lung cancer. N Engl J Med 1992; 327: 1618–24.
2. Johnson BE, Grayson J, Makuch RW et al. Ten-year survival of patients with small-cell lung cancer treated with combination therapy with or without irradiation. J Clin Oncol 1990; 8: 396–401.
3. Fishman AP. Pulmonary Diseases and Disorders (vol 3), 2nd edition. New York: McGraw-Hill 1988; 1945–54.
4. Webb RW. Radiologic evaluation of the solitary pulmonary nodule. AJR 1990; 154: 701–8.
5. Siegelman SS, Khouri NF, Leo FP et al. Solitary pulmonary nodules: CT Assesment. Radiology 1986; 160: 307–12.
6. Cook RM, Miller YE, Bunn PA. Small-cell lung cancer: Etiology, biology, clinical features, staging and treatment. Curr Probl Cancer 1993; XVII(2): 105–41.
7. Gupta NC, Frank AR, Dewan NA et al. Solitary pulmonary nodules: Detection of malignancy with PET with 2-(F-18)-fluoro-2-deoxy-D-glucose. Radiology 1992; 184: 441–4.
8. Patz EF, Lowe VJ, Hoffman JM et al. Focal pulmonary abnormalities: Evaluation with F-18 fluorodeoxyglucose PET scanning. Radiology 1993; 188: 487–90
9. Cummings SR, Lilington GA, Richard RJ. Estimating the probability of malignancy in solitary pulmonary nodules. Am Rev Respir Dis 1986; 134: 449–52.
10. Postmus PE. Staging and Treatment for Small-Cell Lung Cancer. Current Topics in Lung Cancer. Berlin, Heidelberg: Springer-Verlag 1991: 47–60.
11. Hansen HH. Management of small-cell cancer of the lung. Lancet 1992; 339: 846–9.
12. Wahl RL, Quint LE, Greenough RL et al. Staging of mediastinal non-small-cell lung cancer with FDG PET, CT and fusion images, preliminary prospective evaluation. Radiology 1994; 191: 371–7.
13. Rawson NSB, Peto J. An overview of prognostic factors in small-cell lung cancer. Br J Cancer 1990; 61: 597–604.
14. Souhami RL, Bradbury I, Geddes DM et al. Prognostic significance of laboratory parameters measured at diagnosis in small-cell carcinoma of the lung. Cancer Res 1985; 45: 2878–82.
15. Greco FA, Hainsworth JD. Practical approaches to the treatment of patients With extensive stage small-cell lung cancer. Semin Oncol 1994; 21(Suppl 7): 3–6.
16. Murray N, Coy P, Pater JL et al. Importance of timing for thoracic irradiation in the combined modality treatment of limited stage small-cell lung cancer. J Clin Oncol 1993; 11: 336–44.

17. Fox W, Scadding JG. Medical research council comparative trial of surgery and radiotherapy for primary treatment of small-celled or oat-celled carcinoma of the bronchus. Ten year follow-up. Lancet 1973; 2: 63–5.

18. Kreisman H, Wolkove N, Quoix E. Small-cell lung cancer presenting as a solitary pulmonary nodule. Chest 1992; 101: 225–31.

19. Quoix E, Fraser R, Wolkove N et al. Small-cell lung cancer presenting as a solitary pulmonary nodule. Cancer 1990; 66: 577–82.

20. Warren WH, Memoli VA, Jordan AG et al. Reevaluation of pulmonary neoplasms resected as small-cell carcinomas. Cancer 1990; 65: 1003–10.

21. Shields TW, Higgins GA, Matthews MJ et al. Surgical resection in the management of small-cell carcinoma of the lung. J Thorac Cardiovasc Surg 1982; 84: 481–8.

22. Merkle NM, Mickisch GH, Kayser K et al. Surgical resection and adjuvant chemotherapy for small-cell carcinoma. Thorac Cardiovasc Surgeon 1986; 34: 39–42.

23. Østerlind K, Hansen M, Hansen HH et al. Influence of surgical resection prior to chemotherapy on the long term results in small-cell lung cancer. A study of 150 operable patients. Eur J Cancer Clin Oncol 1986; 22: 589-93.

24. Shepherd FA, Evans WK, Feld R et al. Adjuvant chemotherapy following surgical resection for small-cell carcinoma of the lung. J Clin Oncol 1988; 6: 832–8.

25. Karrer K, Shields TW, Denck H et al. The importance of surgery and multimodality treatment for small-cell bronchial carcinoma. J Thorac Cardiovasc Surg 1989; 97: 168–76.

26. Hara N, Ohta M, Ichinose Y et al. Influence of surgical resection before and after chemotherapy on survival in small-cell lung cancer. J Surg Oncol 1991; 47: 53–61.

27. Prasad US, Naylor AR, Walker WS et al. Long term survival after pulmonary resection for small-cell carcinoma of the lung. Thorax 1989; 44: 784–7.

28. Shepherd FA, Ginsberg RJ, Feld R. Surgical treatment for limited small-cell lung cancer. J Thorac Cardiovasc Surg 1991; 101: 385–93.

29. Smit EF, Groen HJM, Timens W et al. Surgical resection for small-cell carcinoma of the lung. Thorax 1994; 49: 20-2.

30. Baker RR, Ettinger DS, Ruckdeschel JD et al. The role of surgery in the management of selected patients with small-cell carcinoma of the lung. J Clin Oncol 1987; 55: 697–702.

31. Williams CJ, McMillan I, Lea R et al. Surgery after Initial chemotherapy for localized small-cell carcinoma of the lung. J Clin Oncol 1987; 5: 1579–88.

32. Shepherd FA, Ginsberg RJ, Patterson GA. A prospective study of adjuvant surgical resection after chemotherapy for limited small-cell lung cancer. A University of Toronto Lung Oncology Group Study. J Thorac Cardiovasc Surg 1989; 97: 177–86.

33. Lad T, Piantadosi S, Thomas P et al. A prospective randomized trial to determine the benefit of surgical resection of residual disease following response of small-cell lung cancer to combination chemotherapy. Chest 1994; 106: 320S-3S.

34. Shepherd FA, Ginsberg R, Patterson GA et al. Is there ever a role for salvage operations in limited small-cell lung cancer. J Thorac Cardiovasc Surg 1991; 101: 196–200.

R. L. Souhami (ed.) The Teaching Cases from Annals of Oncology, 145–149, 1997.

Management of advanced colorectal cancer

C. Bradley[1] & P. Selby[2]

[1] Oncology Department, Bradford Royal Infirmary, Bradford; [2] ICRF Cancer Medicine Research Unit, St James's University Hospital, Leeds, U.K.

Key words: colorectal cancer

Case Report

In February 1989, during a holiday in Gran Canaria, a 55-year-old man was admitted as an emergency to the local hospital following several days of nausea and vomiting associated with absolute constipation. He gave a history of abdominal pain and fullness over the preceding 2 weeks, although there was no anorexia or weight loss. On examination there was generalised abdominal distension and increased bowel sounds. Plain abdominal X-ray showed dilated bowel loops and faecal loading of the ascending and transverse colon. At laparotomy, a stenosing carcinoma of colon was found at the splenic flexure. There was no evidence of disease in the liver or elsewhere in the abdomen. A left hemicolectomy and reanastomosis was performed. Histological examination of the resected specimen showed circumferential involvement with a moderately differentiated adenocarcinoma extending through the full thickness of the bowel wall into surrounding adipose tissue. One of 9 lymph nodes showed malignant infiltration.

His post-operative recovery was uncomplicated. An abdominal CT scan was performed in March 1989 on his return to England and this revealed a 2 cm metastasis in segment 5 of his liver. In May 1989 this was excised, again showing moderately differentiated adenocarcinoma. At surgery several small nodules were noted in the small bowel mesentery which were considered suspicious of tumour but biopsy showed only fibrosis.

A follow-up CT scan was performed in November 1989 which showed several new lesions in the right lobe of liver suspicious of metastases. Liver function tests were normal. As he was asymptomatic, it was considered that there was no immediate need for further therapy and he was simply followed at the clinic without treatment. However a further CT scan in January 1990 showed an increase in the size of the liver lesions and a new soft tissue mass near the anastomosis on the left colon. In view of concern that the anastomotic mass

might cause obstructive symptoms, and the possibility that the liver metastases might still be resectable, a further laparotomy was performed the following month. The operative findings were of a tumour mass in the left paracolic gutter which extended into muscle. The liver was not visible because of adhesions. A complete resection was not considered possible, and a trucut biopsy only was performed to confirm recurrent adenocarcinoma.

He commenced systemic chemotherapy later that month with a combination of 5-fluorouracil (5-FU) and interferon alpha (INF) as part of a randomised clinical trial. 5-FU was given at a dose of 750 mg/m^2 daily for 5 days by continuous intravenous infusion, followed by weekly bolus therapy at 750 mg/m^2. 9MU INF was administered subcutaneously three times weekly starting day 1 [1]. A repeat CT scan after 2 months treatment showed a partial response, with a greater than 50% reduction in the size of the left upper quadrant mass and liver metastases.

A number of toxicities were seen in association with the treatment. These included fatigue, sweating and fevers, leucopenia, alopecia, diarrhoea and mucositis. Severe palmar-plantar erythema, associated with desquamation and fissures developed, but improved with regular pyridoxine [2]. After 8 months treatment he complained of impaired memory and ataxia. CT scan of brain showed some cerebellar atrophy but no other abnormality. In view of these cutaneous and neurological toxicities and of progressive fatigue it was necessary to reduce the dose of 5-FU and ultimately its frequency to every 14 days, with improvement in symptoms. The dose of interferon was not changed. Although there was some evidence of tumour progression on CT scan by October 1991, after 20 months of treatment, he remained extremely well and chemotherapy was continued at reduced dose until June 1992. Treatment was stopped at that time as a result of further enlargement of the liver metastases.

As the liver disease at that time appeared radiologically to be limited to segments 4 to 8, it was decided to attempt a further palliative resection in July 1992. At laparotomy the tumour was noted to transgress slightly into segment 3, and so a non-anatomically extended right hepatic lobectomy was performed, and it was also possible to excise the local recurrence at the splenic flexure. The resection appeared macroscopically and histologically complete, and he made an uncomplicated post-operative recovery. He remained well for several months before again relapsing with liver metastases and ascites in December 1992. He received a single dose of mitomycin C, but his condition continued to deteriorate and he died in January 1993.

Discussion

Our patient presented acutely, requiring emergency laparotomy for bowel obstruction. He had no family history or known risk factors for development of bowel cancer. The circumferential pattern of growth which he demonstrated is more characteristic of left sided tumours, and obstruction is more often a presenting feature. Obstruction has been reported as an adverse prognostic feature for survival, independently of stage, although there is no consistent association between site of primary tumour and prognosis.

A two stage procedure with a defunctioning colostomy is often considered necessary in cases presenting with obstruction, particularly with left sided lesions. There were no post-operative complications associated with the use of a single stage procedure in this case. There was no evidence of liver or other intra-abdominal metastases at laparotomy and the surgical staging was therefore Duke's stage C.

Adjuvant chemotherapy

A role for adjuvant chemotherapy in high risk colon cancer has only become firmly accepted in the past few years. Earlier studies with 5-FU regimens, alone and in combination had been generally negative, or at best inconsistent. A meta analysis of trials did identify a small overall benefit [3] but few clinicians were persuaded to adopt adjuvant chemotherapy as part of the routine management in these cases.

The Intergroup study of Moertel et al. in 1990 was the first demonstration of a substantial benefit from adjuvant treatment in a large well conducted trial [4]. At a median follow up of 3 years, patients with stage C disease treated with 5-FU and levamisole for 12 months had a 41% reduction in risk of recurrence and 33% reduction in risk of death. No benefit was seen for stage B2 patients and levamisole alone had no effect. The results of this trial, which confirmed those of an earlier study [5], were sufficient for an NIH consensus conference in 1990 to recommend that this regimen be standard treatment for all stage C patients who are unable to enter a clinical trial. Doubts have been raised regarding the contribution of levamisole to the combi-

nation in view of the absence of any advantage for 5-FU/levamisole over 5-FU alone in advanced disease [6]. Partly as a result of these concerns, there has not been a general adoption of the regimen in Europe.

Evidence from more recent trials suggests that the combination of leucovorin (LV) with 5-FU may produce a benefit of comparable magnitude to 5-FU/levamisole, although further follow up is needed [7–9]. In these studies an effect was seen in both stage B and stage C patients. The outcome of a series of trials assessing the value of various schedules and combinations of levamisole, LV and INF to 5-FU is awaited with interest. As the liver is the most common site of metastases, post-operative intraportal infusion of 5-FU has been examined as adjuvant treatment. Several trials have indicated a survival benefit, although, surprisingly, not always in association with a reduction in liver metastases, and in the UK this approach is being pursued in the AXIS trial [10]. Our policy is to accept that, although the optimum combination of currently available drugs is not yet known, there is now evidence of a disease-free and overall survival benefit from adjuvant chemotherapy in node-positive patients. Where possible they should be treated in clinical trials.

Treatment of advanced disease

Before embarking upon adjuvant chemotherapy, it is clearly appropriate to perform a series of screening investigations to exclude occult metastases. These should routinely include liver function tests, carcinoembryonic antigen (CEA), chest X-ray and CT scan of abdomen and pelvis. An abdominal CT scan in our patient revealed an unsuspected liver metastasis. The major options for treatment of liver metastases are systemic chemotherapy, regional intrahepatic chemotherapy and surgery. Their relative merits and the optimum combination and timing of each is disputed and we shall consider each in turn. Our patient was treated by resection in the first instance, followed by systemic chemotherapy when a second attempted resection failed, and then by further surgery and finally second-line chemotherapy.

Systemic chemotherapy

Until recently, there had been little genuine development in the chemotherapy of advanced colorectal cancer since the introduction of 5-FU. Response rates to 5-FU have been consistently in the 10%–20% range, although toxicity was relatively minor. None of the more recently developed cytotoxics has had significant activity, and the addition of further agents such as nitrosoureas, mitomycin, methotrexate and cisplatin to 5-FU regimens has been largely unsuccessful. There is some evidence that combination chemotherapy can improve survival and quality of life in advanced colorectal cancer [21] although prolongation of life with current regimens is only measured in months.

Recent interest has focused on biochemical modulation of 5-FU activity, stimulated by increased knowledge of the metabolic pathways involved (Fig. 1). 5-FU is metabolised in cells to 5-FdUMP which binds to and inhibits the key target enzyme thymidylate synthase (TS). The provision of increased amounts of intracellular reduced folates by the use of leucovorin (LV) stabilises the complex between 5-FdUMP and TS, thus prolonging TS inhibition. A series of trials with the combination of 5-FU and LV has confirmed the clinical relevance of this biochemical approach, and a recent report in rectal cancer patients has shown high TS expression in tumour samples to be predictive of poorer disease-free and overall survival [11]. A meta-analysis of 9 randomised trials comparing 5-FU/LV to 5-FU alone has shown a highly significant benefit in terms of response rate (23% vs. 11%), but no improvement in overall survival [12]. There is some evidence that when a higher dose intensity of 5-FU is employed, there may be no further benefit from the addition of LV. The optimum LV dose and schedule has not yet been defined. It is possible that lower (and much less expensive) doses of LV may be as effective as high dose treatment.

A randomised study by Lokich et al. [13] has recently reawakened interest in the use of protracted infusions of 5-FU. They found a clear increase in response rate for continuous low dose infusion of 5-FU compared to bolus therapy (30% vs. 7%). The authors compare the biochemical effect of prolonged TS inhibition from their regimen to the stabilised covalent ternary complex produced by LV. Trials investigating combinations of these approaches are underway.

The other modulatory approach of current interest is the addition of interferon alpha (INF) to 5-FU, as in the regimen received by our patient. Reduction in 5-FU clearance and alterations in TS transcription have been described after INF administration although the precise mechanism of synergy is not known. Although the initial optimistic response rate of 76% reported by Wadler et al. [1] has not been reproduced, there is evidence of improved response rate compared to 5-FU alone [14]. A randomised trial comparing 5-FU/INF and 5-FU/LV has shown no difference in response or survival, although toxicity differed between the two arms with diarrhoea, nausea/vomiting and stomatitis more frequent with LV and fatigue, somnolence and fever more frequent with INF [15]. Interferon alpha has no routine role at present, in our view. Current trials are evaluating new thymidylate synthase inhibitors and prodrugs of 5-FU with some encouraging evidence of modest benefits.

Regional chemotherapy

In view of the propensity of colorectal cancers to metastasise to the liver, often as the only clinically detectable site of disease, there has been considerable interest in regional chemotherapy via hepatic arterial infusion (HAI). The pharmacological basis of this approach is an attempt to maximise intra-tumoural drug concentration whilst reducing systemic exposure and thus toxicity. The high first pass hepatic extraction of 5-FU and particularly of 5-fluoro-2-deoxyuridine (FUdR) makes these fluorinated pyrimidines particularly suitable for this approach. Phase II trials of FUdR, usually as a 14 day infusion, have shown response rates as high as 80%. The few randomised trials of HAI compared to systemic 5-FU/FUdR show a consistent improvement in response rates with the regional approach, but no overall survival benefit [16]. The introduction of implantable pumps has reduced the complications of catheter displacement and infection associated with external catheters and pumps but requires surgical expertise. Biliary toxicity in the form of sclerosing cholangitis is dose limiting and regular monitoring of alkaline phosphatase and bilirubin is necessary for early detection of this complication. Most patients eventually develop extrahepatic metastases, particularly with lung involvement. The use of concurrent systemic treatment is being investigated, as is the use of LV and INF containing regimens. The high level of expertise necessary for HAI has restricted its use to specialised centres. In view of the associated morbidity and expense, wider adoption of this technique will be dependent on stronger evidence of overall patient benefit and a current MRC trial addresses this question.

Surgery

When patients develop locally recurrent or metastatic disease, the only modality of treatment which offers any possibility of cure is surgical resection. For many patients the site or extent of tumour when recurrence is first detected precludes this possibility, although a structured surveillance programme after initial surgery may increase the proportion of relapsing patients who are amenable to salvage surgery. In colorectal cancer, the liver is the first or only site of metastases in less

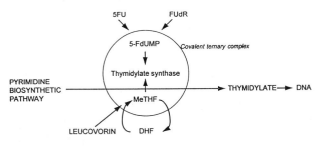

DHF	Dihydrofolate
MeTHF	Methylene tetrahydrofolate
FUdR	5-fluoro-2-deoxyuridine
5-FdUMP	5-fluoro-deoxyuridine monophosphate
5FU	5-fluorouracil

Fig. 1. Biochemical modulation of 5-FU.

148

than 20% of cases. A normal chest CT scan and colonoscopic assessment of the anastomosis seem sensible pre-operative investigations. Complete surgical resection will be possible in only a proportion of those where pre-operative investigation suggests the potential for resection, since some patients will be found to have unsuspected extrahepatic disease or unresectable liver metastases. Intra-operative ultrasound can help exclude additional small liver metastases undetected by palpation or pre-operative scanning. There is uncertainty as to whether the presence of extrahepatic disease is a contraindication to resection.

Resection of up to 3 or 4 metastases, even bi-lobar and 50% or more of the liver, would normally be considered and most series report an operative mortality of less than 5% from major resections and a 5 year survival of 20%–25% [17]. Prognostic features include the number and size of metastases, the resection margin achieved, the presence of extrahepatic disease and the latency between diagnosis of primary and metastases. It is not clear to what extent the long survival of the surgical series is biased by selection of a favourable prognostic group with slow growing, asymptomatic small volume disease, and it is unlikely that a randomised comparison to assess the value of surgery will be performed in cases with resectable disease. The survival curves of reported surgical studies tend to show a plateau after 5 years which suggests a definite benefit from resection [17]. Only a minority of patients subsequently relapse in the liver alone. The lung is a common site of recurrence, whereas diffuse intra-abdominal recurrence is the usual picture if there was extrahepatic disease at the time of surgery. The value of adjuvant chemotherapy after resection of metastases is not known, although the benefits obtained in patients with high risk primary tumours suggests that investigation of this approach may be worthwhile.

Repeated resections, as in our case, are performed only rarely and are most often possible when the initial operation did not require major hepatic resection. There are reports of long survival after a second or even third resection [18]. Resection of metastases at other sites can be as effective as hepatic resection. In a report of 252 resections of recurrent colon cancer, 27% of patients are alive and disease free at a median follow up of 41 months, with no difference between liver, lung, peritoneal or local resections [19].

operations it was possible to perform a complete resection of visible disease, and he obtained a good partial response of 16 months duration from 5-FU/INF. The achievement of complete macroscopic and histological clearance on the latter occasion suggests that the surgeon's judgement was appropriate given an especially high level of technical skill.

It was described not to commence immediate chemotherapy when our patient's liver metastases first recurred. Although a Scandinavian trial has suggested that deferring chemotherapy in patients with advanced disease can adversely affect survival [20], we do not consider the evidence of benefit is sufficiently strong to justify immediate treatment in all asymptomatic patients although the issue of timing needs to be discussed with patients who vary considerably in their views.

Our patient encountered significant toxicity from 5-FU/INF including many of the recognised side effects of the combination. The cutaneous and neurological symptoms, together with cumulative fatigue, were dose-limiting but improved with dose modification and local measures. He attended the outpatient chemotherapy clinic every 1–2 weeks for his treatment, but for much of this time was able to continue at work. Mitomycin C was used as a 'last resort' in spite of its recognised low activity. It was ineffective but there was no noticeable toxicity.

Out patient was an intelligent man with a very positive attitude to his disease and its treatment. He was keen to remain involved in his management at all times and to actively participate in all treatment decisions. His wish at each point was to continue with active treatment whenever possible, despite full knowledge of the limitations of therapies. This characteristic undoubtedly influenced the treatment decisions and contributed to the interventionist nature of his care.

He survived for almost 4 years after the initial diagnosis of liver metastases and it is arguable that this aggressive approach was justified in his case. Even his final operation, which would have appeared at the outset to be of doubtful palliative benefit, allowed him a 5 month disease-free interval of good health and may have prolonged his survival. We would not advocate such an approach in all patients, but for fully informed individuals such as our patient the outcome may be favourably influenced.

Conclusions

By most standards, the treatment approach to our patient would be classed as aggressive. The case illustrates several aspects of an intensive and controversial management of advanced colorectal cancer. He underwent three separate operations to attempt resection of recurrences in the liver and abdomen, in addition to 26 months chemotherapy with 5-FU/INF and a single dose of mitomycin C at final relapse. In two of the

References

1. Wadler S, Schwartz EL, Goldman M et al. Fluorouracil and recombinant alfa-2a-interferon: an active regimen against advanced colorectal cancer. J Clin Oncol 1989; 7(12): 1769–75.
2. Mortimer J, Anderson I. Managing the toxicities to high dose leucovorin and 5-Fluorouracil. Proc Am Soc Clin Oncol 1989; 8: 98.
3. Buyse M, Zeleniuch-Jacqotte A, Chalmers TC. Adjuvant therapy of colorectal cancer: Why we still don't know. JAMA 1988; 259: 3571–8.
4. Moertel CG, Flemming TR, Macdonald JS et al. Levamisole

and fluorouracil for adjuvant therapy of resected colon carcinoma. N Engl J Med 1990; 322: 352–8.

5. Laurie JA, Moertel CG, Flemming TR et al. Surgical adjuvant therapy of large bowel carcinoma: An evaluation of levamisole and the combination of levamisole and fluorouracil. J Clin Oncol 1989; 7: 1447–56.

6. Buroker TR, Moertel CG, Flemming TR et al. A controlled evaluation of recent approaches to biochemical modulation or enhancement of 5-fluorouracil therapy in colorectal carcinoma. J Clin Oncol 1985; 3: 1624–31.

7. O'Connell M, Mailliard J, Macdonald J et al. An intergroup trial of intensive course 5-FU and low dose leucovorin as surgical adjuvant therapy for high risk colon cancer. Proc Am Soc Clin Oncol 1993; 12: 190.

8. Zaniboni A, Erlichman C, Seitz JF et al. FUFA increases disease free survival (DFS) in resected B2C colon cancer (CC): Results of a prospective pooled analysis of three randomised trials (RCTs). Proc Am Soc Clin Oncol 1993; 12: 191.

9. Wolmark N, Rockette H, Fisher B et al. The benefit of leucovorin-modulated fluorouracil as post-operative adjuvant therapy for primary colon cancer: Results from National Surgical Adjuvant Breast and Bowel Project protocol C-03. J Clin Oncol 1993; 11(10): 1879–87.

10. Gray R, James R, Mossman J et al. AXIS – A suitable case for treatment. Br J Cancer 1991; 63: 841–5.

11. Johnston PG, Fisher E, Rockette HE et al. Thymidylate synthase expression is an independent predictor of survival/disease free survival in patients with rectal cancer. Proc Am Soc Clin Oncol 1993; 12: 202.

12. Piedbois P, Buyse M, Rustum Y et al. Modulation of fluorouracil by leucovorin in patients with advanced colorectal cancer: Evidence in terms of response rate. J Clin Oncol 1992; 10(6): 896–903.

13. Lokich JJ, Ahlgren JD, Gullo JJ et al. A prospective randomised comparison of continuous infusion fluorouracil with a conventional bolus schedule in metastatic carcinoma: A Mid-Atlantic Oncology Program study. J Clin Oncol 1989; 7(4): 425–32.

14. York M, Greco FA, Figlin RA et al. A randomised phase III trial comparing 5-FU with or without interferon alfa 2a for advanced colorectal cancer. Proc Am Soc Clin Oncol 1993; 12: 200.

15. The CORFU-A Study Group. Phase III randomised study of two fluorouracil combinations with either interferon alfa-2a or leucovorin for advanced colorectal cancer. J Clin Oncol 1995; 13(4): 921–8.

16. Patt YZ. Regional hepatic arterial chemotherapy for colorectal cancer metastatic to the liver: The controversy continues. J Clin Oncol 1993; 11(5): 815–9.

17. Steele G, Ravikumar TS. Resection of hepatic metastases from colorectal cancer: Biologic perspectives. Ann Surg 1989; 210(2): 127–38.

18. Gouillat C, Ducerf C, Partensky C et al. Repeated hepatic resections for colorectal metastases. Eur J Surg Oncol 1993; 19: 443–7.

19. Moertel C, Fleming T, Macdonald J et al. Recognition and salvage of the patient with recurrent colon cancer. Proc Am Soc Clin Oncol 1993; 12: 224.

20. Nordic Gastrointestinal Tumor Adjuvant Therapy Group. Expectancy or primary chemotherapy in patients with advanced asymptomatic colorectal cancer: A randomised trial. J Clin Oncol 1992; 10(6): 904–11.

21. Scheithauer W, Rosen H, Kornek GV et al. Randomised comparison of combination chemotherapy plus supportive care with supportive care alone in patients with metastatic colorectal cancer. Br Med J 1993; 306: 752–5.

R. L. Souhami (ed.) The Teaching Cases from Annals of Oncology, 151–157, 1997.

Detection and management of advanced gastric cancer

P. Hohenberger & M. Hünerbein

Division of Surgery and Surgical Oncology, Robert-Rössle Hospital and Tumor Institute at the Max-Delbrück Center for Molecular Medicine, Humboldt University of Berlin, Germany

Key words: diagnostic work-up, gastric cancer, staging laparoscopy

Introduction

Although its incidence has decreased significantly in Western countries during the past decade, gastric cancer is still one of the leading causes of death worldwide. The highest incidence is found in Japan where it is the principal type of fatal cancer. In contrast to Japan, the proportion of patients presenting with 'early gastric cancer' (limited to the mucosa and submucosa of the stomach) in Western countries is generally less than 10% to 15%. On the other hand, the number of patients with tumors of the gastric cardia has increased in the past two decades. Both trends are particularly unfortunate because they are associated with a dismal prognosis [1].

The only curative treatment is aggressive surgery to completely remove the tumor. However, most gastric cancers are diagnosed at an advanced stage. Non-resectable local spread and a high incidence of synchronous metastasis often compromise a curative surgical approach. Palliative resections are associated with a significant operative morbidity and mortality. Consequently, exploratory laparotomy should be avoided if not required for palliation. The potential of multimodal treatment to improve prognosis has been evaluated, and preoperative treatment may be useful for improving resectability and curability in patients with advanced tumors.

The case presented here illustrates the problem of identifying advanced gastric cancer and the options of treatment today.

Case report

A 44-year-old man presented with a four-month history of upper abdominal discomfort and mild nausea. He had lost 2 kg of body weight but laboratory tests (white and red cell count, hemoglobin, liver enzymes) revealed no abnormalities. There was no history of prior GI-tract diseases or complaints and no drugs had been prescribed in the previous 20 years. The general practi-

tioner had sent him for gastroscopy, and an ulcerous lesion of 3 to 4 cm in diameter at the border between the gastric body and antrum was diagnosed (Fig. 1). Biopsies proved a malignant lesion of signet-ring cell type. The patient was referred for further therapy.

X-ray of the chest and *abdominal ultrasound* were performed but no metastases were detected. Sonographically a slightly thickening wall but not the typical folding and thickening of the gastric wall was observed. *Laboratory test results* were all within normal

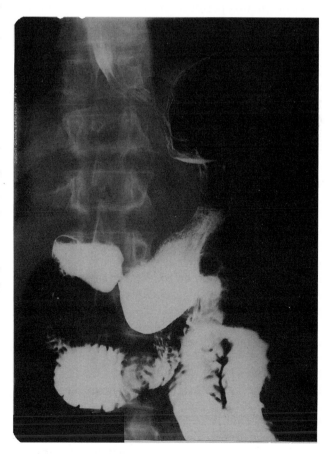

Fig. 1. Contrast study of the stomach showing a gastric carcinoma which infiltrates the corpus of the stomach.

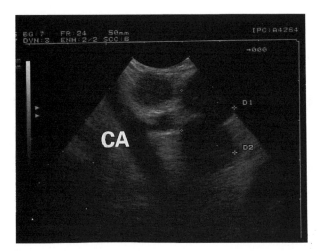

Fig. 2. Endosonography reveals three hypoechoic lymph nodes at the celiac axis (CA).

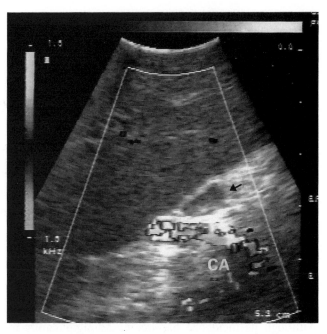

Fig. 3. Laparoscopic ultrasound: Colour coded Doppler ultrasound accurately displays a lymph node (arrow) at the celiac axis (CA).

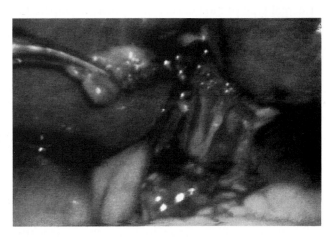

Fig. 4. Laparoscopic view: The lymph node is excised laparoscopically for histologic evaluation of metastatic involvement.

except for a slightly increased CA 72-4 to 6 U/l (normal range up to 4 U/l). *Endoluminal ultrasound* revealed that the tumor was infiltrating all layers of the gastric wall with penetration of the serosa (uT3) and close contact to the left liver lobe, but revealed suspicious hypoechoic lymph nodes at the lesser curvature (uN+) and the left gastric artery at its point of origin in the celiac axis (Fig. 2).

No signs of incurability and/or locally advanced disease were present. Prior to definitive surgery *staging laparoscopy* was performed under general anesthesia. In this procedure a Veress-needle is inserted through the linea alba immediately superior to the umbilicus. Subsequently the abdomen is insufflated with carbon dioxide up to a pressure of 13–15 mmHg. After removal of the needle a 1-cm incision is made for insertion of a 10-mm disposable trocar. If required for further instruments, additional ports can be inserted. The peritoneal cavity is carefully explored with a 45° side viewing laparoscope for free fluid, peritoneal and serosal deposits of tumor and lesions on the surface and undersurface of the liver. Any infiltration of adjacent organs, i.e., liver, diaphragm or pancreas, can be determined by testing the mobility of the stomach with a grasping forceps. Lesser sac exploration is approached by incision of the gastrocolic ligament to exclude retroperitoneal infiltration. In our patient exploration of the lesser sac indicated no infiltration of the pancreas, but did reveal a bulky 2-cm lesion at the serosal site of the gastric fundus. Biopsies obtained showed leiomyoma.

Laparoscopic ultrasound is afterward carried out to improve the results of staging by counteracting the absence of tactile sensitivity of laparoscopic instruments. Introduction of the ultrasound probes with high resolution transducers (7.5 MHz) allows visualization of tumors as small as 5 mm. Since most intra-abdominal lymph nodes are not visible on laparoscopy intra-abdominal ultrasound is particularly valuable, as it can reveal even small nodes. In our patient, lymph nodes at the common hepatic artery (Fig. 3) were enlarged to

2 cm and were suspected of being infiltrated by tumor. The lymph nodes (Fig. 4) were excised and signet cell cancer metastases were seen in frozen sections.

In conclusion, the investigations resulted in a diagnosis of locally advanced primary gastric cancer (T3 lesion). Lymphatic spread was proven to involve the regional nodes at major arteries (N2 node metastases) at the common hepatic artery. The tumor would have been resectable but the patient had to be assigned to stage IIIa according to TNM (Table 1). This stage of disease could qualify the patient for a neoadjuvant treatment study aiming at improved survival and recurrence rate although resection for cure is expected.

Treatment: At laparotomy no intra-abdominal metastases were detected, and frozen sections of the lymph nodes at the liver hilus were negative. However, the tumor spread at the lesser sac invaded the capsule

Table 1. TNM staging of gastric cancer according to the UICC.

Tis	Tumor confined to the epithelial layer without infiltration to lamina propria
T1a	Tumor infiltrates the lamina propria
T1b	Tumor invades to the submucosa
T2	Tumor infiltrates muscularis propria or subserosa
T3	Tumor penetrates serosa (visceral peritoneum)
T4	Tumor infiltrates adjacent structures (spleen, transverse colon, liver, diaphragm, pancreas, abdominal wall, adrenal glands, duodenum, retroperitoneum)
N0	No regional lymph node metastases
N1	Lymph node metastases in perigastric nodes within 3 cm of the border of the primary tumor
N2	Lymph node metastases in perigastric nodes beyond 3 cm of the border of the primary tumor or at the left gastric, common hepatic, splenic or celiac artery
	Regional lymph nodes are: Along the lesser curvature – right cardiac, lesser curvature, suprapyloric nodes Along the greater curvature – left cardiac, left and right greater curvature, infrapyloric
M0/M1	Presence or absence of distant metastases

Stage groups

Stage IA	T1 N0 M0		
Stage IB	T1 N1 M0 or	T2 N0 M0	
Stage II	T1 N2 M0 or	T2 N1 M0 or	T3 N0 M0
Stage IIIA	T2 N2 M0 or	T3 N1 M0 or	T4 N0 M0
Stage IIIB	T3 N2 M0 or	T4 N1 M0	
Stage IV	T4 N2 M0 or	any T any N M1	

Table 2. Purposes and principles of staging with respect to special aspects of gastric cancer.

The category M1 may be specified according to the following notation

PER	Peritoneum
LYM	Lymph nodes
ADR	Adrenals
HEP	Hepatic
OSS	Osseous
PUL	Pulmonary
PLE	Pleura
SKI	Skin
MAR	Bone marrow
BRA	Brain
OTH	Other

Additional descriptors of the TNM classification

u Symbol	Classification determined at ultrasound examination
m Symbol	Multiple primary tumors in a single site
y Symbol	Classification following initial multimodality therapy
r Symbol	Recurrent tumors
a Symbol	Classification determined at autopsy

Histopathological grade (G)
Quantitative assessment of the extent to which a tumor resembles the normal tissue at that site

G1	Well differentiated
G2	Moderately differentiated
G3	Poorly differentiated
G4	Undifferentiated

Histological typing of gastric cancer according to Lauren [43]

Intestinal type	Tendency of malignant cells to form glands, usually well to moderately differentiated; more favourable prognosis
Diffuse type	Lack of organized gland formation, usually poorly differentiated and more common in younger patients; less favourable prognosis

Optional descriptors

L0	No lymphatic invasion
L1	Lymphatic invasion
V0	No venous invasion
V1	Microscopic venous invasion
V2	Macroscopic venous invasion

Residual tumor classification

R0	No residual tumor
R0a	Negative markers after tumor resection for cure
R0b	Persistently elevated marker level after tumor resection for cure
R1	Microscopic residual tumor
R2	Macroscopic residual tumor

Extent of lymphatic dissection during standard gastrectomy

D1 compartment	Removal of perigastric lymph nodes (right and left cardiac, lesser and greater curvature, supra- and infrapyloric)
D2 compartment	Additional removal of lymph nodes along the left gastric, common hepatic, celiac, and splenic artery and at the splenic hilus
D3 compartment	Additional removal of lymph nodes in the hepatoduodenal ligament, at the posterior aspect of the pancreas, the root of the mesenterium, as well as the lower thoracic paraesophageal and diaphragmatic nodes

(the terms D1, D2, and D3 are used in Europe instead of the R1, R2, R3 description of the Japanese Research Society of Gastric Cancer [44])

of the pancreas continuously via the serosa of the gastric wall. A type D2 compartment dissection (Table 2) gastrectomy was performed including removal of the capsule of the pancreas. Reconstruction of the upper GI tract was achieved by construction of a 'neogastric' reservoir (pouch) from small bowel and by Roux-Y anastomosis of the duodenal loop. Due to the invasion of the pancreas capsule (R1 resection) intraperitoneal chemotherapy of 5-FU, mitomycin and cisplatinum was administered via peritoneal catheters starting on day 8 postoperatively.

Histopathological report: pT3 N2 (18/45) M1 PER G3/4 L1 V0 R1, Lauren: diffuse type. (Table 2).

Discussion points

Epidemiology, spread and prognosis of gastric cancer

Generally the prognosis of gastric cancer is poor with less than 20% of the patients surviving for 5 years [2]. The only curative treatment is radical resection. Understanding the pattern of spread and the relation to failure of surgical therapy is of major importance for the development of more efficient therapies. Adenocarcinoma of the stomach spreads by local extension and develops lymphatic, hematogenous or peritoneal metastases. Local extension occurs by intramural growth and by penetration through the gastric serosal layer with infiltration of adjacent structures e.g., omentum, liver, pancreas, or retroperitoneum.

A multicenter study reported data on the epidemiology and treatment of gastric cancer of 2394 patients who underwent laparotomy in 19 university hospitals from 1986 to 1989 [3]. The resectability rate was 82.7%. The proportion of tumors in the proximal stomach was 30%. Seventeen percent of the patients presented with early gastric cancer (pT1), but 16.5% of them had lymph node metastases. In 36% of the patients the tumor was confined to the muscularis whereas in 39% of the tumors serosal infiltration was observed. Infiltration to adjacent organs was confirmed in 8% of the resected tumors.

Lymphatic invasion of gastric cancer occurs early: at the time of resection more than 60% of the patients present with lymph node metastases [3]. A large number of metastatic lymph nodes and involvement of distant lymph nodes indicates a poor prognosis [4]. Peritoneal and distant metastases are found in more than 30% of the patients indicating an extremely poor prognosis. However, 5-year survival after resection of gastric liver metastases has been reported [5].

Generally, survival percentages to be expected at 5 years are 90% for stage IA, 85% for stage IB, about 50% in stage II, 35% in stage IIIA, 20% in stage IIIB and 0% in stage IV.

Although surgery can yield excellent results in early gastric cancer, appropriate treatment of advanced tumors remains a challenge [6]. Even after curative resection 40%–60% of the patients will die of tumor recurrence later in the course of the disease [7], so it has been suggested that the outcome of patients could be improved by adding pre- or postoperative treatment. The choice of a multimodal treatment requires sensitive preoperative staging procedures.

Preoperative staging

General staging procedures involve careful physical examination (medioclavicular (Virchow's) lymph node), endoscopy, upper GI contrast study and abdominal ultrasound. Tumor markers such as CEA, CA19-9 and CA72-4 have not been reliably correlated with extent of disease. Other imaging methods including CT, MRI as well as isotope scanning have been evaluated for preoperative staging, but their resolution is limited to lesions larger than 1 cm. Consequently in a considerable number of patients disseminated disease e.g., small liver metastases, spread to lymph nodes and peritoneum may not be detected. Definite assessment of resectability and curability of cancer of the stomach is frequently achieved only at laparotomy. About 20% to 30% of the patients undergo exploratory laparotomy without resection. Serious complications related to laparotomy have been reported in 15%–20% of patients with gastric cancer, resulting in a mortality rate of more than 10% [8].

In the last few years pre-operative staging of gastric cancer has been improved by the use of endoscopic ultrasonography (EUS) using high-frequency transducers. In a comparative study on 50 patients EUS was superior to CT and MRI in the determination of the T and N categories. An accuracy of 75%–85% in assessment of the depth of tumor infiltration was confirmed by other investigators [9]. The figures for correct assessment of lymph node involvement are less favourable, ranging between 60% and 78%. However, endosonographic evaluation of gastric cancer may be limited by the inability to pass a tumor stenosis in about 14% of the patients [10]. Despite the capability of endosonography to depict small liver metastases and ascites the value of this technique is usually limited to detection of regional tumor spread. Laparoscopy has attracted increasing interest for staging of intra-abdominal tumor dissemination, because sensitive assessment of the viscera and the peritoneal surfaces is possible, since biopsy can be taken under vision [11].

Staging laparoscopy

The objective of laparoscopy is to confirm the histology of suspicious lesions and to precisely define the stage of disease. This includes assessment of local infiltration, and tumor spread by careful examination of the primary, peritoneum, liver and relevant intra-abdominal lymph nodes.

In a series of 369 patients with carcinoma of the esophagus and the gastric cardia intra-abdominal metastases were demonstrated laparoscopically in 24% of 250 patients. Subsequent laparotomy revealed a false negative result in only 4.4% [12]. In the detection of peritoneal metastases laparoscopy showed a sensitivity of 89% while ultrasound and computed tomography (CT) had a sensitivity of 22% and 0%, respectively. In hepatic metastases laparoscopy was more sensitive (96%) than either ultrasound (48%), or CT (56%) [13]. While conventional imaging studies are less invasive than laparoscopy their sensitivity is limited to lesions of 1 cm in diameter or more. Especially small lesions of the peritoneum often escape detection.

Staging laparoscopy can also improve the assessment of resectability in gastric cancer. Advanced and unresectable disease was detected in 27.5% of patients who were considered resectable on the basis of imaging studies including ultrasound and CT. Of patients who subsequently underwent exploratory laparotomy, however, 87% of the tumors could be resected [14].

Although laparoscopy allows detection of small superficial lesions within the abdominal cavity, non-superficial lesions, i.e. intra-parenchymatous metastases and lymph nodes are not always detected. A rate of 26% false negatives for the detection of intra-abdominal lymph nodes by laparoscopy was reported [13]. This is of major importance in gastric cancer because the presence of lymph node metastases at the proper hepatic artery indicates incurability of the disease and consequently radical surgery should be abandoned.

It must be emphasized that laparoscopy is a remarkably safe procedure. In a prospective study there was a complication rate of 2.3% and a mortality rate below 0.5% documented [15]. It is therefore justified to conclude that laparoscopy is safer than explorative laparotomy if tissue diagnosis must be obtained under direct vision. In our own experience [16] with more than 110 patients only four have experienced severe complications: two of them required transfusions due to blood loss, and in both of the other patients laparotomy was mandatory because of bleeding from a major artery after forceps biopsy.

Surgical treatment

The standard treatment in patients assigned to the stages I to III of gastric cancer in our hospital is D2 (Japanese R2) compartment gastrectomy. The procedure includes gastrectomy en bloc with omentectomy, splenectomy, and lymphadenectomy encompassing the nodes of the extragastric N2 level (along the common hepatic, central left gastric, and splenic artery). This type of resection results in substantial change in tumor stage and could account for the different stage-specific survival rates between Japan and the West [17]. There is also evidence that the survival rates are improved [18]. In patients with early gastric cancer proven by endoscopic ultrasound limited endoscopic resection has yielded excellent survival rates [19].

Preoperative chemotherapy

The rationale for *pre-operative chemotherapy* is the induction of tumor regression to improve the local control of subsequent surgery and to eradicate occult metastatic disease. Neoadjuvant treatment may also be a valuable indicator of the responsiveness of the tumor to cytotoxic therapy. Several phase II studies have reported encouraging results in stage III tumors with improved R0 resection rates [20, 21]. The median survival in the chemotherapy group was more than twice of that in the control group. Other authors have observed tumor regression in up to 70% and in some cases even complete eradication of the tumor as evidenced by histopathologic examination [22]. A recent survey of pre-operative chemotherapy summarized seven trials in patients clinically staged as unresectable [23]. However, only two trials were published in full and neither revealed significantly improved survival rates.

Adjuvant and neoadjuvant therapy

Definitive staging of the gastric cancer and identification of patients at high risk for tumor recurrence is only obtained after histopathologic examination of the resected specimen. *Postoperative chemotherapy* offers the chance to eradicate microscopic residual disease when minimal tumor burden is present. The initial study which appeared to improve survival after adjuvant chemotherapy used 5-FU and methyl-CCNU [24]. The 5-year survival rate of patients receiving chemotherapy was 50% compared to 31% in the control group. However two major trials conducted by the ECOG and the VASAG did not confirm these findings. In addition to the questionable efficiency of nitrosurea, there is a considerable risk of treatment-induced leukemia. Sixty-two trials utilizing 5-FU, mitomycin, doxorubicin, methotrexate, nitrosurea and combinations have failed to improve treatment results [25] and other substances capable of overcoming the situation are not yet available [26].

Because peritoneal and lymph node recurrence frequently occur after surgery for gastric cancer *intra-peritoneal chemotherapy* has been favoured in some centres. The rationale is derived from colon cancer in which postoperative intra-peritoneal chemotherapy resulted in a decrease of peritoneal metastases below that of intravenous chemotherapy [27]. However, an Austrian prospective randomized multicenter study involving 67 patients with gastric cancer failed to establish survival advantages in the group receiving intra-peritoneal cisplatin with systemic thiosulfate rescue [28]. Japanese authors favour a carbon-absorbed mitomycin against peritoneal and lymph node recurrence due to its transport in lymphatic vessels [29].

Due to the low radiosensitivity of adenocarcinoma and radiation tolerance of the intestine only few investigators have evaluated *radiotherapy* as an adjuvant to surgical resection. *Intraoperative radiation therapy (IORT)* has been proposed as alternative with a reduced risk of small bowel toxicity. In a non-randomized trial, encouraging survival rates of patients treated with IORT were observed. In patients with stages II, III and IV disease the 5-year survival rate was higher in the IORT than in historic controls treated by surgery alone. Until now, there has been no clear evidence of improved overall survival from the addition of radiation therapy, whether pre-, intra- or postoperatively, nor its combination with chemotherapy [30].

Preliminary data suggested that the effectiveness of radiation can be increased with local *hyperthermia* [31]. Thermotherapy also was added to systemic and intra-peritoneal chemotherapy [32]. However, no definitive conclusions can be drawn as to its value.

Palliative chemotherapy

Agents with at least moderate efficiency include 5-FU, doxorubicin, mitomycin C, epirubicin, BCNU and cis-platinum. Generally the effects of monotherapy are brief and have no significant influence on survival.

In the past decade numerous trials have been conducted to develop more effective *combination chemotherapy* regimen. The FAM regimen (5-FU, doxorubicin, mitomycin), first introduced by MacDonald et al.

[33], induced a partial response (PR) in 42% of the patients and their median survival was 12.5 months. In subsequent studies using FAM a cumulative response rate of 30% and a complete remission (CR) rate of 2% were achieved in more than 600 patients [34]. Although there was no general improvement in disease-free or overall survival, some data indicate that patients with advanced disease may benefit from treatment [35].

Attempts have been made to enhance the cytotoxicity of 5-FU by biochemical modulation with agents such as methotrexate (MTX) that increase the level of ribonucleotides in tumor cells. Initial treatment results using 5-FU, doxorubicin and methotrexate (FAMTX) were encouraging, with a response rate of 59% with 12% of the patients achieving a CR [36]. The median survival was 9 months. Later randomized trials confirmed the superiority of FAMTX with respect to the response rate but a beneficial effect on survival has only been observed in an EORTC study [37].

More recently the combination of etoposide, doxorubicin and cisplatin (EAP) was reported to induce a PR in more than 60% and a CR in up to 10%–20% of the patients [38]. Despite the improved short-term response the median survival after chemotherapy is generally less than 12 months. Severe hematologic toxicity and treatment-related death due to myelosuppression may occur in about 10% of the patients [39]. Therefore EAP therapy cannot be considered as standard treatment. Various other multidrug regimens including modulation of 5-FU with leucovorin and interferon have not demonstrated superiority for combination therapy to 5-FU alone [40]. Regional chemotherapy via the celiac axis also has still to prove its value [41].

In this context, with inconsistent response rates reported, and no definite improvement in survival rates, the quality of life of the patient and economical aspects have to be taken into consideration when deciding to initiate palliative chemotherapy for gastric cancer.

Laparoscopic palliation

In instances of inoperable malignant disease palliative procedures may be performed laparoscopically. In these patients a laparoscopic approach is preferable to open surgery because a significant improvement in the quality of life can be provided with reasonable risk and inconvenience for the patient. Indications for non-resective bowel operations include surgical access for enteral nutrition as well as bowel division and enteric bypass procedures for obstructing gastrointestinal cancer [11].

Percutaneous enteral nutrition is often required in severe dysphagia caused by advanced cancer of the esophagus and the proximal stomach. Percutaneous laparoscopic gastrostomy (PLG) and percutaneous laparoscopic jejunostomy (PLJ) provide an alternative to open surgery if an endoscopic approach is impossible due to the inability to pass the endoscope over the stenosis. While accomplishing the same results as conventional surgery PLG and PLJ are associated with less pain, short ileus and a low infection rate, thus contributing to a rapid postoperative recovery of the patient. After the learning phase the procedure can be performed in less than 45 minutes. All patients advanced to full nutritional support within two days and none of them suffered reflux or aspiration [42]. In non-resectable gastric cancer with gastric outlet obstruction gastrointestinal bypass procedures may be required, and there is already initial experience with laparoscopic gastrojejunostomy.

References

1. Breaux JR, Bringaze W, Chappuis C, Cohn IJ. Adenocarcinoma of the stomach: A review of 35 years and 1,710 cases. World J Surg 1990; 14: 580–6.
2. Akoh JA, Macintyre IM. Improving survival in gastric cancer: Review of 5-year survival rates in English language publications from 1970. Br J Surg 1992; 79: 293–9.
3. Böttcher K, Roder JD, Busch R et al. Epidemiologie des Magencarcinoms aus chirurgischer Sicht. Dtsch. Med Wschr 1993; 118: 729–36.
4. Lee WJ, Lee PH, Yue SC et al. Lymph node metastases in gastric cancer: Significance of positive number. Oncology 1995; 52: 45–50.
5. Ochiai T, Sasako M, Mizuno S et al. Hepatic resection for metastatic tumours from gastric cancer: Analysis of prognostic factors. Br J Surg 1994; 81: 1175–8.
6. Habu H, Saito N, Sato Y et al. Results of surgery in patients with gastric cancer extending to the adjacent organs. Hepato-gastroenterology 1990; 37: 417–20.
7. Moriguchi S, Maehara Y, Korenaga D et al. Risk factors which predict pattern of recurrence after curative surgery for patients with advanced gastric cancer. Surg Oncol 1992; 1: 341–6.
8. Böttcher K, Siewert JR, Roder JD et al. Risk of surgical therapy of stomach cancer in Germany. Results of the German 1992 Stomach Cancer Study. Chirurg 1994; 65: 298–306.
9. Tio TL, Coene PP, Schouwink MH, Tytgat GN. Esophagogastric carcinoma: Preoperative TNM classification with endosonography. Radiology 1989; 173: 411–7.
10. Grimm H, Binmoeller KF, Hamper K et al. Endosonography for preoperative locoregional staging of esophageal and gastric cancer. Endoscopy 1993; 25: 224–30.
11. Cushieri A. Laparoscopic management of cancer patients. J R Coll Surg Edinb 1995; 40: 1–9.
12. Dagnini G, Caldironi MW, Marin G et al. Laparoscopy in abdominal staging of esophageal carcinoma. Report of 369 cases. Gastrointest Endosc 1986; 32: 400–2.
13. Watt J, Stewart J, Anderson D et al. Laparoscopy, ultrasound and computed tomography in cancer of the esophagus and gastric cardia: A prospective comparison for detecting intra-abdominal metastases. Br J Surg 1989; 76: 1036–9.
14. Kriplani AK, Kapur BM. Laparoscopy for pre-operative staging and assessment of operability in gastric carcinoma. Gastrointest Endosc 1991; 37: 441–3.
15. Kane MG, Kreis GJ. Complication of diagnostic laparoscopy in Dallas. A seven year prospective study. Gastrointest Endosc 1984; 30: 237–40.
16. Hünerbein M, Rau B, Schlag PM. Laparoscopy and laparoscopic ultrasound for staging of upper gastrointestinal tumours. Eur J Surg Oncol 1995; 21: 50–5.
17. Bunt AM, Hermans J, Smit VT et al. Surgical/pathologic-stage migration confounds comparisons of gastric cancer survival rates between Japan and Western countries. J Clin Oncol 1995; 13: 19–25.
18. Siewert JR, Böttcher K, Roder JD et al. Prognostic relevance of

systematic lymph node dissection in gastric carcinoma. German Gastric Carcinoma Study Group. Br J Surg 1993; 80: 1015–8.

19. Takekoshi T, Baba Y, Ota H et al. Endoscopic resection of early gastric carcinoma: Results of a retrospective analysis of 308 cases. Endoscopy 1994; 26: 352–8.

20. Yonemura Y, Sawa T, Kinoshita K et al. Neoadjuvant chemotherapy for high-grade advanced gastric cancer. World J Surg 1993; 17: 256–61.

21. Plukker JT, Sleijfer CJ, Verschuren WTA et al. Neo-adjuvant chemotherapy for locally advanced cancer of the cardia. Results of a phase II study with carboplatin, 4-epiadriamycin and tenposide (CET). Proc Am Soc Clin Oncol 1994; 13: 223.

22. Ajani JA, Roth JA, Ryan MB et al. Intensive preoperative chemotherapy with colony stimulating factor for resectable adenocarcinoma of the esophagua or the gastroesophageal junction. J Clin Oncol 1993; 11: 22.

23. Wilke H, Stahl M, Fink U et al. Preoperative chemotherapy for unresectable gastric cancer. World J Surg 1995; 19: 210–5.

24. Gastrointestinal Tumor Study Group. Controlled trial of adjuvant chemotherapy following curative resection for gastric cancer. Cancer 1982; 49: 1116–22.

25. Hermans J, Bonenkamp JJ, Boon MC et al. Adjuvant therapy after curative resection for gastric cancer: Meta-analysis of randomized trials. J Clin Oncol 1993; 11: 1441–7.

26. Douglas HOJ. Adjuvant therapy of gastric cancer: Have we made any progress? Ann Oncol 1994; 5 (Suppl 3): 49–57.

27. Sugarbaker PH, Cunliffe WJ, Belliveau J et al. Rationale for integrating early postoperative intraperitoneal chemotherapy into the surgical treatment of gastrointestinal cancer. Semin Oncol 1989; 16: 83–97.

28. Sautner T, Hofbauer F, Depisch D et al. Adjuvant intraperitoneal cisplatin chemotherapy does not improve long-term survival after surgery for advanced gastric cancer. J Clin Oncol 1994; 12: 970–4.

29. Hagiwara A, Takahashi T, Kojima O et al. Prophylaxis with carbon-adsorbed mitomycin against peritoneal recurrence of gastric cancer. Lancet 1992; 339: 629–31.

30. Budach VG. The role of radiation therapy in the management of gastric cancer. Ann Oncol 1994; 5 (Suppl 3): 37–48.

31. Shchepotin IB, Evans SR, Chorny V et al. Intensive preoperative radiotherapy with local hyperthermia for the treatment of gastric carcinoma. Surg Oncol 1994; 3: 37–44.

32. Kaibara N, Hamazoe R, Iitsuka Y et al. Hyperthermic peritoneal perfusion combined with anticancer chemotherapy as prophylactic treatment of peritoneal recurrence of gastric cancer. Hepatogastroenterology 1989; 36: 75–8.

33. Macdonald JS, Schein PS, Woolley PV. 5-FU, mitomycin C and adriamycin (FAM): A new chemtherapy regimen for advanced gastric carcinoma. Ann Int Med 1980; 93: 533.

34. Preusser P, Achterrath W, Wilke H. Chemotherapy of gastric cancer. Cancer Treat Rev 1988; 15: 257–77.

35. Coombes RC, Schein PS, Chilvers CE et al. A randomized trial comparing adjuvant fluorouracil, doxorubicin, and mitomycin with no treatment in operable gastric cancer. International Collaborative Cancer Group. J Clin Oncol 1990; 8: 1362–9.

36. Klein HO. Wickramanayke PD, Dieterle F et al. Chemotherapieprotokoll zur Behandlung des fortgeschrittenen Magenkarzinoms. Dtsch Med Wschr 1982; 107: 1708.

37. Wils JA, Klein HO, Wagener DJ et al. Sequential high-dose methotrexate and fluorouracil combined with doxorubicin – a step ahead in the treatment of advanced gastric cancer: A trial of the European Organization for Research and Treatment of Cancer Gastrointestinal Tract Cooperative Group. J Clin Oncol 1991; 9: 827–31.

38. Preusser P, Wilke H, Achterrath W. Phase II study with the combination of etoposide, doxorubicin and cisplatin in advanced measurable gastric cancer. J Clin Oncol 1989; 7: 1310–7.

39. Kelsen D, Atiq OT, Saltz L et al. FAMTX versus etoposide, doxorubicin, and cisplatin: A random assignment trial in gastric cancer. J Clin Oncol 1992; 10: 541–8.

40. Cullinan SA, Moertel CG, Wieand HS et al. Controlled evaluation of three drug combination regimens versus fluorouracil alone for the therapy of advanced gastric cancer. North Central Cancer Treatment Group. J Clin Oncol 1994; 12: 412–6.

41. Stephens FO. The role of regional chemotherapy in gastric cancer. Eur J Surg Oncol 1994; 20: 187–8.

42. Sangster W, Swanstrom J. Laparoscopic guided feeding jejunostomy. Surg Endosc 1993; 7: 308–10.

43. Lauren P. The two histological main types of gastric carcinoma, diffuse and so-called intestinal type carcinoma. Acta Pathol Microbiol Scand 1965; 64: 31–49.

44. Japanese Research Society of Gastric Cancer. The general rules for the gastric cancer study in surgery and pathology. Jpn J Surg 1981; 11: 127–45.

R. L. Souhami (ed.) The Teaching Cases from Annals of Oncology, 159–164, 1997.
© *1997 Kluwer Academic Publishers. Printed in the Netherlands.*

High grade soft tissue sarcoma

G. F. McLeay & W. P. Steward

Beatson Oncology Centre, Western Infirmary, Glasgow, U.K.

Key words: diagnosis, biopsy, soft tissue sarcoma, management of soft tissue sarcoma

Case history

In May 1987 a 50-year-old male fire-officer presented to his General Practitioner with a 2-week history of increasing pain, tenderness and thickening in the lateral aspect of the right wrist. There was no history of recent trauma. On examination there was marked local tenderness and swelling over the area which was the site of a scar from prior surgery. The patient was otherwise completely asymptomatic. There was no significant family history and he was on no medication.

In 1983 he had sustained a traumatic injury to the same area of the right wrist. On examination at that time he was tender over the scaphoid tuberosity and a clinical diagnosis of a scaphoid fracture was made. Plain radiology was normal. His forearm and hand were immobilised in a plaster-of-Paris cast. The x-ray was repeated two weeks later and again no fracture was seen. He continued to have discomfort over the lower radius and a diagnosis of tenosynovitis was made and treated with local infiltrations of Marcaine and hydrocortisone.

The wrist was eventually explored in July 1983. Thickening of the sheath of flexor carpi radialis was discovered, split and excised and the patient was symptom free five months later. The pain recurred in the same site in May 1985 and the wrist was re-explored. The dorsal branch of the radial nerve was exposed and the tendon sheath of the long extensors was opened. The pain worsened after this procedure and he was unable to return to work. A combination of physiotherapy, carbamazepine and referral to the pain clinic did not result in any improvement.

At the time of exacerbation of pain in 1987 he was referred back to the orthopaedic surgeon in a local hospital. A pulsatile mass measuring 3 × 2 cm was noted in the painful area and was thought to represent a radial artery aneurysm resulting from his original trauma. An angiogram failed to demonstrate either an aneurysm or arterio-venous malformation but the radial artery was displaced to the ulnar side by a mass. The area was subsequently explored in November 1987 using an incision which extended proximally along the original scar and from radial to ulnar aspect of the wrist. A large 'well encapsulated' swelling was found which had dis-

placed most of the structures of the wrist to the ulnar aspect and extended 5 cm proximally from the distal wrist crease. This was dissected free of the radial artery and median nerve and the tumour was excised, although 'gelatinous material' was noted to be invading neighbouring muscle and bone.

Histology was reported as showing a spindle cell tumour with a high mitotic count (Fig. 1a). Most of the resection margins contained tumour. The cytoplasmic contents varied considerably from cell to cell and there was a large amount of glycogen in many cells – features consistent with a diagnosis of leiomyosarcoma. Electron microscopy revealed the nuclei to be composed mainly of euchromatin and to have prominent often multiple nucleoli.

As the excision margins were not clear, further exploration of the wrist was performed in March 1988. Pre-operative CT scans of the chest and wrist revealed no evidence of metastases or of visible residual disease. An attempt was made to remove tissue from the previous excision margins and an area of radial cortex which appeared eroded was removed. Histology revealed tissue from all areas to be involved with leiomyosarcoma – including bone cortex and underlying marrow (Fig. 1b).

An isotope bone scan was performed and revealed the only area of abnormal uptake to be in the right wrist. The patient was referred for post-operative radiotherapy. He received 6000cGy in 30 fractions as a parallel pair, sparing a strip of skin on the ulnar side of the wrist to try and prevent late onset oedema.

He was well until November 1988, when an x-ray showed an ill-defined defect in the distal radius with surrounding sclerosis, thought to be due to a combination of surgery and radiotherapy. By March 1989 there was worsening pain and there was an ill-defined swelling palpable at the site of his original surgery. A repeat x-ray of the wrist showed increasing sclerosis which would have been consistent with further healing. An incision biopsy of the swelling was made and histology confirmed recurrent tumour.

A CT scan of the chest, biochemical profile and isotope bone scan revealed no evidence of metastases. Further conservative surgery was not possible and an above elbow amputation was therefore performed in

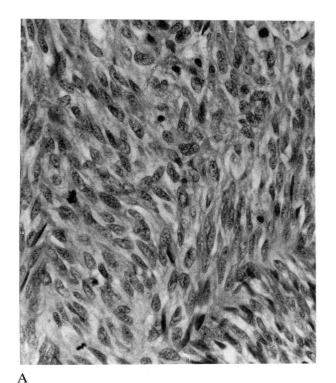

A

B

Fig. 1. Histological sections of leiomyosarcoma. (a) shows a highly cellular tumour with spindle shaped cells arranged in fascicles. Numerous mitotic figures are present. (b) shows tumour surrounding a trabecula of lamellar bone from the medullary canal of the radius.

May 1989. Extensive local recurrence involving bone and soft tissues was reported on histological section.

The patient made a good post-operative recovery, remaining asymptomatic when seen every 3 months for clinical examination and a chest x-ray. Unfortunately in October 1990 the films revealed a mass at the right hilum. CT imaging of the thorax demonstrated three metastases; one in the right upper lobe (4 cm × 4 cm), one in the right lower lobe (1 cm × 1 cm), and one in the left upper lobe (0.6 cm × 0.5 cm) (Fig. 2).

The patient was referred to a cardiothoracic sur-

geon for consideration of metastasectomy. An isotope bone scan and liver ultrasound revealed no evidence of disease outside the thorax and pulmonary function tests were normal. The metastases were excised using segmental resections during bilateral thoracotomies in February 1991. All three specimens contained spindle cell tumour of high mitotic rate in keeping with the original diagnosis of leiomyosarcoma, and all were described as having been completely excised.

Routine follow-up included two-monthly chest x-rays and in June 1991 a metastasis measuring 2 cm × 2 cm was noted in the mid zone of the left lung. Further surgery was contemplated but a CT scan revealed multiple pulmonary nodules in both lung fields which were not operable. As the patient was initially asymptomatic a watch policy was maintained but by August 1991 he complained of increasing dyspnoea on exertion. The chest x-ray confirmed marked progression (Fig. 3) and he was offered chemotherapy.

Single agent epirubicin (50 mg/m^2 daily for three days repeated every 21 days) was given according to an EORTC study which compared the effects of different doses and schedules of anthracyclines in advanced sar-

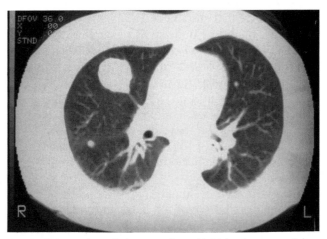

Fig. 2. CT scan through thorax at time of initial pulmonary relapse. Two metastases are seen on the right and one on the left.

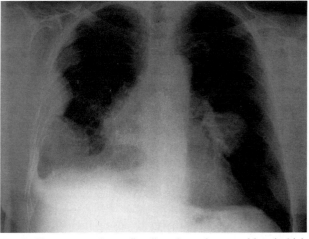

Fig. 3. Chest x-ray prior to first-line chemotherapy with epirubicin showing large bilateral pulmonary metastases.

comas. He received five cycles before treatment was discontinued because of severe mucositis and neutropenia. Despite the side effects, he achieved a partial response (Fig. 4) with reduction in the size of all metastases and resolution of his respiratory symptoms.

The patient remained well until February 1992 (3 months after the last course of epirubicin), when he again developed respiratory symptoms with increasing breathlessness, a troublesome cough and chest pain. A chest x-ray showed further progression of his metastases, and second-line chemotherapy was instituted using single agent ifosfamide (5 g/m²). He tolerated this well with no major toxicities. The metastases showed a further partial response with accompanying resolution of his symptoms after the second course and treatment continued to five cycles. Unfortunately his clinical condition deteriorated again in July 1992 and was associated with rapid progression of his pulmonary metastases. He was managed symptomatically in a hospice and died in September 1992.

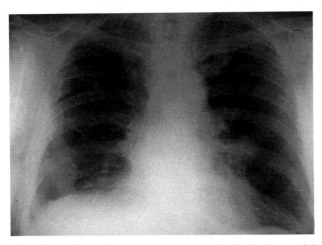

Fig. 4. Chest x-ray after three courses of epirubicin showing partial remission of pulmonary metastases.

Discussion

This history illustrates several of the decisions which may have to be taken during the course of managing patients with soft tissue sarcomas. Although this is a relatively rare neoplasm (0.7% of all cancers) it is essential that clinicians are aware of the possibilities for therapy as optimal management can have a significant impact on outcome. In specialist centres where there is close collaboration between orthopaedic surgeons, pathologists, radiologists and oncologists who are all experienced in the management of these tumours, approximately 70% of patients should be curable. Unfortunately care is often suboptimal and the overall 5-year survival rate is only 45% in most countries of Western Europe and North America [1]. Several treatment decisions which were taken during the care of our patient are open to question and their potential impact on his survival are discussed below.

Presentation — was the diagnosis delayed too long?

There was a six month delay between the onset of pain and swelling of the wrist and a biopsy being performed on this patient. Such delays in diagnosis are a frequent source of confusion and distress for patients with sarcomas. They usually arise (as in this case) as a result of investigations and treatment being carried out for another presumed benign cause of the symptoms – most frequently a recent traumatic injury. Although trauma is a common part of the history of such patients, it is likely that this merely brings a pre-existing lesion to their attention and is not related to the aetiology of their tumour. The delays which occur result in an increase in size of the primary lesion which reduces the ease of performing adequate conservative surgery. There will be an increased risk of developing metastases with consequent reduction in the chance of long-term survival. In this patient the 6 month delay in performing a biopsy was particularly disturbing as he was already under specialist care. It is important to biopsy such swellings early if they continue to grow or do not resolve after 3–4 weeks as there are no reliable clinical signs which differentiate benign from malignant soft tissue masses.

Diagnosis — was the biopsy procedure correct?

Soft tissue sarcomas grow radially, compressing surrounding tissues into a pseudocapsule. The tumour infiltrates widely along tissue planes and invariably penetrates the pseudocapsule. It was therefore inevitable that following a 'shelling out' of the mass in this patient, the resection margins would contain tumour which infiltrated surrounding muscle. The nature of the biopsy is an important aspect of the overall management of soft tissue sarcomas. If a sarcoma is suspected, the patient should be referred for the biopsy to be performed by a surgeon who is experienced in such techniques so that the correct procedure is performed, the tissue is properly processed and examined by a specialist pathologist and definitive surgery, if necessary, can be planned.

An incisional biopsy is usually the appropriate diagnostic procedure. The surgeon must be aware that disturbances of the pseudocapsule and haematoma formation results in the spread of neoplastic cells – the tract of an incision will therefore have to be removed when definitive surgery is performed. This is particularly important in lesions of extremities where a longitudinal incision should be made so as not to compromise muscle group excision which may be necessary later. Unfortunately both longitudinal and lateral incisions were made in this patient, potentially contaminating the whole of the flexor compartment. Needle aspirate cytology gives inadequate material for correct histopathological classification but needle biopsy using a biopsy gun may give adequate tissue and in the case of round cell sarcomas allow chemotherapy to begin before excision of the mass. Excisional biopsy should be avoided since subsequent surgery may then be very difficult (see below).

Interpretation of biopsy specimens requires expert pathologists to differentiate histological subtypes and grade of tumour. In this case the full histological diagnosis was only made because there was adequate tissue to allow electron microscopy to be performed. Although leiomyosarcomas only comprise 6%–10% of all sarcomas they are an important subgroup arising from smooth muscle of blood vessel walls and viscera and may be found anywhere in the body. They are usually of high grade and therefore have an aggressive natural history [2].

Primary management — was local excision and radiotherapy optimal?

Once a diagnosis is made, definitive treatment is planned. It should be based on the extent of local disease and presence or absence of distant metastases. Local spread is best assessed by plain radiography and MR imaging (or CT scanning if MR is not available) of the affected region. Pulmonary metastases are shown by chest radiography and CT scanning of the thorax, and liver metastases by biochemical investigations, liver ultrasonography or CT imaging. At the time of presentation >90% of patients with extremity sarcomas will have no detectable metastatic disease. Two staging systems (Table 1) are widely used [3] and take a number of variables into account including the histological grade of the tumour – the most important single factor to predict the likelihood of local recurrence and length of survival. Other factors which affect prognosis are listed in Table 2.

Optimal management of the primary tumour involves radical local excision (removal of tumour along with all tissues in the compartment occupied by the primary) or a wide excision removing all gross tumour with a margin of normal surrounding tissue in continuity with the primary. Amputation may be necessary to gain local control. In some situations amputation may be avoided by radical excision combined with endoprosthetic replacement of bone – an area of specialist surgical management. This patient underwent excision biopsy alone and unfortunately a large percentage of patients are sill treated in the same fashion. Local recurrence is inevitable with such a procedure (and will be associated with the development of concurrent distant metastases in 40% of cases) so that, if this procedure has been carried out, a decision must then be taken to offer more treatment which may involve both further surgery and radiotherapy.

Soft tissue sarcomas are radiosensitive tumours but treatment has to be aggressive (with doses of 60–80 Gy) to obtain maximum control. The timing of radiotherapy is controversial – it is usually given post-opera-

Table 1. Schemes for staging soft tissue sarcomas.

a) System described by American Joint Committee for Cancer Staging and End Results (AJC).

Stage	Tumour type
Ia	Grade I tumour <5 cm
Ib	Grade I tumour ≥5 cm
IIa	Grade II tumour <5 cm
IIB	Grade II tumour ≥5 cm
IIIa	Grade III tumour <5 cm
IIIB	Grade III tumour ≥5 cm

No regional node involvement or distant metastases

IIIc	Tumour of any grade or size with involvement of the regional lymph nodes, but not distant metastases
IVa	Tumour of any grade that grossly invades bone, a major blood vessel or a major nerve, with or without regional node involvement, but no distant metastases
IVb	Tumour with distant metastases

b) System described by Enneking et al. [3]

Stage	Grade	Site
Ia	Low (G1)	Intracompartmental (T1)
Ib	Low (G1)	Extracompartmental (T2)
IIa	High (G2)	Intracompartmental (T1)
IIb	High (G2)	Extracompartmental (T2)
III	Any (G) Regional or distant metastases	Any (T)

Table 2. Factors of prognostic significance for patients with soft tissue sarcomas.

Histological grade
Site (proximal vs. distral; extremity vs. trunk)
Size
Lymph node involvement

tively, but there are theoretical advantages for preoperative administration and some centres claim better results with this. The results of radical surgery in terms of local control are superior to those of local excision plus radiotherapy. Wide excisions are associated with local recurrences in approximately 50% of patients and this figure is improved to only 14% local failure rates with compartmental excisions, amputation or endoprosthetic replacement [4]. In specialist centres local control may reach 80% in patients with small (<5 cm) extremity tumours using radical radiotherapy (usually pre- and post-operatively) with wide local excision [5]. Post-operative radiotherapy should not, however, be considered as a salvage procedure for inadequate initial surgery.

The problems of inadequate initial surgery are highlighted in this patient. An incisional biopsy could have allowed subsequent imaging to delineate the extent of the tumour and radical definitive surgery with preservation of the limb may have been possible. Unfortunately, following an excisional biopsy, the extent of residual tumour could not be determined and amputation was the only practical radical alternative. Instead of this, however, the patient was managed with an attempt at a wide excision followed by radiotherapy. Despite a maximum tolerable dose of radiotherapy, recurrence occurred within the radiation field 18 months later (80% of relapses occur within 2 years of treatment of the primary).

Should adjuvant chemotherapy have been offered?

Even with a wide excision of the primary lesion, up to 50% of patients will develop a local recurrence and 30%–60% will develop distant metastases. Several studies have therefore been performed in soft tissue sarcomas to examine the potential role of adjuvant chemotherapy. Unfortunately, because of the rarity of this disease, historical untreated controls have often been used and have shown improvements of disease free survival with treatment [6, 7]. Such studies have a major flaw in that concurrent controls at the NCI have been shown to have a significantly better survival than historical controls taken from a previous trial in the same centre [8]. Improvements in surgical and radiotherapy techniques almost certainly explain these changes. Only 4 adjuvant studies have been randomised and 3 have shown no benefit from chemotherapy [for review see 9]. A small study (65 patients) from the NCI [10] showed improved survival for extremity sarcomas with adjuvant doxorubicin, cyclophosphamide and methotrexate but a much larger series from the EORTC has shown no survival benefit from cyclophosphamide, vincristine, doxorubicin and DTIC (CyVADIC) in over 400 patients [11]. The literature would therefore not have supported the routine use of adjuvant chemotherapy for this patient – its use must be limited to carefully controlled randomised trials.

Treatment of recurrent disease — was amputation justified?

At the time the patient developed local recurrence, full staging investigations were performed to exclude sites of possible metastases. For extremity sarcomas, 90% of distant metastases occur in the lungs and <10% in the liver [12]. Staging should therefore include pain radiography and CT scanning of the thorax, liver function tests and, if possible, CT scanning or ultrasonography of the liver and clinical examination of the draining lymph nodes (though these are involved in <5% of patients). For those patients who undergo resection of apparently isolated local recurrences, the 5-year survival rates in most series are 40%–50% [4]. The only practical surgical procedure in this patient was an amputation, and even though this would cause significant disability, the chance of success was high enough to make this a justifiable procedure.

Pulmonary metastases — was thoracotomy justifiable?

The appearance of pulmonary metastases two years after amputation led to referral for a thoracic opinion and subsequent resection of the three lesions which were demonstrated on a CT scan. The results of several series of patients treated by pulmonary metastasectomy have ben published [13]. Three factors appear to correlate with a favourable outcome – low number of lesions, small size and prolonged period from surgery to first appearance [14]. Five year survival rates in different series are between 20%–35%. The NCI reported a 3-year survival rate of 22% for 29 patients undergoing second thoracotomies for recurrent pulmonary metastases [15]. These operations carry minimal mortality and are accompanied by acceptable morbidity. Given the two year latency period between prior surgery and appearance of 3 metastases (albeit that one was relatively large), thoracotomy was a reasonable approach for this patient.

Chemotherapy for advanced disease — when and what?

Unfortunately the patient developed inoperable extensive pulmonary relapse shortly after surgery. As he was initially asymptomatic, no active treatment was indicated – there is no evidence that chemotherapy or radiotherapy for inoperable metastatic disease prolong survival and intervention was only justifiable when he subsequently became severely dyspnoeic. The most active single chemotherapy agent in soft tissue sarcomas is doxorubicin. Response rates between 9%–70% have been reported but for most large series approximately 30% of patients will achieve a partial remission and 5%–10% will achieve a complete response [16]. Survival for responders is usually a median of 12–18 months. There is a clear dose-response relationship for doxorubicin in this disease and this may partly explain the wide variation of results in different series. Optimal results are obtained with a dose-intensity >70 mg/m^2 every 3 weeks [17]. In an attempt to overcome the risk of cardiotoxicity, analogues of doxorubicin have been examined in this disease and epirubicin is currently being evaluated in two different doses and schedules as part of a large randomised study of the EORTC Sarcoma Group.

The only other agent with >20% single agent activity in soft tissue sarcomas is ifosfamide [18]. This patient initially responded well to epirubicin but relapsed shortly afterwards. His symptoms could not be controlled with simple procedures including steroids and analgesics and so he received ifosfamide as part of an ongoing EORTC phase II study examining different schedules of this agent. Again he responded but only for a short duration. No other active chemotherapy drugs were available and he was cared for with symptomatic measures alone.

Combination chemotherapy is still widely used to

treat soft tissue sarcomas. There is, however, no evidence that this is superior to either of the two active agents used alone at optimal dose intensity – indeed combinations compromise the dose of either drug which can safely be given and add to the toxicity of treatment. The EORTC Sarcoma Group recently completed a large randomised study comparing single agent doxorubicin with CyVADIC and the combination of doxorubicin and ifosfamide. The CyVADIC arm was closed early because of significantly greater toxicity and results in terms of response rates and survival were similar for all treatments [19]. A recent EORTC study has combined higher doses of doxorubicin and ifosfamide with the haemopoietic growth factor Granulocyte-Macrophage Colony-Stimulating Factor (GM-CSF) and shown a 45% response rate with 16 month median survival which is higher than has been seen previously by the Sarcoma Group [20]. This regimen is now being compared with standard dose treatment in a prospective trial.

Patients with inoperable symptomatic soft tissue sarcomas for whom chemotherapy is deemed appropriate should therefore be treated in a clinical trial whenever possible. If no such trial is available, single agent doxorubicin (75 mg/m^2) should first be considered. Ifosfamide 5 g/m^2 is a reasonable alternative. Treatment of patients who fail first-line, or at most second-line therapy should be simple palliation.

Summary

The management of our patient was similar to that of many patients with soft tissue sarcomas. His primary care was in a General Hospital where the surgeon had no specialist experience of these tumours and did not anticipate such a diagnosis. As a result the diagnostic procedure was inappropriate and compromised the chances of success of further more radical conservative surgery. Radiotherapy was unable to prevent local recurrence and amputation became necessary. Pulmonary metastases developed and were resected but within a short space of time extensive inoperable metastases recurred. Although these responded to chemotherapy, the response duration was short and the patient died soon afterwards. The major lessons to be learned are the need to have a high index of suspicion about a possible neoplastic cause of increasing soft tissue swellings and to refer patients for biopsy to a specialist centre where there is experience of all aspects of the management of these rare but potentially curable malignancies.

References

1. Simon MA, Enneking WF. The management of soft tissue sarcomas of the extremities. J Bone Joint Surg 1976; 58: 317.
2. Wile AG, Evans HL, Romsdahl MM. Leiomyosarcoma of soft tissue: A clinicopathologic study. Cancer 1981; 48: 1022.
3. Enneking WF, Spanier SS, Goodman MA. The surgical staging of musculoskeletal sarcoma. J Bone Joint Surg 1980; 62: 1027–30.
4. Shiu MH, Castro EB, Hajdu SI et al. Surgical treatment of 297 soft tissue sarcomas of the lower extremity. Ann Surg 1975; 182: 597.
5. Tepper JE, Suit HD. Radiation therapy of soft tissue sarcomas. Cancer 1985; 55: 2273–7.
6. Sordillo PP, Magill GB, Shiu MH et al. Adjuvant chemotherapy of soft part sarcomas with ALOMAD (S4). J Surg Oncol 1981; 18: 345–52.
7. Das Gupta TK, Patel MK, Chaudhuri PK et al. The role of chemotherapy as an adjuvant to surgery in the initial treatment of primary soft tissue sarcomas in adults. J Surg Oncol 1982; 19: 139–44.
8. Rosenberg SA, Chang AE, Glatstein E. Adjuvant chemotherapy for treatment of extremity soft tissue sarcomas: Review of National Cancer Institute experience. Cancer Treat Symp 1985; 3: 83–8.
9. Baker LH. Adjuvant therapy for soft tissue sarcomas. In Ryan JR, Baker LH (eds): Recent Concepts in Sarcoma Treatment. Kluwer Academic Publishers: Dordrecht 1987.
10. Rosenberg SA, Tepper J, Glatstein E et al. Prospective randomised evaluation of adjuvant chemotherapy in adults with soft tissue sarcomas of the extremities. Cancer 1983; 52: 424–34.
11. Bramwell V, Rouesse J, Steward WP et al. European experience of adjuvant chemotherapy for soft tissue sarcoma: Interim report of a randomised trial of CyVADIC versus control. In Ryan JR, Baker LH (eds): Recent Concepts in Sarcoma Treatment. Kluwer Academic Publishers: Dordrecht 1987.
12. Potter DA, Glenn J, Kinsella T et al. Patterns of recurrence in patients with high grade soft tissue sarcomas. J Clin Oncol 1985; 3: 353–66.
13. Lawrence W Jr, Donegan WL, Nachimuth N et al. Adult soft tissue sarcomas. A pattern of care survey of the American College of Surgeons. Ann Surg 1987; 205: 349–59.
14. Roth JA, Putnam JB, Wesley MN et al. Differing determinants of prognosis following resection of pulmonary metastases from osteogenic and soft tissue sarcoma patients. Cancer 1985; 55: 1361–6.
15. Rizzoni WE, Pass HI, Wesley MN et al. Resection of recurrent pulmonary metastases in patients with soft tissue sarcomas. Arch Surg 1986; 121: 1248–52.
16. Pinedo HM, Kenis Y. Chemotherapy of advanced soft tissue sarcoma in adults. Cancer Treat Rev 1977; 4: 67–86.
17. O'Bryan RM, Baker LH, Gottlieb JE et al. Dose response evaluation of adriamycin in human neoplasia. Cancer 1977; 39: 1940–8.
18. Stuart-Harris CA, Gowing HE, Wiltshaw E. High-dose alkylating therapy using ifosfamide infusion with mesna in the treatment of adult soft tissue sarcomas. Cancer Chemother Pharmacol 1983; 11: 69–72.
19. Santoro A, Rouesse J, Steward W et al. A randomized EORTC study in advanced soft tissue sarcomas (STS): ADM vs. ADM + IFX vs. CYVADIC. Proc Am Soc Clin Oncol 1990; 9: 1196.
20. Steward WP, Verweij J, Somers R et al. Granulocyte-macrophage colony-stimulating factor allows safe escalation of dose-intensity of chemotherapy in metastatic adult soft-tissue sarcomas. J Clin Oncol 1993; 11: 22–8.

R. L. Souhami (ed.) The Teaching Cases from Annals of Oncology, 165–170, 1997.
© 1997 *Kluwer Academic Publishers. Printed in the Netherlands.*

Management of desmoid tumours including a case report of toremifene

J. R. Benson, K. Mokbel & M. Baum

Key words: desmoid tumours, surgery, radiotherapy, anti-oestrogens

Case history

A previously fit 17-year-old female presented with a swelling in the left loin region. This was associated with episodes of moderately severe pain of a constant nature, but no other symptoms. Clinical examination revealed a smooth, fixed mass in the left upper abdominal quadrant. A CT scan (Fig. 1) showed an extensive left-sided retroperitoneal soft-tissue mass extending posteriorly between the psoas muscle and vertebrae. The mass was in close apposition to the left side of the abdominal aorta, and encased almost the entire circumference of the common iliac artery and part of the corresponding vein on that side. There was infiltration of the mesentery and psoas muscle with obstruction of the left ureter and a grossly hydronephrotic kidney (Fig. 2). An IVU confirmed the latter finding, though a DPTA scan demonstrated preservation of renal function (differential function approx. 50 : 50).

A laparotomy, an extensive, rather hard, homogeneous lesion was found, whose contiguity to vital structures precluded any surgical extirpation. Multiple biopsies were taken, and histological examination revealed sheets of spindle shaped cells with vesicular nuclei and small nucleoli, but no pleiomorphism. There was negative staining for S100 and focal positivity for SMA. These features are characteristic of fibromatosis.

An attempt was subsequently made to pass a left

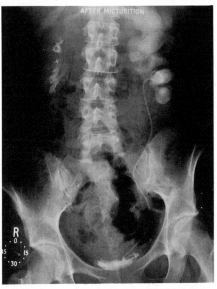

Fig. 2. Intravenous urogram showing an obstructed, grossly hydronephrotic left kidney.

ureteric stent endoscopically, but this was unsuccessful and complicated by pyelonephritis. A nephrostomy was placed to drain the infected system and intravenous antibiotics administered. Following complete resolution of this infective episode, a definitive drainage procedure was performed (ureterolysis and modified Culp pyeloplasty), and a double J-stent placed across the site of anastomosis.

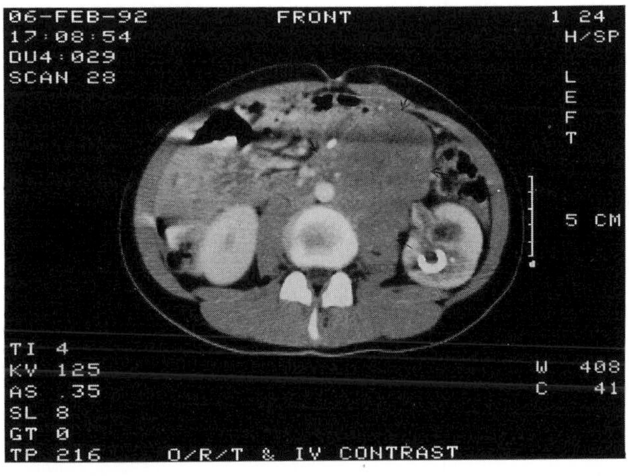

The patient was commenced on toremifene (200 mg daily) 4 months after surgery. Within 2 weeks of starting this agent, a repeat CT scan (Fig. 3) showed a dramatic reduction in tumour size compared with initial films. This response was maintained on films taken at a further 3 and 9 months (Figs. 4 and 5 respectively). A repeat CT scan taken after a further 12 months follow-up revealed minimal increase in tumour size and the patient remains clinically well since discontinuation of medication.

Discussion

Desmoid tumours are a benign proliferative lesion of soft tissue fibroblasts, frequently derived from musculo-aponeurotic structures, which may account for

Fig. 1. CT scan showing extensive retroperitoneal mass on presentation (arrowed).

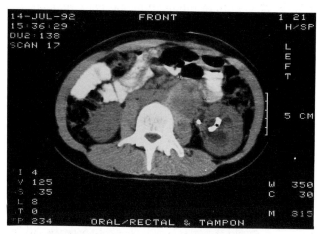

Fig. 3. CT scan appearance 2 weeks after commencing toremifene therapy. Note dramatic reduction in size of tumour.

their name (Gr. *desmos* = band-like [1]. These lesions, though benign and hence non-metastatic, behave in a locally aggressive manner which may render the management of both primary and recurrent lesions difficult, leading to a fatal outcome in many cases.

They are relatively uncommon tumours with an estimated incidence of 2–4 per million of the population [7]. Desmoids constitute only 0.03% of all neoplasms and 3.5% of fibrous tissue tumours usually occurring as

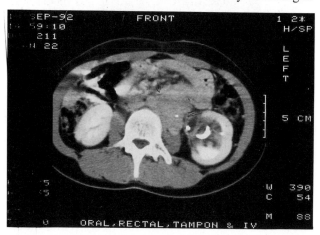

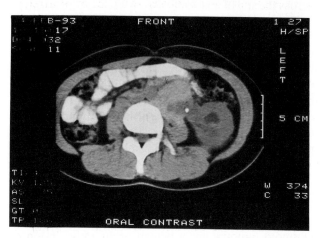

Figs. 4 & 5. CT appearance after 3 months (Fig. 4) and 9 months (Fig. 5) showing maintenance of initial response to toremifene.

solitary lesions, but an important association is with gastrointestinal polyps in Gardner's syndrome [2, 3]. Between 3.5% and 29% of patients with Gardner's syndrome have desmoid tumours [4], which are usually mesenteric in location (55%–72%) and characteristically develop as a delayed (2–3 years) response to surgery [5, 6]. In addition to occurring within the mesentery, the intra-abdominal desmoid may also involve vital retroperitoneal structures as in the case cited. This aspect can limit surgery as a treatment option and render the condition potentially lethal.

The intra-abdominal variety, though of clinical importance, constitutes only 10% of desmoid tumours. The majority (appox. 50%) occur in the trunk musculature, namely the anterior abdominal wall, and the remaining 40% in the extremities.

Desmoid tumours may occur following surgery, but others forms of less deliberate trauma (e.g., working in the gym) may have an aetiological role as an initiating event (a reliable history tends to be elusive). These tumours affect a wide age group, being most common between 20–40 years of age. Reitamo [7] in a relatively large series of 89 patients noted a distinct age and sex distribution. In childhood extra-abdominal desmoids predominated with a female to male ratio of 3:1. In young adults and middle age abdominal wall tumours were most common. Females of fertile age were twice as affected as males, but this evened out in middle age. In older patients, no particular type or sex distribution was evident.

Extra-abdominal desmoids usually present clinically with a mass, typically of the proximal upper limb girdle region [8]. The most commonly affected sites are the upper arm, shoulder and axillary/pectoral areas (see Table 1 and Fig. 6). When the mass, which may reach gross proportions (up to 17 kg [9]) interferes with muscle mobility or disrupts a joint, pain is experienced. Intra-abdominal desmoids may present with a palpable mass per abdomen, but more importantly, such patients may develop bowel obstruction or renal failure from bilateral ureteric obstruction. Intra-abdominal des-

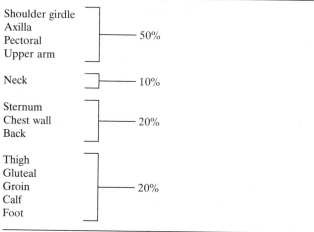

Table 1. Common sites of occurrence of demoid tumours.

Shoulder girdle	
Axilla	
Pectoral	50%
Upper arm	
Neck	10%
Sternum	
Chest wall	20%
Back	
Thigh	
Gluteal	
Groin	20%
Calf	
Foot	

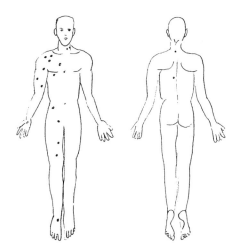

Fig. 6. Scattergram showing common sites of occurrence of extra-abdominal desmoids.

moids may be confused clinically with retroperitoneal fibrosis or lympoma, and extra-abdominal lesions to a lesser extent with hernias (Speigelian or incisional [10]). A rectus sheath haematoma can readily mimic a desmoid and it may too be associated with preceding trauma. Diagnosis of intra-abdominal desmoids is best made with CT scan and confirmed with percutaneous biopsy.

Desmoid tumours, as predicted from their locally invasive behaviour, are poorly defined lesions with no well demarcated boundary or pseudo-capsule. Microscopically, they are composed of bundles of collagen with interspersed spindle and sarcolemmic giant cells. Only normal mitoses are seen, this serving to distinguish desmoids from low-grade fibrosarcomas.

The differential sex and age distribution of these tumours has some bearing on their behaviour and biology. Growth rates are higher in pregnancy, in pre- compared with post-menopausal women, and in females overall relative to men [7]. Moreover, 80% of tumours occur in women [3]. Thus these tumours may be hormonally responsive, their growth rates being dependent on endogenous oestrogen levels. Desmoid tumours have been induced experimentally in guinea-pigs following prolonged oestrogen administration [11] and have occurred in patients treated with oestrogens for prostatic cancer (regressing with subsequent orchidectomy). Spontaneous regression is also more likely post menopause. These tumours may thus be amenable to ablative oestrogen therapy. Indeed, they can bind oestrogens with similar affinity to conventional target tissues. However, overall they are oestrogen receptor (ER) poor with at most one-third of tumours being E.R. positive, these mainly occurring in pre-menopausal women [12].

Only 4% of desmoid tumours regress spontaneously [3]. Though non-malignant with no capacity to metastasize, these tumours are locally aggressive and many infiltrate surrounding tissues extensively. They can also spread subclinically along tissue planes, thwarting

efforts at complete eradication. Surgery remains the principle method of treatment, though its extent with respect to size and location of individual tumours remains ill-defined. Recurrence rates following surgery vary from 20%–70%, with typical values between 40% [13] and 60% [14].

Earlier papers stressed the importance of adequate surgical resection for primary tumours in preventing recurrence [13, 14]. Though infiltrative, desmoids tend to be circumscribed lesions associated with a particular aponeurotic structure. Ideally, resection should include the tumour together with a cuff of surrounding tissue such that surgical margins are clear. As these tumours characteristically spread along skeletal muscles by infiltrating between the fibres, the whole muscle should be resected. Sometimes a 'muscle group resection' is indicated where muscles are in a close anatomical and functional relationship.

Such procedures for extra-abdominal desmoids may lead to significant functional impairment, particularly as the most commonly affected site is the shoulder girdle. Where removal of a whole muscle (e.g., deltoid), or muscle group (e.g., gluteal) would lead to a severe functional defect, surgical excision can be compromised – desmoid tumours do not metastasize and residual disease does not invariably progress to overt clinical recurrence. MacKinnon [15] found recurrence rates of only 4.5% with clear resection margins. However, others have found no correlation with 'cleanliness' of surgical margins [7]. Multiple local resections for recurrent disease may in some circumstances be more acceptable than an extensive and mutilating procedure ab initio.

Surgery may be limited not just to removal of a major muscle or muscle group; ex-articulation and amputations (including fore- and hind-quarter) have been carried out for these tumours. Das Gupta et al. [13] emphasised that aggressive surgery may be indicated, and where so should be executed accordingly, so minimising the chance of recurrence. They reported relatively low recurrence rates of 19% following wide local excision, and not one of four patients undergoing major limb amputation showed evidence of recurrence at a maximum follow-up of 51 months. Others concur that wide extirpation significantly reduced the chance of recurrence compared with lesser surgical procedures. Kofoed et al. [14] reported a recurrence rate overall of 60% in a series of 15 patients, but none of the cases for whom en bloc resection was performed had any recurrence at an average of 55 months of follow-up.

Apart from cases where more radical forms of primary surgery have been adopted, recurrence rates are high overall. In an effort to reduce these, and possibly obviate the need for aggressive primary surgical therapy, other treatment modalities have been investigated in recent years. These include radiotherapy and various forms of medical therapies.

It has been stated that repeated re-excision is

168

worthwhile because the chance of recurrence after a second and third resection is equal to or less than after the first [15]. However, Reitamo [7] reported that up to 45% of tumours recurred after a second operation and 36% following a third.

Radiotherapy has increasingly been employed not only as an adjunct to surgery to reduce rates of local recurrence, but also as primary therapy alone. Since Pack and Erhlich [16] first reported response of desmoid tumours to radiotherapy, opinions on the efficacy of this form of treatment in both these capacities has been mixed. Some have even reported that radiotherapy combined with surgery may actually increase rates of recurrence and predispose to malignancy [7]. Conflicting reports may reflect differing dosages of administration. Nowadays, doses of over 50 gy are generally used, which were previously unattainable with orthovoltage machines. Kiel and Suit [17] reported encouraging results from the use of radiotherapy both alone, and combined with surgery in the management of desmoid tumours. Eight out of 10 patients receiving primary radiotherapy achieved either a complete or partial response with stabilisation of disease. Three patients receiving adjuvant radiotherapy following incomplete surgical excision with gross residual disease showed no evidence of recurrence at a minimum of 27 months follow-up. Planned combination therapy with both pre- and post-operative radiotherapy was similarly successful in preventing recurrence. It was considered that adjuvant radiotherapy was not indicated where only 'minimal' disease was evident at tumour resection margins (and follow-up facilities were good). However, Plukker et al. [18] have recently analysed treatment outcome in a group of abdominal and extra-abdominal desmoid tumours. Of 32 cases managed with wide excision alone, 19 were free of recurrence at a mean follow-up of 72 months. Only 6 of these tumours had histologically negative margins, of which 33% recurred compared with 42% of tumours with positive or indeterminate margins. A selected group of 5 primary tumours with incomplete surgical resection and 9 with recurrent disease were given adjuvant radiotherapy of 50 gy over a 5–6-week period. More than 90% (13/14) of these tumours achieved local control during this period of follow-up. These results suggest that adjuvant radiotherapy may be appropriate for a sub-group of patients with residual disease following incomplete surgical extirpation.

Radiotherapy is effective as a treatment for recurrent lesions in addition to its role as an adjuvant in prevention of recurrence [19–21]. Keur and Bartelink [19] obtained local control of recurrent desmoid tumours in nineteen out of 21 patients with a disease-free survival of 90% at 5 years. All patients had previously experienced at least one recurrence (macro- or microscopic residual disease) which had been treated by surgery alone. Eight patients received radiotherapy because they were deemed at high risk of recurrence on account of narrow (<1 cm) resection margins.

Kiel and Suit [17] reported a favourable response of extra-abdominal desmoid tumours to high dose radiotherapy, with a 59% complete and 18% partial response rates. Such therapy may obviate the need for mutilating surgery, but in an adjuvant capacity may render any further surgery for recurrent lesions more difficult.

Radiotherapy therefore permits more limited primary surgery by eradicating residual disease for which complete surgical extirpation might involve extensive mutilation and accompanying functional impairment. It may also be employed to achieve regression of inoperable desmoid tumours, and possibly where surgery is declined by the patient. Some desmoid tumours will continue to grow/recur despite surgical and radiotherapeutic intervention. Moreover, the intra-abdominal and mesenteric forms may not be amenable to either of the aforementioned therapies at the outset.

A variety of medical therapies based on several rationales have been tried, either as an alternative to, or an adjunct to surgery. Conventional chemotherapy has minimal effect on these tumours, which in contrast to malignant lesions have a low mitotic index, thus precluding therapy based on selective cell-cycle kinetics. Prostaglandin antagonists, e.g., sulindac, have been reported to induce regression of desmoid tumours [22, 23].

Of greatest interest and success in medical therapy are the anti-oestrogens. Many reports have now accrued on the effectiveness of tamoxifen in management of desmoid tumours [24–26]. However, response rates do not correlate well with measured E.R. levels in tumours. There is a parallel here with results of clinical trials' overviews indicating that response to tamoxifen is independent of E.R. status [27, 28]. This observation has led to the hypothesis that tamoxifen and related triphenylethylenes such as toremifene, may exert their effects in part, independently of the E.R. [29]. According to this hypothesis, anti-oestrogens may stimulate stromal fibroblasts to produce TGFbeta, a negative paracrine growth factor for neighbouring (malignant) epithelial cells. Secretion of this is induced 3-30 fold in foetal fibroblasts in vitro [29], and in breast tumour fibroblasts in vivo [30]. Desmoid tumours, consisting of purely mesenchymal elements might be expected to respond to anti-oestrogens based on such an hypothesis. Brookes et al. [31] found a dramatic response of desmoid tumours to toremifene, a chlorinated analogue of tamoxifen which has induced a response in up to a third of patients who have relapsed on tamoxifen [32]. However, the mechanism of action in desmoid tumours is elusive and it is difficult to reconcile with the induction of TGFbeta in fibroblasts. TGFbeta increases synthesis and secretion of matrix proteins by fibroblasts – i.e., is trophic to stromal elements. Perhaps tamoxifen and toremifene may act on desmoid tumours via a cytotoxic mechanism, or somehow alter the balance of growth factors such that a negative effect on fibroblasts ensues, with regression of the tumours. Fibroblasts in desmoids may be phenotypically different to 'normal' fibroblasts and respond to anti-oestrogens in a manner dictated by altered gene expression. A common genetic abnormality may underlie desmoid tumours, which are either not associated with familial adenomatous polyposis or which are (in cases of Gardner's syndrome) [33]. Of interest, anti-oestrogen binding sites have been identified in up to 79% of desmoid tumours, including E.R. negative ones [34]. Correlation between clinical response and levels of AEBS have as yet not been investigated.

Despite the relative inefficacy of conventional chemotherapy, some of the newer agents may be successful in cases which have failed to respond to other medical interventions, including triphenylethylenes. Lynch et al. [35] have reported a complete response to a combination of doxorubicin (90 mg/m^2) and dacarbazine (900 mg/m^2) in 2 cases of intra-abdominal desmoids which were unresponsive to tamoxifen therapy. In common with other chemotherapy schedules, these agents are not without side-effects, and indeed cardiotoxicity precluded continued use of doxorubicin in one patient. We would suggest that toremifene is employed under these circumstances, having previously been shown to be effective either as 1st or 2nd line anti-oestrogen therapy [31].

In conclusion, whatever the mechanism of action, oestrogen antagonism is an effective treatment for desmoid tumours, particularly the mesenteric variety for which surgical extirpation is likely to be incomplete, but for which bowel or ureteric obstruction may demand surgical intervention. For extra-abdominal desmoids, primary surgical treatment with wide local excision and clear margins of resection (short of a mutilating procedure) is optimal. Where considerable function could be spared by a lesser procedure, consideration of combination therapy with surgery and adjuvant radiotherapy is indicated. Anti-oestrogen therapy may be reserved for recurrent lesions for which further surgery or radiotherapy have either proved unsuccessful or would risk damage to vital structures.

References

1. Muller J. Ueber den feirnern bau and formen der krankhaften geschwulste. Berlin: G Reimer 1838; 60.
2. Gardner EJ. Am J Human Genetics 1951; 3: 167.
3. MacAdam WAF, Goligher JC. The occurrence of desmoids in patients with familial polyposis coli. Br J Surg 1970; 57: 618–31.
4. Naylor EW, Gardner EJ, Richards RC. Desmoid tumours and mesenteric fibromatosis in Gardners syndrome. Arch Surg 1979; 114: 1181–5.
5. Richards RC, Rogers SW, Gardner EJ. Spontaneous mesenteric fibromatosis in Gardner's syndrome. Cancer 1981; 47: 597–601.
6. Bulow S. Incidence of associated diseases in FPC. Semin Surg Oncol 1987; 3: 84–7.
7. Reitamo JJ, Scheinin TM, Hayry P. The desmoid syndrome. Am J Surg 1986; 151: 230–7.
8. Cole NM, Guiss LW. Arch Surg 1969; Chicago 98: 530.
9. Rokitansky KW (1880). Cited in Stewart MJ, Mouat TB. Br J Surg 1924; 12: 355.
10. Easter EW, Halasz NA. Recent trends in the management of desmoid tumours. Summary of 19 cases and review of the literature. Ann Surg 1989; 210: 765–9.
11. Lipschutz A, Jadrijevic D, Girardi S et al. Antifibromatogenic potency of 9-fluoro derivatives of progesterone. Nature 1956; 178: 139.
12. Biron P, Meckenstock R, Bobin JY et al. Presence of hormone receptors on desmoid tumours (Meeting abstract). Proc Am Meet Am Soc Clin Oncol 1990; 9: 1107.
13. Das Gupta TK, Brasfield RD, O'Hara J. Extra-abdominal desmoids – a clinico-pathological study. Ann of Surgery 1969; 170: 109–22.
14. Kofoed H, Kamby C, Anagnostaki L. Aggressive fibromatosis. Surg Gynae & Obstetrics 1985; 160: 124–7.
15. McKinnon JG, Neifeld JP, Kay S et al. Management of desmoid tumours. Surg Gynae Obst 1989; 169: 104–6.
16. Pack GT, Erhlich HE. Neoplasms of the anterior abdominal wall with special consideration of desmoid tumours: Experience with 391 cases and a collective review of the literature. Int Abst Surg 1944; 79: 177–84.
17. Kiel KD, Suit HD. Radiation therapy in the treatment of aggressive fibromatoses. Cancer 1984; 54: 2051–5.
18. Plukker JTh, van Oort I, Vermey A et al. Aggressive fibromatosis (non-familial desmoid tumour): Therapeutic problems and role of adjuvant radiotherapy. Br J Surg 1995; 82: 510–4.
19. Keur R, Bartelink H. The role of radiotherapy in the treatment of desmoid tumours. Radiother Oncol 1986; 7: 1–5.
20. Greenberg HM, Goebel R, Weichselbaum RR et al. Radiation therapy in the treatment of aggressive fibromatoses. Int J Radiat Oncol Biol Phys 1983; 7: 305–10.
21. Leibel SA, Wara WM, Hill DR et al. Desmoid tumours: Local control and patterns of relapse following radiation therapy. Int J Radiat Oncol Biol Phys 1983; 9: 1167–71.
22. Belliveau P, Graham AM. Mesenteric desmoid tumour in Gardners syndrome treated by Sulindac. Dis Col Rectum 1984; 27: 53–4.
23. Tsukada K, Church JM, Jagelman DG et al. Non-cytotoxic drug therapy for intra-abdominal desmoid tumour in patients with FAP. Dis Col Rectum 35: 29–33.
24. Kinzbrunner B, Ritter S, Domingo J et al. Remission of rapidly growing desmoid tumours after tamoxifen therapy. Cancer 1983; 52: 2201–4.
25. Proctor H, Singh L, Baum M. Response of multi-centric desmoid tumours to tamoxifen. Br J Surg 1987; 74: 401.
26. Mukherjee A, Malcolm A, De La Hunt M, Neal DE. Pelvic fibromatosis (desmoid) – treatment with steroids and tamoxifen. Br J Urol 1995; 75: 559–60.
27. Nolvadex Adjuvant Trial Organisation. Controlled trial of tamoxifen as a single adjuvant agent in the management of early breast cancer. Br J Cancer 1987; 57: 608.
28. Early Breast Cancer triallists Collaborative Group. Effects of adjuvant tamoxifen and of cytotoxic therapy on the mortality in early breast cancer: An overview of 61 randomised trials amongst 28,896 women. Lancet 1992; 339: 1–15; 71–5.
29. Colletta A, Wakefield LM, Howell FV et al. Anti-oestrogens induce the secretion of active transforming growth factor beta from human foetal fibroblasts. Br J Cancer 1990; 62: 405–9.
30. Butta A, Maclennan K, Flanders KC et al. Induction of transforming growth factor beta in human breast cancer in vivo following tamoxifen treatment. Cancer Res 1992; 52: 4261–2.
31. Brooks MD, Ebbs SR, Colletta AA et al. Desmoid tumours treated with triphenylethylenes. Eur J Cancer 1992; 28: 1014–8.
32. Ebbs SR, Roberts J, Baum M. Response to toremifene therapy in tamoxifen failed patients with breast cancer. J Steroid Biochem 1990; 36: 239.
33. Benson JR, Baum M. Breast cancer, desmoid tumours and Familial Adenomatous Polyposis – a unifying hypothesis. The Lancet 1993; 342: 848–50.

34. Lim CL, Walker MJ, Menta RR et al. Oestrogen and anti-oestrogen binding sites in desmoid tumours. Eur J Cancer Clin Oncol 1986; 22: 583–7.

35. Lynch H, Fitzgibbons R, Chong S et al. Use of doxorubicin and dacarbazine for the management of unresectable intra-abdominal desmoid tumours in Gardner's syndrome. Dis Colon Rectum 1994; 37: 260–7.

R. L. Souhami (ed.) The Teaching Cases from Annals of Oncology, 171–177, 1997.
© 1997 Kluwer Academic Publishers. Printed in the Netherlands.

Primitive neuroectodermal tumour of the chest wall

M. von Schlippe & J. S. Whelan

The London Bone Tumour Service, The Middlesex Hospital, London, U.K.

Key words: Askin tumour, primitive neuroectodermal tumour

Case history

A 30-year-old woman developed a cough and a mass over her posterior left ribs in February 1993. She was otherwise well, with no relevant past medical or family history, and was not investigated at this time as she was in her fourth pregnancy. Two months later, she developed left sided chest pain radiating around the back, and was thought to have a left pleural effusion. She had a spontaneous vaginal delivery of a healthy girl, after which she had a bronchoscopy and open lung biopsy. The initial diagnosis was of a non-Hodgkin's lymphoma, but the clinical picture was felt to be inconsistent. Therefore, a further biopsy was performed, and a small round cell tumour of the Ewing/PNET type was diagnosed. She was then referred to a specialist centre.

On examination, she had a mass over her left eighth rib in the posterior axillary line measuring 8 cm × 8 cm, with reduced air entry at the left base. The chest X-ray at presentation is shown in Fig. 1. CT scan of the chest showed a large left chest wall mass, occupying much of the left hemithorax; the diaphragm was indistinguishable, and the stomach and spleen were displaced (Fig. 2a). Bone scan showed this to be an isolated

(a)

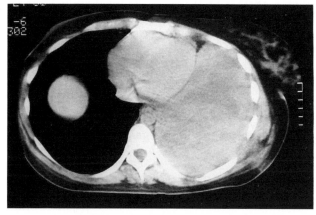

(b)

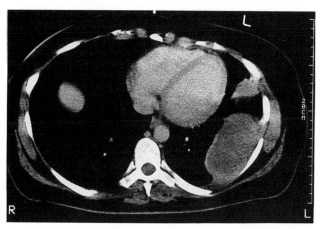

Fig. 2. (a) CT scan of the chest at presentation, on soft tissue settings, showing large mass in the left hemithorax, with soft tissue extension between the ribs into the chest wall, and lymphoedema of the left breast. (b) CT scan of the chest at a comparable level after 5 cycles of chemotherapy, showing decrease in the size of the mass in the left hemithorax and resolution of the lymphoedema of the breast.

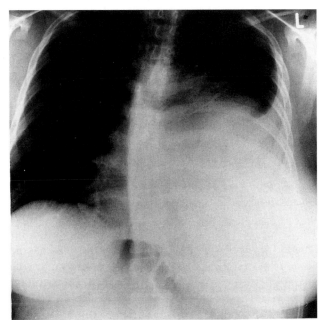

Fig. 1. Chest X-ray at presentation, showing large mass in the left hemithorax.

lesion, with diffuse uptake throughout the ninth rib (Fig. 3).

She was treated initially with chemotherapy devised for patients with poor prognosis Ewing's sarcoma. Five drugs were used: etoposide, vincristine, ifosfamide, and doxorubicin alternating with actinomycin D (Fig. 4). Her pain resolved rapidly, and the chest wall mass decreased in size. Her CT scan confirmed her improvement (Fig. 2b).

After five cycles of chemotherapy, a left thoracotomy was performed. A residual mass arising from the ninth rib was found, contiguous with lung, pericardium, diaphragm and spleen. Her seventh to tenth ribs were removed, along with the associated muscles, left phrenic nerve and central portion of the diaphragm. A chest wall prosthesis of Marlex and methyl methacrylate was inserted. She made a rapid recovery, and had her sixth cycle of chemotherapy 12 days after the operation. Examination of the resection specimen revealed that the excision margin was narrowest at the deep surface, with viable tumour still present.

In view of the marginal excision, hyperfractionated radiotherapy to her chest wall was given concurrently with cycles 8 to 10 of chemotherapy. She received a total of 49.6 Gy in 31 twice daily fractions in 3 blocks, with a 10-day gap scheduled after the first and second blocks. The first 45 Gy were given in two 14-day blocks to large (19 cm × 18 cm) antero-posterior fields. The second block was delayed by one week because of pain

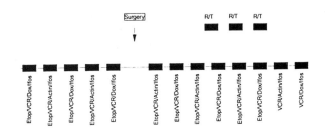

Fig. 4. EVAIA chemotherapy – Arm C of a multinational prospective randomised study of Ewing's sarcoma, EICESS 92. Etop = etoposide, 150 mg/m²/day days 1, 2, 3: VCR = vincristine, 1.5 mg/m² (maximum 2 mg) day 1; Dox = doxorubicin, 20 mg/m²/day days 1, 2, 3 during odd cycles: Actin = actinomycin D, 0.5 mg/m²/day days 1, 2, 3 during even cycles; Ifos = ifosfamide 2 g/m²/day days 1, 2, 3. Mesna uroprotection is given with ifosfamide.

around the prosthesis. Ultrasound of her chest revealed fluid which was inaccessible to a needle because of the prosthesis, and she improved with no specific therapy. Her final block of radiotherapy (4.6 Gy) was given to a smaller field of 14 cm × 7 cm, as planned.

She had severe toxicity during her treatment. WHO grade 3–4 mucositis was a recurring problem, she had two episodes of febrile neutropenia, and required blood transfusion after every cycle of chemotherapy, despite dose reductions. The worst toxicity accompanied cycles given with radiotherapy. She required a platelet transfusion after her eleventh cycle, and etoposide was omitted for the rest of her treatment. By the end of her treatment, she was receiving 60% of her initial doses of ifosfamide, actinomycin D and doxorubicin. She remained amenorrhoeic for five months after completion of chemotherapy. Since completion of chemotherapy, she has also developed cough and haemoptysis, with consolidation around the prosthesis, and is practising postural drainage.

She completed chemotherapy in May 1994, at which stage a CT scan of her chest showed some increased soft tissue shadowing along the internal surface of her prosthesis, with no evidence of tumour. In October 1995, a single 3-cm right-sided pulmonary metastasis was identified. Isotope bone scanning revealed a further metastasis in the left parietal bone. There was no evidence of recurrence at the site of the original tumour. Further chemotherapy has been initiated and consolidation with high-dose melphalan and etoposide is planned, should a further remission be achieved.

Discussion

The concept of primitive neuroectodermal tumour (PNET) has been evolving for many years, as has its nomenclature. It was first described as a tumour arising in peripheral nerve, when it was called neuroepithelioma [1]. These tumours are part of the differential diagnosis of malignant small round cell tumours, which include Ewing's sarcoma, rhabdomyosarcoma, neuroblastoma and lymphoma, and which appear as sheets of

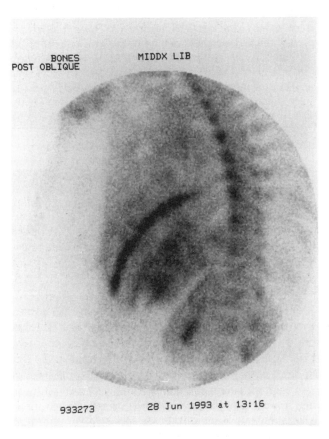

BONES
POST OBLIQUE   MIDDX LIB

933273   28 Jun 1993 at 13:16

Fig. 3. Bone scan at presentation, showing diffuse uptake of tracer throughout the ninth rib.

monotonous small round cells on light microscopy, staining dark blue with haematoxylin and eosin. In the 1970's, reports of tumours displaying neural features introduced new terms such as primitive neuroectodermal tumour and peripheral neuroectodermal tumour. A relationship to the undifferentiated primitive neuroectodermal tumours of the central nervous system in children was assumed by the title of these tumours, although it was recognised that they were not necessarily related to peripheral nerves.

In 1979, Askin described a series of patients with malignant small cell tumours of the chest wall which showed neural differentiation, but which bore a resemblance to Ewing's tumour [2]. Later, this tumour was also diagnosed at other sites, and became identified with the previously described neuroepitheliomas, but the names multiplied, e.g. peripheral neuroepithelioma, peripheral neuroblastoma, Askin tumour, and peripheral PNET. The term 'primitive neuroectodermal tumour' is used in this article. Cytogenetic studies have confirmed that it forms part of a spectrum with both classical and atypical Ewing's tumour [3].

Presentation

The incidence of Ewing's sarcoma in the West is 2 per million per year in people under 16, peaking at 4–6 per million between the ages of 16 and 22 [4]. The incidence of PNET is more difficult to determine, as its distinction from Ewing's sarcoma is often arbitrary, based on the degree of neural differentiation, but retrospective studies suggest that it occurs less frequently. PNETs occur in children and young adults, and are rarely diagnosed after the age of 30. Askin reported a female preponderance, but this has not been consistently borne out in subsequent series of PNET, whatever the site. The chest wall is the most common site (around 40%), followed by the pelvis, extremities and abdomen. PNET was originally described as a soft tissue tumour, but bone involvement is common (74% in one series [5]), and it may indeed arise in bone [6]. PNET of the chest wall often erodes rib, and frequently encroaches on the lung and diaphragm; a pleural effusion may also be seen. PNET may be associated with peripheral nerves, but rarely appear to arise from them or invade them.

Patients usually present with a mass, with or without pain. There may be systemic symptoms as well as specific ones, for example breathlessness from a pleural effusion or weakness from nerve compression [7]. Posterior chest wall tumours may invade the spinal canal, causing pain and neurological signs. Up to 50% of patients present with metastases, usually to the lungs or bones; the bone marrow may also be involved, and lymph node and liver metastases occur less frequently [8–10]. Patients with chest wall primaries often have dissemination of tumour around the pleural cavity [2], but their incidence of metastases at presentation is lower.

Radiology

Plain X-rays of the more common soft tissue PNETs may be normal, or show a soft tissue mass or bone erosion. In the case of chest wall tumours, the chest X-ray may be grossly abnormal, showing a large mass with or without a pleural effusion. Primary PNET of bone may be indistinguishable from Ewing's on plain X-ray, with a permeative destructive lesion and periosteal reaction being present. The tumour may be further demonstrated by CT scanning, but MRI may be more informative, showing tumour and peritumoural oedema on T2 weighted images, as well as altered marrow signal on T1 weighted images if the bone marrow is involved.

Tissue diagnosis

A diagnosis can be made on material obtained by core needle biopsy in almost all cases [11]. The techniques employed include light and electron microscopy, immunohistochemistry, fluorescent in situ hybridisation, and cytogenetic analysis. With so many approaches now available for tissue diagnosis, all of which have a role, it is important that an adequate biopsy be taken, and that the samples be stored and distributed appropriately.

On light microscopy, rosettes are usually seen. These are the Homer-Wright pseudorosettes originally described in neuroblastoma, often poorly formed, with a centre filled with the fibrillary cytoplasmic extensions of surrounding cells. There may be dense clumping of the nuclei with many mitotic figures, unlike in extraosseous Ewing's sarcoma, where the nuclei are more uniform and mitoses are scarce [12]. There is little or no intracellular glycogen, which may be shown rapidly on tumour imprints. On electron microscopy, further evidence of neural differentiation is seen, with dense core granules, and elongated cellular processes containing filaments and microtubules.

Immunocytochemistry usually confirms neuroectodermal differentiation, as the cells are usually positive for neurone-specific enolase (the γγ subunit of enolase) and protein gene product 9.5 [13]. PNET also expresses choline acetyl transferase, unlike neuroblastoma, which expresses enzymes involved in catecholamine synthesis [14]. MIC2, which is a marker for Ewing's sarcoma, is also overexpressed in PNET [15] and may be detected by the monoclonal antibodies 12E7 [16] and HBA-71 [17]. It codes for the membrane sialoglycoprotein p30/32, which is a cell adhesion molecule on the surface of erythrocytes and T cells [18]; it has been suggested that overexpression of this adhesion molecule may contribute to the propensity of the Ewing's family of tumours to metastasis widely [15]. Some of the immunocytochemical and cytogenetic markers used in the differential diagnosis of small round cell tumours are listed in Table 1.

Cytogenetic analysis of Ewing's sarcoma shows a

174

Table 1. Differential diagnosis of small round cell tumours: immunohistochemical and cytogenetic markers. Most important positive results obtained with a panel of antibodies and by cytogenetic methods. NSE = neurone-specific enolase.

Tumour type	Immunohisto-chemistry	Cytogenetics
Ewing's sarcoma	MIC2	t(11;22)(q23;q12)
Primitive neuro-ectodermal tumour	MIC2, NSE	t(11;22)(q23;q12)
Rhabdomyosarcoma	Desmin	t(2;13)q(35;q14) Loss of hetero-zygosity 11p
Neuroblastoma	NSE	1p
Lymphoma	Leucocyte common antigen	Various
Small cell osteo-sarcoma	Alkaline phos-phatase	–

non-random balanced translocation between chromosomes 11 and 22: t(11;22)(q23;q12) [19, 20]. This translocation was observed in 83% of cases of Ewing's sarcoma in one series, with some other related or complex cytogenetic abnormalities also found [21]. Whang-Peng et al. described the same translocation in PNET and in Askin's tumour [3, 22]. The translocation can also be demonstrated in interphase nuclei by fluorescent in situ hybridisation [23], which is particularly useful in cases where a metaphase spread cannot be prepared. Even when no chromosomal translocation is seen, the transcribed message for a hybrid product can be detected by reverse transcriptase polymerase chain reaction in 95%–98% of cases [24].

Cloning of the breakpoint regions on chromosomes 11 and 22 revealed that the translocation found most commonly resulted in the fusion of the N′ terminal of the EWS gene on chromosome 22 with the C′ terminal of the FLI1 gene on chromosome 11. The EWS gene is related to RNA polymerase II; in the t(11;22) translocation, its promoter region is retained and is linked to the DNA binding domain of FLI1 (a transcription factor and the human analogue of Friend leukaemia integration site 1, a murine oncogene) [25]. The exact breakpoint varies, and a similar translocation, found in some cases of Ewing's sarcoma, links EWS to ERG, which belongs to the same family of genes as FLI1. The EWS/FLI1 chimeric protein can behave as a transcriptional activator [26], and some of these fusion genes have been shown to transform cells in vitro [27]; these properties may give rise to tumorigenesis. No correlation has been found as yet between the type of translocation and tumour behaviour [28].

Staging

Assessment of the patient includes staging of the tumour and identification of prognostic markers. Plain X-rays are taken of the tumour, supplemented by CT or MRI. Tumour volume is an important prognostic factor in Ewing's sarcoma, but any correlation in PNET is, as

yet, undefined, although small distal tumours of a limb, which are rarely encountered, have a better prognosis [9]. If an attempt has been made to remove the tumour, the adequacy of resection is classified by Enneking's criteria [29]. Chest X-ray, CT scan of the lungs, radionuclide bone scan, and bone marrow aspiration and trephine are performed in a search for metastases. Serum lactate dehydrogenase may be elevated, and is associated with a poor prognosis in some series of Ewing's sarcoma, but the significance in PNET is still unclear.

Treatment

PNET is a highly aggressive but curable tumour, and planned multimodality therapy should therefore be offered to all patients with this condition, preferably in specialist centres. Because of the diverse presentation and the developing recognition of these rare tumours, treatment strategies and results have been inconsistent. Most analyses of results are retrospective, although prospective studies, such as IESS-III and EICESS 92, are now in progress. When planning treatment of PNETs, it appears reasonable to extrapolate from the results of trials of the management of Ewing's sarcoma. Treatment is therefore given, where possible, within studies of Ewing's sarcoma; this will identify differences in the behaviour and clinical response of the tumours included.

Surgery

Many patients have an attempt made to resect the tumour, either at biopsy or following the diagnosis. Because the tumour is often extensive and in a difficult anatomical site, resection is usually incomplete, and a large surgical field is contaminated with tumour. In a series of 11 chest wall PNETs, seven of 10 attempted excisions were incomplete, and at least one apparently complete resection specimen contained vascular invasion [30]. In a prospective series of PNET at all sites, Miser found that 10 of 17 patients had had previous attempts at total excision of tumour, and only one of these attempts was successful [9]. The recommended approach now, as with Ewing's sarcoma, is to delay surgery (after an initial needle biopsy) until induction chemotherapy is complete: not only may systemic micrometastases be treated, but the tumour may become more easily resectable, and previously inoperable tumours may become operable [31]. A report from the Memorial Sloan-Kettering Cancer Center suggested that survival was worse in patients with localised PNET if surgery was performed more than three months from diagnosis [10]; however, it is unwise to generalise from this experience as only 18 of the 54 patients in the series received chemotherapy.

Chest wall PNETs are frequently very large at presentation, and surgery, even after previous chemotherapy, may still be extensive, requiring the resection of one or more ribs as well as of soft tissue structures.

Chest wall reconstruction may then be required [31]. Limb salvage procedures, with resection of affected bone and endoprosthetic replacement, are employed wherever possible in PNETs of the extremities. In all these cases, previous scars, whether from biopsies, drains or larger procedures, must be excised, to reduce the risk of local recurrence.

Chemotherapy
There is little information on chemotherapy specifically in PNET, either of single agent data or prospective studies; there are also, as yet, no randomised studies. When PNETs first began to be treated with chemotherapy, they were mostly treated as neuroblastoma, in view of their neuroectodermal markers. Later, when they were placed in the Ewing family of tumours, the introduction of alkylating agents and doxorubicin led to an improvement in the response rates and survival. The most active drugs are cyclophosphamide and ifosfamide, vincristine, doxorubicin and actinomycin D; carboplatin is also active, as is etoposide, whose role is currently being evaluated. Methotrexate, bleomycin and carmustine have also been used, usually in the context of a study of Ewing's sarcoma.

In a large retrospective European series, Jürgens et al. studied 42 patients with PNET treated between 1980 and 1986; 10 had metastases at presentation [5]. Twenty-four had had alternative diagnoses made, usually Ewing's sarcoma. Thirty-three had been treated as Ewing's sarcoma, two as rhabdomyosarcoma, and five as neuroblastoma. Relapse was seen in four of the 12 treated with VACA (vincristine, doxorubicin, cyclophosphamide, actinomycin D), four of the 15 treated with VAIA (vincristine, doxorubicin, ifosfamide, actinomycin D), and all three patients given neuroblastoma-type chemotherapy (which was cisplatin-based). A 56% 3-year disease-free survival was seen in the patients with localised PNET, whereas all of the patients with metastases had disease progression or recurrence during this time, a median of 10 months following their diagnosis. In the same year, Miser et al. reported the early results of a prospective study of 17 newly-diagnosed patients with PNET, eight with metastases at presentation, at the National Cancer Institute and the Children's Hospital, Philadelphia [9]. These patients were all treated with VADRIAC (vincristine, doxorubicin and cyclophosphamide), and complete remission was achieved in sixteen. By 18 months, six patients had relapsed (three with residual disease at referral and three with metastases at presentation); disease-free survival was not significantly different between these two groups. Unusually, Marina et al. [8] in their review of 26 patients treated at the St. Jude Children's Research Hospital found that results of treatment were better in patients with PNET treated on neuroblastoma protocols (12/16) responses than by VAIA (4/6 responses).

The prognosis of PNET has been compared with that of Ewing's sarcoma in some studies. Miser et al.

found similar rates of survival and disease-free survival in patients with high-risk Ewing's sarcoma or PNET [9]. However, it was found in a retrospective study of 119 patients with Ewing's sarcoma and PNET on the Kiel Pediatric Tumor Registry that 54% of patients with PNET died of their disease compared with 35% of patients with Ewing's sarcoma, with a minimum follow-up period of two years [32]. The question as to whether the prognosis of these tumours really is different will be addressed in the current studies in which patients with Ewing's sarcoma or PNET are treated on the same protocol.

Radiotherapy
Radiotherapy may be used as the primary method of local control or in an adjuvant setting where surgical excision is incomplete. Radical radiotherapy is usually given to a dose of 55–60 Gy, in daily fractions of about 1.8 Gy. Miser et al., for example, used 45 Gy to the tumour and a surrounding 2 cm margin when treating PNET of the chest wall, giving a 10 Gy boost to the soft tissue mass; there were no local recurrences in the radiation field, although there were three pleural recurrences [9]. Doses of adjuvant radiotherapy vary more widely. In Jürgens' series, 21 patients received adjuvant radiotherapy at doses of 20–60 Gy. Eight patients relapsed, seven of them locally (only one of these had had 60 Gy, all the rest had had a maximum of 46 Gy) [5]. This is in line with other reports of the propensity of PNET to recur locally, and suggests that radiation dose and fractionation is important in local control.

Classical Ewing's sarcoma is relatively radiosensitive, with radiotherapy, often given concurrently with modern chemotherapy, producing good rates of local control. There is no evidence that PNET responds differently. Radical surgery of the primary is preferred where possible because of concern about late second malignancy, but, where this is not feasible or would give a poor functional result, radical radiotherapy may be given. Radical radiotherapy is used in an adjuvant setting where there is a high risk of recurrence because of residual microscopic disease, marginal resection (as in this case) or probable tumour contamination from previous fracture or surgery. Chest wall tumours produce specific problems because of pleural contamination and the proximity of lung, myocardium and spinal cord. Radiation and surgery need to be part of a multi-disciplinary approach to treatment in centres with considerable experience of these rare diseases.

Intensification in patients with a poor prognosis
Patients with metastases at presentation have a poorer prognosis compared with those with localised disease, with a disease-free survival of less than a year from diagnosis and virtually no chance of cure with conventional treatment [5, 8, 10]. In such patients, intensification with a high dose procedure (total body irradiation or high-dose chemotherapy) with either autologous bone marrow transplantation (ABMT) or peripheral

blood stem cell support may be of value, as it is in Ewing's sarcoma [33]. Miser et al. gave consolidation treatment with total body irradiation and ABMT to eight patients who had had gross residual disease or metastases at the start of chemotherapy and who were in complete remission. Three had relapsed by the end of the study, which had a median follow-up of 18 months [9]. Stefanko et al. treated four patients with PNET, three of the chest wall, with high dose chemotherapy and ABMT; only one was alive at four years, but no response to second line chemotherapy was seen in at least one of the other three, and it is unclear whether the others were treated when in remission or at the time of progression [30].

Summary

Primitive neuroectodermal tumours are rare malignant small round cell tumours biologically closely related to classical Ewing's sarcoma. A readily distinguishable subgroup of patients presents with primary chest wall tumours. Diagnosis, ideally using material obtained by needle biopsy, requires considerable pathological expertise, and morphological studies should be supplemented with immunocytochemistry and, where possible, by cytogenetic and molecular studies of t(11;22) and related translocations. The therapeutic implications of the distinction from Ewing's sarcoma are as yet unclear; the inferior prognosis apparent from the literature may simply reflect changes in diagnostic pattern and inadequate treatment. All patients with PNET should be treated on protocol, in a centre experienced in the intensive multimodality therapy of sarcomas. Currently, neo-adjuvant chemotherapy is used to gain control of the disease, and the primary tumour is then treated, preferably by radical excision which may be facilitated by the preceding chemotherapy. If there is residual disease or the tumour is unresectable, the site is then irradiated with curative doses, given, if possible, concurrently with adjuvant chemotherapy. The place of high-dose procedures in PNET remains to be defined. Novel approaches to treatment may stem from further study of the characteristic disease markers MIC2 and t(11;22). Prospective studies, currently underway, will provide valuable new information to guide treatment strategies in the future.

Acknowledgments

We are grateful for advice given by Dr. A. M. Cassoni, Dr. M. Smith, and Professor R. L. Souhami.

References

1. Stout AP. A tumor of the ulnar nerve. Proc NY Path Soc 1918; 18: 2–12.
2. Askin FB, Rosai J, Sibley RK et al. Malignant small cell tumor of the thoracopulmonary region in childhood. A distinctive clinicopathologic entity of uncertain histogenesis. Cancer 1979; 43: 2438–51.
3. Whang-Peng J, Triche TJ, Knutsen T et al. Chromosome translocation in peripheral neuroepithelioma. N Engl J Med 1984; 311: 584–5.
4. Stein RC, Cannon S, Cassoni A et al. Clinical oncology: Case presentations from oncology centres 1 Ewing's sarcoma. Eur J Cancer 1991; 27: 1525–33.
5. Jürgens H, Bier V, Harms D et al. Malignant peripheral neuroectodermal tumors. A retrospective analysis of 42 patients. Cancer 1988; 61: 349–57.
6. Jaffe R, Santamaria M, Yunis EJ et al. The neuroectodermal tumor of bone. Am J Surg Pathol 1984; 8: 885–98.
7. Saifuddin A, Robertson RJH, Smith SEW. The radiology of Askin Tumours. Clin Radiol 1991; 43: 19–23.
8. Marina NM, Etcubanas E, Parham DM et al. Peripheral primitive neuroectodermal tumor (peripheral neuroepithelioma) in children. A review of the St Jude experience and controversies in diagnosis and management. Cancer 1989; 64: 1952–60.
9. Miser JS, Kinsella TJ, Triche TJ et al. Treatment of peripheral neuroepithelioma in children and young adults. J Clin Oncol 1987; 5: 1752–8.
10. Kushner BH, Hajdu SI, Gulati SC et al. Extracranial primitive neuroectodermal tumors. The Memorial Sloan-Kettering Cancer Center experience. Cancer 1991; 67: 1825–9.
11. Stoker DJ, Cobb JP, Pringle JAS. Needle biopsy of musculoskeletal lesions. A review of 208 procedures. J Bone Joint Surg (Br) 1991; 73B: 498–500.
12. Dehner LP. Primitive neuroectodermal tumor and Ewing's sarcoma. Am J Surg Pathol 1993; 17: 1–13.
13. Carter RL, Al-Sam SZ, Corbett RP et al. A comparative study of immunohistochemical staining for neuron-specific enolase, protein gene product 9.5 and S-100 protein in neuroblastoma, Ewing's sarcoma and other round cell tumours in children. Histopathol 1990; 16: 461–7.
14. Thiele CJ, McKeon C, Triche TJ et al. Differential protooncogene expression characterizes histopathologically indistinguishable tumors of the peripheral nervous system. J Clin Invest 1987; 80: 804–11.
15. Kovar H, Dworzak M, Strehl S et al. Overexpression of the pseudoautosomal gene MIC3 in Ewing's sarcoma and peripheral primitive neuroectodermal tumor. Oncogene 1990; 5: 1067–70.
16. Levy R, Dilley J, Fox RI et al. A human thymus leukemia antigen defined by hybridoma monoclonal antibodies. Proc Natl Acad Sci USA 1979; 76: 6552–6.
17. Hamilton G, Fellinger EJ, Schratter I et al. Characterization of a human endocrine tissue and tumor-associated Ewing's sarcoma antigen. Cancer Res 1988; 48: 6127–34.
18. Gelin C, Aubrit F, Phalipon A et al. The E2 antigen, a 32 kd glycoprotein involved in T-cell adhesion processes, is the MIC2 gene product. EMBO J 1989; 11: 3253–9.
19. Aurias A, Rimbaut C, Buffe D et al. Chromosomal translocations in Ewing's sarcoma. N Engl J Med 1983; 309: 496–7.
20. Turc-Carel C, Philip I, Berger M-P et al. Chromosomal translocations in Ewing's sarcoma. N Engl J Med 1983; 309: 497–8.
21. Turc-Carel C, Aurias A, Mugneret F et al. Chromosomes in Ewing's sarcoma. I. An evaluation of 85 cases and remarkable consistency of t(11;22)(q24;q12). Cancer Genet Cytogenet 1988; 32: 229–38.
22. Whang-Peng J, Triche TJ, Knutsen T et al. Cytogenetic characterization of selected small round cell tumors of childhood. Cancer Genet Cytogenet 1986; 21: 185–208.
23. Taylor C, Patel K, Jones T et al. Diagnosis of Ewing's sarcoma and peripheral neuroectodermal tumour based on the detection of t(11;22) using fluorescence in situ hybridisation. Br J Cancer 1993; 67: 128–33.
24. Delattre O, Zucman J, Melot T et al. The Ewing family of tumors – a subgroup of small-round-cell tumors defined by specific chimeric transcripts. N Engl J Med 1994; 331: 294–99.

25. Delattre O, Zucman J, Plougastel B et al. Gene fusion with an *ETS* DNA-binding domain caused by chromosome transloca-tion in human tumours. Nature 1992; 359: 162–5.

26. Ohno T, Rao VN, Reddy ESP. EWS/Fli-1 chimeric protein is a transcriptional activator. Cancer Res 1993; 53: 5859–63.

27. May WA, Gishizky ML, Lessnick SL et al. Ewing sarcoma 11;22 translocation produces a chimeric transcription factor that requires the DNA-binding domain encoded by *FLI1* for transformation. Proc Natl Acad Sci USA 1993; 90: 5752–6.

28. Zucman J, Melot T, Desmaze C et al. Combinatorial genera-tion of variable fusion proteins in the Ewing family of tumours. EMBO J 1993; 12: 4481–7.

29. Enneking WF, Spanier SS, Goodman MA. A system for the surgical staging of musculoskeletal sarcoma. Clin Orthop Rel Res 1980; 153: 106–20.

30. Stefanko J, Turnbull AD, Helson L et al. Primitive neuroecto-dermal tumors of the chest wall. J Surg Oncol 1988; 37: 33–7.

31. Shamberger RC, Tarbell NJ, Perez-Atayde AR et al. Malig-nant small round cell tumor (Ewing's-PNET) of the chest wall in children. J Ped Surg 1994; 29: 179–85.

32. Schmidt D, Herrmann C, Jürgens G et al. Malignant peripheral neuroectodermal tumor and its necessary distinction from Ewing's sarcoma. Report from the Kiel pediatric tumor regis-try. Cancer 1991; 68: 2251–9.

33. Burdach S, Jürgens H, Peters C et al. Myeloablative radio-chemotherapy and hematopoietic stem-cell rescue in poor-prognosis Ewing's sarcoma. J Clin Oncol 1993; 11: 1482–88.

R. L. Souhami (ed.) The Teaching Cases from Annals of Oncology, 179–184, 1997.

Management of head and neck cancer

U. Tirelli,[1] G. Franchin,[2] S. Morassut[3] & L. Barzan[4]

[1] Division of Medical Oncology and AIDS; [2] Division of Radiotherapy; [3] Department of Radiology; [4] Division of Otolaryngology; Centro di Riferimento Oncologico, Aviano, Italy

Key words: head and neck cancer, neo-adjuvant chemotherapy

Malignancies arising in the head and neck area are heterogeneous diseases, each with its own natural history and prognosis. Cancer of the larynx, for example, has a better prognosis than cancer of the hypopharynx [1]. However, due to the relatively low number of cases in each anatomic site, and because the predominant lesion is squamous cell carcinoma, they are usually considered together in clinical trials.

A consistent chromosomal abnormality has been identified at 11q 13 [2]. Analysis of molecular genetic changes and expression of growth factors, and other tumour secretory products may provide determinants of progression of disease and of response to therapy.

Overall, one-third of patients with head and neck cancer present with localized disease. The remaining two-thirds have loco-regionally advanced disease, with only a few patients presenting with distant metastases [1]. Treatment of patients may be complicated by their excess smoking and alcohol consumption, with consequent poor function of the lungs, heart or liver. Retinoids have been shown to reduce the risk of a second primary tumor after therapy of head and neck tumors [3]. However, the side effects and the cost of the treatment render this approach not yet suitable for routine use. The following case report indicates some of the difficulties in management.

Case report

C.B., a 59-year-old woman, was referred with a large pharyngeal mass. She had a 6-month history of odynophagia, dysphonia and cough. Her past medical history was unremarkable and she denied smoking or consuming an excessive amount of alcohol. Physical examination revealed an enlarged (2 cm) lymph node in the upper right cervical region.

ENT examination demonstrated a large vegetating lesion in the angle between the right lateral and the posterior pharyngeal walls, extending from the upper pole of the palatine tonsil to the entire pyriform sinus,

also involving the valleculae, epiglottis, right aryepiglottic fold, right ventricular band and right vocal cord (with immobility of the right hemilarynx). The biopsy showed a poorly differentiated squamous cell carcinoma. CT scan demonstrated invasion of the parapharyngeal space (Fig. 1a & 1b). Chest x-ray and panendoscopy revealed no abnormalities. The tumor was staged as T4 N1 MO. Because of the extent of the tumor and its grade, neo-adjuvant chemotherapy was started with cisplatin 100 mg/m^3 i.v. day 1 and 5-FU 1000 mg/m^2 continuous infusion (from d.1 to d.5). After 3 courses of chemotherapy a dramatic improvement was noted, the vegetating lesion disappeared and only a small infiltrating lesion of the right aryepiglottic fold with impaired mobility of the right hemilarynx was detectable (see Fig. 2a & 2b). The patient experienced grade 3 hematologic toxicity and grade 3 alopecia.

Fifty-five days after the last cycle of chemotherapy the tumor was resected, with the initial limits of the tumor being taken into account. A total laryngectomy was performed extending to the right lateral oro- and hypo-pharyngeal wall and to the right half of the posterior pharyngeal wall from the level of the soft palate to the pharyngoesophageal joint, en bloc with right hemithyroidectomy, bilateral neck dissection (from level I to level V, with preservation of both internal jugular veins, both spinal accessory nerves and the sternocleidomastoid muscle of the left side). A food passage of appropriate caliber was reconstructed by a right pectoralis major myo-cutaneous flap. The postoperative period was uneventful. Pathologic examination of the specimen showed residual microfoci of moderately differentiated squamous cell carcinoma inside the aryepiglottic fold and the paraglottic space, with resection margins free of disease, and involvement of one lymph node at the second level of the right side (pR1 N1 according to TNM; G2 according to WHO). The patient attended a rehabilitation course and acquired a fair esophageal voice. She is free of disease after a follow-up of 29 months. Unfortunately, she has quite a poor esophageal voice and refuses prosthetic rehabilitation.

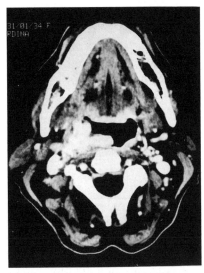

Fig. 1a. CT scan of the neck shows a distinct soft-tissue mass in the bed of the right tonsil deforming the mesopharynx.

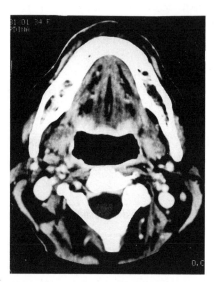

Fig. 2a. Post-treatment scan, performed at the same level as Fig. 1, demonstrates complete resolution of the tumor.

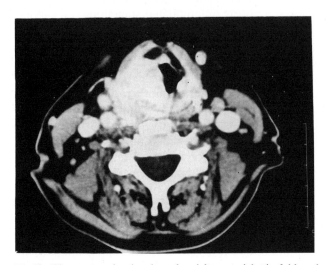

Fig. 1b. The tumor also involves the right aryepiglottic fold and pyriform sinus. No metastatic lymph nodes are seen.

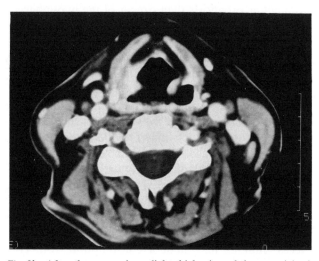

Fig. 2b. After therapy, only a slight thickening of the aryepiglottic fold is still detectable.

Standard treatment

Standard therapy is based on surgery and radiotherapy, which reflects the predominantly localized presentation of the majority of these malignancies.

The choice of local treatment, i.e., surgery or radiotherapy, depends on the patient's general condition, the stage (i.e., the size of the tumoral mass) the localization of the tumor, the side effects of each modality, the cosmetic and functional outcome, and the oncological expertise at the institution in question. For example, radiotherapy is better than surgery for a small laryngeal cancer because of the significant reduction of side effects, in particular the impairment of laryngeal function. On the other hand, surgery may be preferred for a small lesion of the tongue, in order to avoid the toxic effects of radiotherapy, which include mucositis, xerositis, xerostomia and loss of taste. With either surgery or radiotherapy, cure can be achieved in the majority of patients and 60% to 90% of patients will be without

any evidence of disease after two years [1]. In patients with locally advanced disease, the standard therapy is surgery followed by radiotherapy, at least in those with resectable disease, such as our case report patient. Surgery and radiation are therefore frequently employed together and, as a general guideline, in the absence of clinically identifiable lymph node disease, T1 or T2 lesions are equally well managed by either surgery or radiation and the choice is usually based on relative morbidity and physician experience. For large primary tumors with clinically evident lymph node disease, combined treatment with radiation and surgery is indicated. In these patients the aim of therapy is also to cure, although despite the use of the two treatment modalities available, this can be achieved only in a minority of patients, and less than 30% of these patients are alive at five years [4–8]. The majority of these patients will die of recurrent loco-regional disease, while only a minority will develop distant metastasis, usually in lungs, bones or liver.

Patients with head and neck cancer are also at risk of second malignancies, especially from those tumors related to excess cigarette smoking and alcohol consumption. These are second tumors of the head and neck, cancers of the lung and esophagus [5–9]. This is true especially for patients cured of head and neck cancer who are at higher risk of second malignancy because of the longer follow-up period. Patients with distant metastasis or those developing recurrent disease after prior therapy with surgery and/or radiotherapy are candidates for chemotherapy, with the goal of palliation of symptoms. In fact, survival is not clearly improved by the use of chemotherapy in this setting. This may be due to a diminished efficacy of chemotherapy in locally-recurrent disease in areas previously submitted to surgery and radiotherapy. Objective responses to chemotherapy are observed in 30%–50% of patients with advanced disease, but usually these responses are partial and of only 3- to 6-months' duration. However, chemotherapy can produce significant benefit, since it may result in relief of pain and other symptoms. The side effects of chemotherapy should, however, be considered. Methotrexate remains the standard agent against which newer drugs are evaluated [10–18]. Cisplatin is another standard drug [14–16]. Carboplatin can be administered more easily and can be given on an outpatient basis [17–19]. Cisplatin has shown activity similar to that of Methotrexate in randomized comparisons.

Other active drugs are 5-fluorouracil (5-FU), with substantially higher activity when administered as a 5-day continuous infusion [20], bleomycin [10–13], hydroxyurea, cyclophosphamide, doxorubicin and mitomycin C. The last four drugs have not yet been fully evaluated. Overall, methotrexate and cisplatin in conventional doses are still the most active single agents, yielding average partial response rates of 30%–50%. Higher doses of cisplatin may increase the response rate, but this question is still under evaluation. Combination chemotherapy regimens have not resulted in a significant prolongation of survival, while their is toxicity is increased [1]. Newer combinations including that of cisplatin and 5-FU have shown promise in some pilot studies. Further studies to identify additional active drugs and combinations are needed. Finally, the combination of cisplatin and the 5-day continuous infusion of 5-FU appears to be one of the most active combination chemotherapy regimens [21–24] and is under evaluation in randomized studies in comparison with older regimens.

In patients with advanced unresectable head and neck cancer, chemotherapy alternating with radiotherapy increases the median survival and may increase the three-year survival over those with radiotherapy alone [25].

Newer uses of chemotherapy

Neoadjuvant chemotherapy

Neoadjuvant chemotherapy has been introduced in order to improve loco-regional tumor control, and to eradicate microscopic metastases which are present in a large number of patients with advanced loco-regional disease at the time of diagnosis. It involves the administration of cycles of chemotherapy in previously untreated patients with locally advanced head and neck cancer prior to surgery and/or radiotherapy given with curative intent, i.e., standard local therapy. This requires a careful, well organised, multidisciplinary approach involving surgeons, radiation therapists and medical oncologists. With neoadjuvant chemotherapy it may be possible to preserve organ function, i.e., to administer subsequent radiotherapy rather than ablative surgery. Many pilot [26–31] and some randomized trials [32–40] have been carried out, but except in one study [41] randomized trials have yet to show that this approach can improve the survival of patients with locally advanced head and neck cancer. However, the best available chemotherapy regimens have rarely been employed in these studies, so the absence of survival benefit cannot thus far be considered conclusive, and further studies are needed. An important new study was recently published by Paccagnella et al. [41], showing that effective neoadjuvant chemotherapy significantly improves local control and long-term survival in inoperable patients. In 171 inoperable patients, combined cisplatin + 5-fluorouracil followed by radiotherapy achieved a 44% complete remission rate vs. 29% for radiotherapy alone. The 2-year and 3-year overall survivals were, respectively, 28% vs. 19% and 24% vs. 10%.

Overall, neoadjuvant chemotherapy has resulted in high response rates in pilot studies, but its precise effect on survival and disease-free survival remains unknown. The inability of neoadjuvant chemotherapy to improve the survival of many patients, in spite of good local response, is due to the inability of chemotherapy to kill enough cells. A good partial or complete remission induced by neoadjuvant chemotherapy is actually a reduction in cell number by only one or two logarithms.

Induction of a good tumor response after neoadjuvant chemotherapy is also consistent with subsequent relapse. This explains the short median duration of response in these patients if they do not receive radiation or surgery [42, 43].

The administration of neoadjuvant chemotherapy has the theoretical advantage of limiting surgery to non-responsive patients only, whereas patients who respond to chemotherapy (partial response greater than 50% or complete response) could be managed by radical radiotherapy. However, as mentioned above, most randomized studies comparing loco-regional treatment with or without neoadjuvant chemotherapy have shown no advantage in terms of disease-free and overall survival; the Paccagnella et al. study is an exception [41].

New approaches in combined radiotherapy and chemotherapy

The most effective combination of radiotherapy and chemotherapy for the treatment of stages III and IV head and neck cancer, is still not known. The combination of radiotherapy and chemotherapy in concomitant regimens offers advantages different from those obtained when the same combination is used in alternating regimens.

The simultaneous administration of chemotherapy and radiotherapy averts protraction of the radiotherapy, as happens with sequential treatment. Simultaneous radiotherapy and chemotherapy, in addition, allows for possible synergistic effects of the two modalities.

However, on the negative side, simultaneous chemotherapy and radiotherapy has the disadvantage of increased toxicity, which usually requires a decrease in the doses of both radiotherapy and chemotherapy. With the alternating regimen there is no reduction in doses, the radiosensitivity of chemically-treated cells may be increased during repopulation and the degree of treatment-induced toxicity is less. The most serious disadvantage of an alternating regimen lies in the reduced efficacy of radiotherapy due to the split-course schedule.

Randomized studies comparing the combination of simultaneous chemotherapy and radiotherapy have shown better disease-free and overall survivals for the following combinations: radiotherapy plus bleomycin [44–46], radiotherapy plus 5-FU [47, 48], radiotherapy plus MTX [49], or plus cis-platinum [50] but only an increased disease-free survival for the combination of radiotherapy and mitomycin C [51]. However, none of these combinations have reduced the incidence of distant metastases.

Randomized studies comparing alternating radiotherapy and chemotherapy regimens versus neoadjuvant chemotherapy followed by radiotherapy [52, 53] have obtained higher disease-free and overall survival rates with the alternating regimen despite interruptions in the radiation therapy schedule. These data suggest that chemotherapy counteracts the diminished efficacy of a split-course radiation treatment.

Reconstruction after ablative surgery

The possibilities offered by the various types of flaps (particularly pedicled mucocutaneous flap, and free flap with vascular microanastomosis), have widened the scope of ablative surgery and emphasized the functional and aesthetic importance of reconstruction. One of the most complex types of reconstruction, allowing restoration of a sensate oral cavity lining and of mandi-

bular bone, was described by Urken [54]. The follow-up is short and the survival is not reported, but the technique is undoubtedly promising.

The possibility of using CO_2 laser endoscopic surgery (+/− radiotherapy) was reported by Steiner [55] as being as effective as conventional surgery for both early and advanced laryngeal and pharyngo-laryngeal tumors, avoiding tracheotomy and ablative techniques. Unfortunately, similar results are not reported by other authors. Early (T1, T2 NO) laryngeal tumors are treated by radiotherapy or by conservative surgery, with an increasing popularity of radiotherapy, which is judged to give better function with regard to quality of voice. A recent report [56] stresses that endoscopic laser surgery for early vocal cord tumors may result in a better quality of voice, with a treatment which is shorter and cheaper.

Moderately advanced laryngeal tumors ('large' T2, T3) may be treated by subtotal reconstructive laryngectomies, avoiding tracheostomy, and with acceptable oncological and functional results [57]. A precise selection of patients is required to avoid aspiration pneumonia and other post-operative complications.

Discussion of case report

Our stage IV pharyngeal cancer patient was treated with an investigational type of therapy, i.e., neoadjuvant chemotherapy followed by surgery. Three courses of neoadjuvant chemotherapy consisting of cisplatin and 5-FU, both in continuous infusion for 5 days, were delivered, with complete clinical remission, but with residual malignant cells in the pathology material after surgery. Due to bone marrow toxicity, chemotherapy somewhat delayed the scheduled time of surgery, otherwise as radical as though no neoadjuvant chemotherapy had been delivered. We think that our patient can be considered cured; however, the functional outcome is unsatisfactory. Using the current protocols at our Institution, this patient would have been treated with radiotherapy instead of surgery with the aim of organ preservation.

This female patient is unusual, in that the male/female ratio for head and neck cancer is about 3/1 to 4/1. Moreover our patient is a non-smoker and does not drink alcohol. The standard therapy for this patient would normally have been combined surgery and radiotherapy. However, this investigational approach was chosen in an attempt to improve the quite poor prosnosis of this patient, since cure can be achieved in less than one-third of patients with this disease stage. Neoadjuvant chemotherapy may allow delivery of chemotherapy with the patient in good condition, resulting in increased compliance, tolerance of higher doses of chemotherapy and improvement of response. For these reasons, chemotherapy might be more effective both locally and for metastases [58, 59]. There are, however, some disadvantages, i.e., the toxic effects of chemotherapy, and the time required for administration of the neoadjuvant chemotherapy. This can result in a significant prolongation of the overall treatment time and, in patients who fail to respond to chemotherapy, lead to decreased chances of curative local therapy [60]. In our patient, grade III hematologic toxicity occurred, delaying the subsequent surgical treatment, which was undertaken 55 days after the end of the last cycle of chemotherapy. Moreover, a total laryngectomy was carried out of the same extent as if surgery had been undertaken before chemotherapy. The resection specimen showed no pathologic complete remission, since microfoci of moderately differentiated squamous cell carcinoma were present. The pathologic examination showed disease-free resection margins and only one intranodal metastasis, and so no radiotherapy was given. Radiation could still be employed if relapse occurs. In conclusion, this approach is still experimental and further randomized studies are needed to determine whether the preliminary positive results reported by Paccagnella et al. [41] can be confirmed. It is possible that radiation therapy can be used initially in order to avoid the mutilation of total laryngectomy.

References

1. Vokes EE. Head and neck cancer. In Perry MC (ed): The chemotherapy Source Book. Baltimore: Williams & Wilkins 1992; 918–31.
2. Kao-Shan CS, Fine RL, Whang-Peng J et al. Increased fragile sites and sister chromatid exchanges in bone marrow and peripheral blood of young cigarette smokers. Cancer Res 1987; 47: 6278–82.
3. Hong WK, Lippman SM, Itri LM et al. Prevention of second primary tumors with isotretinoin in squamous-cell carcinoma of the head and neck. N Engl J Med 1990; 323: 795–801.
4. Marcial VA, Pajak TF, Kramer S et al. Radiation Therapy Oncology Group (RTOG) studies in head and neck cancer. Semin Oncol 1988; 15: 39–60.
5. Goepfert H. Are we making any progress? Arch Otolaryngol Head Neck Surg 1984; 110: 562–3.
6. Cachin Y, Eschwege F. Combination of radiotherapy and surgery in the treatment of head and neck cancers. Cancer Treat Rev 1975; 2: 177–91.
7. Marcial VA, Pajak TF. Radiation therapy alone or in combination with surgery in head and neck cancer. Cancer 1985; 55: 2259–65.
8. Mendenhall WM, Parsons JT, Amdur RJ et al. Squamous cell carcinoma of the head and neck treated with radiation therapy. The impact of neck stage on local control. Int J Radiat Biol Phys 1988; 14: 249–52.
9. Jesse RH, Sugarbaker EL. Squamous cell carcinoma of the oropharynx: Why we fail. Am J Surg 1976; 132: 435–8.
10. Wittes RE. Chemotherapy of head and neck cancer. Otolaryngol Clin North Am 1980; 13: 515–20.
11. Mead GM, Jacobs C. Changing role of chemotherapy in treatment of head and neck cancer. Am J Med 1982; 73: 582–95.
12. Hong WK, Bromer R. Chemotherapy in head and neck cancer. N Engl J Med 1983; 308: 75–9.
13. Al-Sarraf M. Head and neck cancer: Chemotherapy concepts. Semin Oncol 1988; 15: 70–85.
14. Wittes RE, Cvitkovic E, Shah J et al. Cis-dichlorodiammineplatinum (II) in the treatment of epidermoid carcinoma of the head and neck. Cancer Treat Rep 1977; 61: 359–66.
15. Wittes R, Heller K, Randolph V et al. Cis-dichlorodiammineplatinum (II)-based chemotherapy as initial treatment of advanced head and neck cancer. Cancer Treat Rep 1979; 63: 1533–8.
16. Jacobs C, Bertino JR, Goffinet DR et al. 24-hour infusion of cisplatinum in head and neck cancers. Cancer 1978; 42: 2135–40.
17. de Andres Basauri L, Lopez Pousa A, Alba E et al. Carboplatin, an active drug in advanced head and neck cancer. Cancer Treat Rep 1986; 70: 1173–6.
18. Al-Sarraf M, Metch B, Kish J et al. Platinum analogs in recurrent and advanced head and neck cancer: A Southwest Oncology Group and Wayne State University study. Cancer Treat Rep 1987; 71: 723–6.
19. Eisenberger M, Hornedo J, Silva H et al. Carboplatin (NSC-241-240): An active platinum analog for the treatment of squamous-cell carcinoma of the head and neck. J Clin Oncol 1986; 4: 1506–9.
20. Tapazoglou E, Kish J, Ensley J et al. The activity of a single-agent 5-fluorouracil infusion in advanced and recurrent head and neck cancer. Cancer 1986; 57: 1105–9.
21. Kish JA, Weaver A, Jacobs J et al. Cisplatin and 5-fluorouracil infusion in patients with recurrent and disseminated epidermoid cancer of the head and neck. Cancer 1984; 53: 1819–24.
22. Rowland KM, Taylor SG, O'Donnel MR et al. Cisplatin and 5-FU infusion chemotherapy in advanced recurrent cancer of the head and neck: An Eastern Cooperative Oncology Group pilot study. Cancer Treat Rep 1986; 70: 461–4.
23. Creagen E, Ingle J, Schutt A et al. A phase II study of cisdiaminedichloroplatinum and 5-fluorouracil in advanced upper aerodigestive neoplasms. Head Neck Surg 1984; 7: 1020–3.
24. Choksi AJ, Hong WK, Dimery IW et al. Continuous cisplatin (24-hour) and 5-fluorouracil (120-hour) infusion in recurrent head and neck squamous cell carcinoma. Cancer 1988; 61: 909–12.
25. Merlano M, Vitale V, Rosso R et al. Treatment of advanced squamous-cell carcinoma of the head and neck with alternating chemotherapy and radiotherapy. N Engl J Med 1992; 327: 1115–31.
26. Hong WK, Shapshay SM, Bhutani R et al. Induction chemotherapy in advanced squamous head and neck carcinoma with high-dose cisplatinum and bleomycin infusion. Cancer 1979; 44: 19–25.
27. Spaulding MB, Kahn A, De Los Santos R et al. Adjuvant chemotherapy in advanced head and neck cancer. An update. Am J Surg 1982; 144: 432–6.
28. Ervin TJ, Clark JR, Weichselbaum RR et al. An analysis of induction and adjuvant chemotherapy in the multidisciplinary treatment of squamous-cell carcinoma of the head and neck. J Clin Oncol 1987; 5: 10–20.
29. Rooney M, Kish J, Jacobs J et al. Improved complete response rate and survival in advanced head and neck after three-course induction therapy with 120-hour 5-FU infusion and cisplatin. Cancer 1985; 55: 1123–118.
30. Vokes EE, Moran WJ, Mick R et al. Neoadjuvant and adjuvant methotrexate, cisplatin, and fluorouracil in multimodal therapy of head and neck cancer. J Clin Oncol 1989; 7: 838–45.
31. Vogl SE, Lerner H, Kaplan BH et al. Failure of effective initial chemotherapy to modify the course of stage IV (MO) squamous cancer of the head and neck. Cancer 1982; 50: 840–4.
32. Knowlton AH, Percapio B, Bobrow S et al. Methotrexate and radiation therapy in the treatment of advanced head and neck tumors. Radiology 1975; 116: 709–12.
33. Fazekas JT, Sommer C, Kramer S. Adjuvant intravenous methotrexate or definitive radiotherapy alone for advanced squamous cancers of the oral cavity, oropharynx, supraglottic larynx, or hypopharynx. Int J Radiat Oncol Biol Phys 1980; 6: 533–41.
34. Stell PM, Dalby JB, Strickland P et al. Sequential chemotherapy and radiotherapy in advanced head and neck cancer. Clin Radiol 1983; 34: 463–7.

184

35. Schuller DE, Metch B, Mattox D et al. Preoperative chemotherapy in advanced resectable head and neck cancer: Final report of the Southwest Oncology group. Laryngoscope 1988; 98: 1205–11.

36. Stolwijk C, Wagener DJT, Van Den Broeck P et al. Randomized neo-adjuvant chemotherapy trial for advanced head and neck cancer. Neth J Med 1985; 28: 347–51.

37. Holoye PY, Grossman TW, Toohill RJ et al. Randomized study of adjuvant chemotherapy for head and neck cancer. Otolaryngol Head Neck Surg 1985; 93: 712–7.

38. Toohill RJ, Anderson T, Byhardt RW et al. Cisplatin and fluorouracil as neoadjuvant therapy in head and neck cancer. Arch Otolaryngol Head Neck Surg 1987; 113: 758–61.

39. Taylor SG, Applebaum E, Showel JL et al. A randomized trial of adjuvant chemotherapy in head and neck cancer. J Clin Oncol 1985; 3: 672–9.

40. Head and Neck ContRacts Program. Adjuvant chemotherapy for advanced head and neck squamous carcinoma. Cancer 1987; 60: 301–11.

41. Paccagnella A, Orlando A, Marchiori C et al. A phase II trial of neoadjuvant chemotherapy in head and neck cancer. Abs 894, ASCO 1993.

42. Tannock IF. Combined modality treatment with radiotherapy and chemotherapy. Radiother Oncol 1989; 16: 83–101.

43. Tannock IF, Hill RP (eds): The basic science of oncology, ed 2. New York: McGraw-Hill 1992.

44. Shanta V, Krishnamurthi S. Combined bleomycin and radiotherapy in oral cancer. Clin Radiol 1980; 31: 617.

45. Fu KK, Phillips TL, Silverberg IJ et al. Combined radiotherapy and chemotherapy with bleomycin and methotrexate for advanced inoperable head and neck cancer: Update of a Northern California Oncology Group randomized trial. J Clin Oncol 1987; 5: 1410.

46. Parvinen LM, Parvinen M, Nordman E et al. Combined bleomycin treatment and radiation therapy in squamous cell carcinoma of the head and neck region. Acta Radiol 1985; 24: 487.

47. Lo TCM, Wiley AL Jr, Ansfield FJ et al. Combined radiation therapy and 5-Fluorouracil for advanced squamous cell carcinoma of the oral cavity and oropharynx: A randomized study. Am J Roentgenol 1976; 126: 229.

48. Ansfield FJ, Ramirez G, Davis HL Jr et al. Treatment of advanced cancer of the head and neck. Cancer 1970; 25: 78.

49. Gupta NK, Pointon RCS, Wilkinson PM. A randomized clinical trial to contrast radiotherapy with radiotherapy and methotrexate given synchronously in head and neck cancer. Clin Radiol 1987; 38: 575.

50. Al Sarraf M, Pajak TF, Marcial VA et al. Concurrent radiotherapy and chemotherapy with cisplatin in inoperable squamous cell carcinoma of the head and neck. Cancer 1987; 59: 259.

51. Weissberg JB, Son YH, Papac RJ et al. Randomized clinical trial of mytomicin-C as an adjunct to radiotherapy in head and neck cancer. Int J Radiat Oncol Biol Phys 1989; 17: 3.

52. Merlano M, Rosso R, Sertoli MR et al. Randomized comparison of two chemotherapy, radiotherapy schemes for stage III and IV unresectable squamous cell carcinoma of the head and neck. Laryngoscope 1990; 100: 531.

53. Clifford P, Durden-Smith DJ, Peto J. A randomized trial of combined multidrug chemotherapy and radiotherapy in advanced squamous cell carcinoma of the head and neck. An interim report from the SECOG participants. Eur J Surg Oncol 1986; 12: 289.

54. Urken M, Weinberg H, Vickery C et al. The combined sensate radial forearm and iliac crest free flaps for reconstruction of significant glossectomy-mandibulectomy defects. Laryngoscope 1992; 102: 543–58.

55. Ambrosch P, Steiner W. Treatment of NO neck in patients with lasermicrosurgically resected carcinoma of the larynx. International symposium diagnosis and treatment of the NO neck of carcinomas of the upper aerodigestive tract. Goettinge, 17–18 sept 1992.

56. Cragle SP, Brandenburg JH. Laser cordectomy or radiotherapy: Cure rates, communication, and cost. Otolaryngol Head and Neck Surg 1993; 108: 648–54.

57. Piquet J, Chevalier D. Subtotal laryngectomy with crico-hyoidoepiglotto-pexy for the treatment of extended glottic carcinoma. Am J Surg 1991; 162: 357–61.

58. Kotwall C, Sako K, Razack MS et al. Metastatic patterns in squamous cell cancer of the head and neck. Am J Surg 1987; 154: 439–442.

59. Zbaeren P, Lehmann W. Frequency and sites of distant metastases in head and neck squamous cell carcinoma. Arch Otolaryngol Head Neck Surg 1987; 113: 662–4.

60. Van Putten LM, Kram LKJ, Van Dierendonck HHC et al. Enhancement by drugs of metastatic lung nodule formation after intravenous tumor cell injection. Int J Cancer 1975; 15: 588–95.

R. L. Souhami (ed.) The Teaching Cases from Annals of Oncology, 185–189, 1997.
© 1997 Kluwer Academic Publishers. Printed in the Netherlands.

The management of bladder cancer — a case history

A. P. M. Lydon, S. J. Harland & G. M. Duchesne

Department of Oncology, University College London Medical School, The Middlesex Hospital, London, U.K.

Key words: bladder cancer, staging of bladder cancer, muscle-invasive disease

Introduction

Bladder cancer is a common disease, accounting worldwide for approximately 3.5% of all new cancers. It manifests a wide spectrum of disease, ranging from a solitary, papillary, non-invasive lesion, through to solid, fixed tumours, invading through the bladder wall and into local structures with metastatic disease a common accompaniment. Treatment varies for each patient, depending on the stage and grade of the tumour, as well as patient characteristics. The following case-history illustrates a number of management problems for a patient with bladder cancer, and discusses the possible therapeutic options for each stage of the disease.

Case history

A sixty-seven year old man presented with a three month history of painless haematuria. He admitted to smoking thirty cigarettes per day for the last forty years. There was no history of chronic urinary tract infection, or exposure to known industrial carcinogens. He had a myocardial infarction five years previously, and had mild irreversible obstructive airways disease for which he was on no regular medication. On examination, he was obese, and had an early expiratory wheeze throughout the chest. Investigations, which included full blood count, plasma electrolytes and creatinine, liver function tests, urine microscopy and cytology and chest x-ray were within normal limits.

An intravenous urogram was obtained prior to cystoscopy, which revealed a filling defect on the left of the bladder (Fig. 1) but no lesion elsewhere in the renal tracts. Cystoscopy was performed, which revealed a 1.5 cm papillary lesion on the left bladder wall which was macroscopically completely resected, and histological examination revealed a moderately differentiated transitional cell carcinoma, with invasion of the lamina propria but no muscle invasion. Random biopsies taken near the tumour and at other macroscopically normal looking sites were negative.

At the initial follow up cystoscopy three months after diagnosis, no tumour was seen, and urine cytology was negative. However, six months later urine cytology revealed malignant cells. At cystoscopy, abnormal mucosa was seen around the trigone which on histology was found to be carcinoma-in-situ. Random biopsies revealed a further area of carcinoma-in-situ in the lateral wall of the bladder. Treatment with weekly intravesical B.C.G. for six weeks was instituted, and check

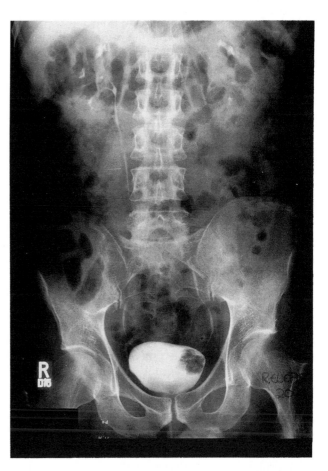

Fig. 1. Intravenous urogram at presentation revealing filling defect in the left side of the bladder, suggesting the presence of a tumour.

186

cystoscopy six weeks later revealed no residual tumour; urine cytology and regular cystoscopies remained normal for the next three years.

Four years after the initial presentation, he again noticed haematuria. Urine cytology was negative, but cystoscopy revealed an extensive tumour involving the bladder base and posterior wall and the left ureteric orifice could not be identified. The tumour was resected, but a mass was still palpable after resection. Histology confirmed a poorly differentiated transitional cell carcinoma invading deep muscle (stage T3a). Computerised tomography of abdomen and pelvis showed an obstructed left ureter with preservation of the renal cortex (Fig. 2). No extra-vesical disease or lymphadenopathy was found, and screening for metastases was negative. A left percutaneous nephrostomy was inserted, followed by a double J ureteric stent, to relieve the ureteric obstruction. It was elected to treat with radical external beam irradiation, using a three-field technique to treat the bladder and perivesical tissues, avoiding the rectum and making no attempt to treat the pelvic lymph nodes. A tumour dose of 64 Gy treating with daily fractions of 2 Gy was delivered. Cystoscopy three months later revealed no residual tumour and subsequent cystoscopies showed only a small area of telangiectasia in the posterior bladder wall, but no recurrent disease.

Despite primary control and a negative metastatic screen at the time of developing muscle-invasive disease, he developed pulmonary and bone metastases 18 months later, and received palliative systemic chemotherapy with cisplatin, vinblastine and methotrexate; he achieved a good partial response after six cycles of chemotherapy (Fig. 3a and b) which was maintained for seven months prior to his death from progressive metastatic disease.

Discussion points

1. Stage, grade and prognosis in bladder cancer

Ninety percent of bladder cancers are transitional cell cancers, six percent are squamous and one percent are adenocarcinomas. The remaining three percent comprise a mixture of sarcomas, lymphomas, phaeochromocytomas and carcinoid tumours.

U.I.C.C. staging [1] of the primary tumour is based on the degree of invasion through mucosa or muscle and correlates closely with the development of nodal metastases and prognosis (Table 1). Transitional cell cancers are sub-divided on the basis of cellular differentiation and mitotic activity into grades 1–3. There is a strong correlation between increasing grade and increasing depth of invasion and for superficial tumours grade also predicts the risk of progression to invasive disease (Table 2). Carcinoma-in-situ, particularly if multifocal, is a serious disease with a significant risk of progression to invasive bladder cancer and death.

2. Management of high grade superficial bladder cancer

It is always distressing when a patient with a curable condition progresses to being incurable despite expert management. Sadly this happens not uncommonly to

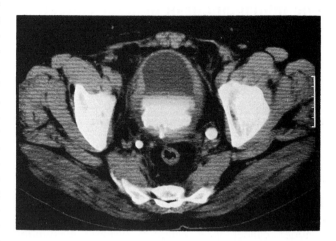

Fig. 2. Axial CT scan of pelvis at the time of diagnosis of muscle-invasive disease showing extensive tumour of the posterior and lateral bladder wall, together with an obstructed left ureter.

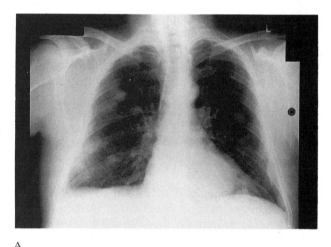

A

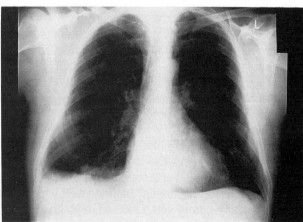

B

Fig. 3. The development of multiple pulmonary metastases (a), treated with four courses of combination chemotherapy (CMV) which resulted in almost complete clearing of the visible lesions (b).

Table 1. Staging and prognosis in bladder carcinoma.

	TNM	% nodal involvement	% 5 year survival
In situ	Tis	0	85
Papillary non-invasive	Ta	0	95
Submucosa	T1	5	75
Superficial muscle	T2	30	60
Deep muscle	T3a	50	35
Perivesical fat	T3b	60	
Prostate/uterus/vagina	T4a	80	30
Other pelvic organs	T4b	60	<10
Lymph nodes	N1–3		
Distant metastases	M1	–	<10

Table 2. Tumour grade and the risk of stage progression in superficial bladder cancer.

Histology grade	Risk of progression (%)
Grade 1	2
Grade 2	11
Grade 3	45

patients with superficial bladder cancer. Eighty percent of patients with bladder cancer present with superficial (pTa and pT1) disease and in most large series 15%–20% of these patients eventually develop muscle-invasive disease and then only a minority can be salvaged. These supervised disasters could be avoided by a liberal policy of prophylactic cystectomy, but most of these major operations would be performed unnecessarily.

Predicting those patients likely to progress is a vital part of the urological management of superficial bladder cancer and the well known indices of tumour size, stage, grade (Table 2), multiplicity and rate of recurrence are used for this purpose. Intravesical chemotherapy is frequently given with the dual aims of reducing the frequency of tumour recurrence in the bladder and preventing progression. There is almost no evidence that it is successful in the latter aim, though failure of this modality to clear the bladder of recurrences is one of the strongest predictors of tumour progression [2, 3]. Freedom from recurrence, however, brings its own hazards as this may be interpreted as a low likelihood of progression requiring only low intensity surveillance. This is inappropriate since the effect of chemotherapy is nearly always temporary. Radical external beam radiotherapy may have a role in the treatment of grade 3 pT1 lesions: in the series reported by Quilty and Duncan [4] there was a 56% recurrence-free rate at five years. The relative roles of chemotherapy, radiotherapy and radical surgery are still debated.

The presence of widespread carcinoma in situ (CIS) was until recently considered an absolute indication for cystectomy because progression was seen in 60%–80% of cases and the results of surgery in terms of long-term survival were excellent. As intravesical BCG can produce remissions in a high proportion of cases, bladder conservation is now the usual practice. Longer term studies have shown that recurrence of CIS occurs in the majority of cases within $2\frac{1}{2}$–5 years and deaths from transitional cell carcinoma are not infrequent [5, 6], with tumours often arising from the prostatic ducts or ureters – areas not exposed to the BCG – in addition to the bladder. Radical cystectomy is now reserved for those in whom remission is not achieved or at the time of recurrence, although this policy carries a risk that invasive disease and metastasis may occur. Radiotherapy has little place in the management of carcinoma in situ.

3. Management of muscle-invasive disease

Muscle-invasive bladder cancer may be managed by either radical cystectomy or radical radiotherapy and the relative merits of these two modalities remain hotly disputed. Many now advocate radical cystectomy as the treatment of choice, with five-year relapse-free rates following radical cystectomy of 75 percent for (pathologically staged) T2 and T3a lesions, 44 percent for all pT3 tumours, and 16 percent for pT4 or node-positive patients [7]. Comparison with the results of radical radiotherapy [8] suggests that radiotherapy may produce somewhat lower figures overall, with five-year survival rates of 40 percent for T2, 26 percent for T3, and 12 percent for T4 tumours but these were clinically staged patients and undoubtedly would have had more 'advanced' disease stage for stage than the surgical series. Long-term survival after radiotherapy depends on achieving complete remission and a policy of early salvage cystectomy for residual disease or local relapse in selected patients may provide equivalent survival rates to radical surgery [9]. Combined preoperative radiotherapy with planned cystectomy also has its advocates and may in certain patients be superior to either modality used alone [10].

The results of radical radiotherapy may be improved firstly by careful patient selection to exclude those likely to have occult metastatic disease and by identifying those patients whose tumours are unlikely to respond to radiotherapy: for example, those with bulky disease, incomplete macroscopic resection and ureteric obstruction [8, 11, 12]. Alternative treatments such as surgery, chemotherapy or combined modality approaches would be preferable in these patients. Secondly, the use of innovative dose-fractionation schedules designed to reduce late normal tissue damage or to combat the effects of tumour cell proliferation during protracted radiotherapy courses may improve local response rates and therefore the chance of cure. Reduction in fraction size may reduce toxicity to late tissues and allow an increase in the total tumour dose for equivalent late tissue damage. An early report [13] suggested that a hyperfractionation schedule of 1 Gy three times daily to a total tumour dose of 84 Gy gave significantly improved local control and survival rates over standard treatment, without increase in late bowel toxicity. An alternative approach is to 'accelerate' radiotherapy, using short overall treatment times to reduce the extent of tumour cell proliferation during treatment. Accelerated schedules, with or without hyperfractionation, and treating over two, three or four weeks are currently being evaluated [14].

Patient preference both for the type of treatment itself and for the associated side effects should also be considered. Morbidity is lessening for radical cystectomy with the development of continent diversion techniques along with nerve-sparing procedures to preserve potency. The incidence of late radiation damage to bowel or bladder increases with time, and may be expected in up to 10 percent of survivors, although the percentage developing serious complications requiring surgical intervention is much lower than this. The risk of late damage depends critically on volume: treating the pelvic nodes will significantly increase early and late morbidity, without improving survival for the majority of patients as those with involved pelvic nodes will usually die with metastatic disease. The current trend towards irradiating smaller target volumes together with improvements in planning techniques should reduce the incidence of late morbidity and make radical radiotherapy an eminently recommendable alternative to radical cystectomy.

4. Neoadjuvant chemotherapy for muscle-invasive tumours

Radical treatments for muscle-invasive bladder cancers apparently confined to the bladder are successful in only about a third of cases and median survival for patients who have nodal disease is only fifteen months. Of patients who die of their disease the majority have metastases which must have been present in subclinical form at the time of diagnosis. In order to improve the survival of these patients a systemic treatment is necessary and a policy of giving chemotherapy as soon as possible after diagnosis is a logical one. Studies in metastatic bladder cancer suggest that the most active agents in this disease are methotrexate and cisplatin. In fact, both these agents have been tested individually in adjuvant fashion in T2-T3 bladder cancer in randomised controlled studies. Their influence on survival has been shown to be insignificant in both cases [15, 16], and early data from an international randomised trial of neoadjuvant chemotherapy do not look promising. When given as initial treatment for bladder tumours impressive responses are seen with complete tumour disappearance in 20%–30% of cases [17]. When histological examination of the cystectomy specimen is included in the criteria for complete remission the incidence is at the lower end of the range. It is possible that patients attaining complete remission are those who would have had a good outcome with standard treatments. Many more complete remissions are seen in T2 disease (40%) than in T4 disease (6%). The converse is certainly true: patients who respond poorly to chemotherapy have a very poor prognosis despite radiotherapy or surgery [18]. More effective chemotherapeutic agents will need to be developed if the survival rates are to be improved.

5. Management of metastatic disease

Most patients who die from bladder cancer die as a result of metastatic disease. Prognosis for those with extra-nodal disease is very poor, with five percent of patients alive one year after diagnosis. Accumulated series suggest that cisplatin and methotrexate have single agent response rates in metastatic bladder cancer of the order of 30% [19]. The vinca alkaloids, adriamycin, mitomycin C and 5-fluorouracil also have significant activity but less. The most successful combinations have included both methotrexate and cisplatin, the most widely used being 'M-VAC' (with adriamycin and vinblastine) and CMV (with vinblastine). In the original series of 92 patients treated with M-VAC there was an overall response rate of 70% with 30% of patients entering complete remission. Furthermore, the median survival of these patients was almost 4 years [20]. The experience in a second centre was less good with overall and complete response rates of 40% and 13%. The median survival of the whole group was only 10 months. The authors also noted that 54% of patients required hospitalisation for management of toxic complications despite a median patient age of only 56 years [21].

The question of whether combination chemotherapy is superior to cisplatin alone has been tested in a randomised study involving over 250 patients. Thirty-nine percent of patients responded to M-VAC, only 12% responding to cisplatin ($p < 0.0001$) [22]. The low response rates underline the difference between the results of a specialist centre and those seen in multi-centre studies – presumably a reflection on characteristics of the patient populations – and the problem of extrapolating single institution results. Nonetheless, the superiority of combination chemotherapy has been demonstrated both in terms of response rate and survival, with median survivals of 12.5 and 8.2 months for the combination and single agent groups respectively ($p = 0.0002$). The ideal components of a combination regimen have yet to be determined. The demonstration that the CISCA regimen (cisplatin, cyclophosphamide and adriamycin) is inferior to M-VAC [23] suggests that this would be of some importance.

Who should be given combination chemotherapy given the short overall survival of patients with metastatic bladder cancer and the significant toxicity, particularly alopecia, neutropenic sepsis and renal toxicity, of the treatment? Selection based on prognostic factors would seem sensible. Negative prognostic factors include extranodal disease, weight loss and poor performance status [20, 22]. Such selection has not yet been widely adopted.

References

1. UICC TNM classification of malignant tumours. 4th edition 1987. Springer Verlag.
2. Riddle PR, Khan O, Fitzpatrick JM et al. Prognostic factors influencing survival of patients receiving intravesical epodyl. J Urol 1982; 127: 430–2.
3. Mufti GR, Virdi JS, Hall MH. Long-term follow up of intravesical epodyl therapy for superficial bladder cancer. Br J Urol 1990; 65: 32–5.
4. Quilty P, Duncan W. Treatment of superficial T1 tumours of the bladder by radical radiotherapy. Br J Urol 1986; 58: 147–52.
5. Brosman S. The influence of Tice strain BCG treatment in patients with transitional cell carcinoma in situ. In: Progress in Clinical and Biological Research 1989; 30; EORTC. Genitourinary Group Monograph 6: BCG in Superficial Bladder Cancer.
6. Harland SJ, Charig CR, Highman W et al. Outcome in carcinoma in situ of the bladder treated with intravesical Bacille Calmette-Guerin. Br J Urol 1992; 70: 271–5.
7. Skinner DG, Lieskovsky G. Contemporary cystectomy with pelvic node dissection compared to preoperative radiation therapy plus cystectomy in management of invasive bladder cancer. J Urol 1984; 131: 1069–72.
8. Duncan W, Quilty P. The results of a series of 963 patients with transitional cell carcinoma of the urinary bladder primarily treated by radical megavoltage x-ray therapy. Radiother Oncol 1986; 7: 299–310.
9. Jenkins BJ, Caulfield MJ, Fowler CG et al. Reappraisal of the role of radical radiotherapy and salvage cystectomy in the treatment of invasive (T2/T3) bladder cancer. Br J Urol 1988; 62: 343–6.
10. Parsons JT, Million RR. Planned preoperative irradiation in the management of clinical stage B2-C (T3) bladder carcinoma. Int J Rad Oncol Biol Phys 1988; 14: 797–810.
11. Babiker A, Shearer RJ, Chilvers CE. Prognostic factors in a T3 bladder cancer trial. Co-operative Urological Cancer Group. Br J Cancer 1989; 59: 441–4.
12. Gospodarowicz MK, Hawkins NV, Rawlings GA et al. Radical radiotherapy for muscle invasive transitional cell carcinoma of the bladder: Failure analysis. J Urol 1989; 142: 1448–54.
13. Edsmyr F, Andersson L, Esposti PL et al. Irradiation therapy with multiple small fractions per day in urinary bladder cancer. Radiother Oncol 1985; 4: 197–203.
14. Horwich A. Treatment of muscle invasive (T2/T3) carcinoma of the bladder: The role of radiotherapy. In Alderson AR, Oliver RTD, Hanham IWF, Bloom HJG (eds): Urological Oncology: Dilemmas and developments. Chichester. John Wiley & Sons 1991; 137–44.
15. Shearer RJ, Chilvers CED, Bloom HJG et al. Adjuvant chemotherapy in T3 carcinoma of the bladder. Br J Urol 1988; 62: 558–64.
16. Wallace DMA, Raghavan D, Kelly KA et al. Neo-adjuvant (pre-emptive) cisplatin therapy in invasive transitional cell carcinoma of the bladder. Br J Urol 1991; 67: 608–15.
17. Scher HI. Chemotherapy for invasive bladder cancer: Neo-adjuvant versus adjuvant. Semin Oncol 1990; 17: 555–65.
18. Splinter TA, Scher HI, Denis L et al. The prognostic value of the pT category after combination chemotherapy for patients with invasive bladder cancer who underwent cystectomy. EORTC-GU group. Prog Clin Biol Res 1990; 353: 219–24.
19. Yagoda A. Chemotherapy of urothelial tract tumours. Cancer 1987; 60: 574–85.
20. Sternberg CN, Yagoda A, Scher HI et al. M-VAC (methotrexate, vinblastine, doxorubicin and cisplatin) for advanced transitional cell carcinoma of the urothelium. J Urol 1988; 139: 461–69.
21. Tannock I, Gospodarowicz M, Connolly J et al. M-VAC (methotrexate, vinblastine, doxorubicin and cisplatin) chemotherapy for transitional cell carcinoma: The Princess Margaret Hospital Experience. J Urol 1989; 142: 289–92.
22. Loehrer PJ, Einhorn LH, Elson PJ et al. A randomised comparison of cisplatin alone or in combination with methotrexate, vinblastine and doxorubicin in patients with metastatic urothelial carcinoma: A co-operative group study. J Clin Oncol 1992; 10: 1066–73.
23. Logothetis CJ, Dexeus FH, Finn L et al. A prospective randomised trial comparing MVAC and CISCA chemotherapy for patients with metastatic urothelial tumours. J Clin Oncol 1990; 8: 1050–5.

Subject index